Health, Illness,
and the Social Body

Health, Illness, and the Social Body

A Critical Sociology

Peter E. S. Freund

Montclair State College

Meredith B. McGuire

Trinity University

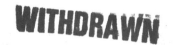

PRENTICE HALL
Englewood Cliffs, New Jersey 07632

Library of Congress Cataloging-in-Publication Data

Freund, Peter E. S.
    Health, illness, and the social body : a critical sociology /
Peter E.S. Freund and Meredith B. McGuire.
        p.   cm.
    Includes bibliographical references and indexes.
    ISBN 0-13-818717-7
    1. Social medicine.   2. Sick--Psychology.   3. Medical care.
I. McGuire, Meredith B.
RA418.F753 1991
306.4'61--dc20

90-39699
                                                                 CIP

Editorial/production supervision: Tara Powers-Hausmann
Interior design: Karen Buck
Cover design: Ben Santora
Manufacturing buyer: Mary Anne Gloriande

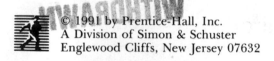

© 1991 by Prentice-Hall, Inc.
A Division of Simon & Schuster
Englewood Cliffs, New Jersey 07632

Printed in the United States of America
10 9 8 7 6 5 4 3 2 1

ISBN   0-13-818717-7

Prentice-Hall International (UK) Limited, *London*
Prentice-Hall of Australia Pty. Limited, *Sydney*
Prentice-Hall Canada Inc., *Toronto*
Prentice-Hall Hispanoamericana, S.A., *Mexico*
Prentice-Hall of India Private Limited, *New Delhi*
Prentice-Hall of Japan, Inc., *Tokyo*
Simon & Schuster Asia Pte. Ltd., *Singapore*
Editora Prentice-Hall do Brasil, Ltda., *Rio de Janeiro*

Contents

Chapter Six
The Social Meanings of Sickness   129

Chapter Seven
The Illness Experience   153

Chapter Eight
Seeking Health and Help   179

Chapter Nine
The Social Construction of Medical Knowledge   203

Chapter Ten
Modern Biomedicine: Knowledge and Practice   230

Chapter Eleven
Stratification and Power in Health Care Systems   259

Chapter Twelve
Economic Interests and Power in Health Care   282

Preface

Human bodies as well as ideas and perceptions about those bodies are profoundly influenced by their social and political contexts. To convey the complex interrelationships of body, mind, and society in producing health and illness, we have selected key themes in the sociology of health and illness, rather than writing a comprehensive text. While we describe various interpretive approaches and review much conventional literature in several related disciplines, our primary aim is to present a critical, holistic interpretation that emphasizes *power* as a key social-structural factor in health and in societal responses to illness.

This book is best used as a core of essays around which instructors can build a course and assign related articles, monographs, or readings to complement their own emphasis. Chapter One is an introduction that outlines relevant problems and key concepts in the field, and especially shows how this text links materialist and social-constructionist theories of health and illness through the unifying theme of power. Chapter Two introduces students to social epidemiology, and outlines broad patterns of morbidity and mortality. Chapters Three through Five describe the social production of unhealthy bodies and develop interpretations of the nature of connections among mind, body, and society. Chapters Six through Nine discuss the social context of ideas and experiences of health and illness. Chapters Ten through Twelve examine social and cultural factors in the medical system's treatment of sick persons and the political economy of health care in the United States.

While presented in an orderly arrangement, the book's chapters may be used in a different sequence. Each chapter introduces relevant key concepts and a limited number of sociological theorists or researchers. For reasons of practical flexibility, we have reiterated explanations of a few key terms in more than one chapter. Authors mentioned by name in the text have been generally selected for the importance of their theoretical contributions. Others are cited in the recommended readings and references, which have been included both to acknowledge our intellectual debts and to provide students with extensive useful references for further research.

Each chapter ends with an annotated list of some recent recommended readings. Two appendices suggest further useful materials. Appendix A outlines major resources for a search of the literature in the field. Students preparing term papers or theses will find these resources essential. The book's extensive bibliography should also be invaluable for researchers. Appendix B is an annotated list of film and video resources. We have found good visual presentations to be invaluable aids in concretizing and illustrating points that are often far from students' personal experiences, as well as for stimulating discussion.

As a set of core essays, this text does not attempt to cover several themes that some instructors may wish to discuss. The topics of aging or AIDS are, for example, not treated in separate sections, although related material is spread across several chapters. We have avoided a separate discussion of mental health and illness for two important reasons. First, a central theme of the text is that mind and body are interrelated, and we wish to avoid the conception that mind problems are utterly separate from body problems. Second, our main points about the professions and the social construction of illness apply equally to what have been called "physical" and "mental" illnesses, but we prefer to use as many examples as possible of "physical" conditions, because they make a stronger case about the social construction of illness and bodies.

The discipline of sociology of health and illness is not clearly delineated, fixed, or methodologically unified. There is wide diversity of opinion as to the proper scope of the subject matter and how to approach it. The field is undergoing significant reconceptualization; as its paradigms shift, so do its boundaries. Writing a text in a rapidly changing field involves choosing whether to limit ourselves to materials "acceptable" to all in the field or to open possibilities and incorporate materials that might not be conventionally considered appropriate. We have chosen to do the latter. We use data to describe available evidence but also as a springboard for stimulating various ways of thinking about health and illness.

In writing this book, we have received help from many people, whose assistance we gratefully acknowledge: Virginia Black, Barbara Chasin, John Donahue, Miriam Fisher, Richard Franke, Harriet Klein, Laura Kramer, George Martin, Evelyn Savage, and Steve Tucker. Also very welcome were the advice and encouragement of our editors, Bill Webber and Nancy Roberts, and reviewers Jon Darling and Susan Gore. We want to express our special appreciation to Susan Goscinski for her helpful comments and care in the preparation of the manuscript; Rachel McGuire's assistance with word processing was also greatly appreciated. Finally, we want to thank our families, Miriam Fisher, and Daniel, Rachel, and Kieran McGuire, for putting up with us during the writing of this book and for illustrating by their very lives why sociologists should care about health.

Chapter One

A Sociological Perspective on Health, Illness, and the Body

When we think of health and illness, we usually think of eating properly and other healthy habits, of institutions such as hospitals, and of health professionals such as doctors and nurses. While we may be dimly aware that health has its social dimensions, we may not think of health as a topic for social scientists.

Sociological analysis emphasizes that the occurrence of illness is not random. Eckholm (1977: 18–19) notes:

> Individuals who enjoy good health rightly think of themselves as fortunate: But luck has little to do with the broad patterns of disease and mortality that prevail in each society. The striking variations in health conditions among countries and cultural groups reflect differences in social and physical environments. And increasingly the forces that shape health patterns are set in motion by human activities and decisions. Indeed, *in creating its way of life, each society creates its way of death* [emphasis added].

The sociology of health and illness studies such issues as how social and cultural factors influence health and people's perceptions of health and healing, and how healing is done in different societies. Social structures and cultural practices have concrete consequences for people's lives.

We like to think that a newborn infant is as yet untouched by these abstract forces and has possibilities for health limited only by the child's genetic makeup. Even at birth, however, these abstract forces have begun to inscribe themselves on the baby's body. The very life chances of this infant, including the probabilities that she will live, be well, acquire the skills for success in her culture, and achieve and maintain that success, are powerfully influenced by all of the social circumstances and forces she will encounter throughout her life. In short, the baby's life chances, including possibilities for health and long life or sickness and death, are shaped or constructed by society itself.

The baby's birth weight, for example, is influenced by her mother's diet, which in turn is partly a product of her society, her culture, and her social class. Other features of the mother's social context have direct consequences for the newborn's health, including the mother's smoking or drug habits, the housing and sanitary conditions in which the infant is born, and the like. Later, whether the baby is a victim of cholera, bubonic plague, schistosomiasis, or lead poisoning depends upon public health measures taken in her environment. What other factors in the baby's home life and environment will shape her sense of self and self-esteem, and her ability to cope with stress and manage her environment? As she matures, how will her gender, race, ethnicity, and social class influence her life chances?

Later in life, her experiences as a worker will place her in various physical environments and social relationships that will affect her health. Her culture will shape what she likes to eat, how she experiences stress, whether she drinks alcohol, and how she feels about her body. How she experiences the process of giving birth will be shaped by her culture's meanings of childbirth as well as by the social context of birth, such as whether it takes place in a hospital under the supervision of an obstetrician trained in Western notions of pregnancy as a medical problem.

The infant is born into a social structure and culture that also powerfully influence what will be considered illness and how that illness will be treated. When this person gets sick, social forces play an important role in determining her chances of becoming well. How does she decide when she is sick and needs help? If she is sick, for example with a bad cold, how will others respond? If she develops multiple sclerosis, how will the attitudes and responses of others, and the quality of her social and physical environment affect her very life chances? What will happen if she develops a stigmatizing illness, such as leprosy or AIDS?

What resources are available to her in dealing with her needs when ill? If she approaches the medical system for help, how does she pay for it? How do her social class, age, race, and ability to pay influence the quality of her medical care? How does the institutional context of her medical care (for example, a public versus a for-profit private hospital, or a nursing home compared to a hospice or home care) help determine its quality? In addition to the quality of life, even the quality of death is linked with such social contexts.

Medical systems involve concrete organizations that reflect the economic interests of such groups as doctors and other professionals, insurance companies, pharmaceutical industries, manufacturers of medical equipment, hospitals, research organizations, government agencies, and medical schools. They all compete for resources, influence policy, and try to set health care and research agendas. Health care systems differ greatly from society to society in how they define and meet the needs of individual citizens. The baby's life chances are, therefore, intimately intertwined with these seemingly remote, social organizations.

The fates of individual bodies are thus linked to the workings of the social body. A person's life chances are not some deterministic fate nor a purely accidental, random result. Rather, a person's chances for illness and successful recovery are very much the result of specifiable social arrangements, which are in turn products of human volition and indeed deliberate policy choices made by identifiable groups and individuals. In large part, illness, death, health, and well-being are socially produced.

THE SOCIAL CONSTRUCTION OF THE BODY

To construct is to make or build something. Clearly, societies do not literally make or produce bodies, but they can influence, shape, and misshape them. Just as an artist can mold clay to construct an object (which is constrained by the physical properties of the clay), social groups and the cultures they share can shape members' bodies. Obvious examples of the deliberate cultural shaping of the human body include the foot binding practiced in traditional Chinese society, the cradle boards used to shape infants' heads among the Kwakiutl Indians, the stays and corsets worn by nineteenth-century middle-class European and American women, and the high heels and pierced earrings favored today. Similarly, having to live in a polluted environment or to sit at a desk, to work on an assembly line, or to bend over all day in a mine shaft are examples of social conditions that can indirectly shape the body and in turn the body's health.

Those things that happen to human bodies are closely related to the working and anatomy of the social body. Illness is not merely a physical experience but also a social experience. The sick body is not simply a closed container, encased in skin, that has been invaded by germs or traumatic blows but is also open and connected to the world that surrounds it. Thus the human body is open to the social body. Similarly, our material (or physical) environment, such as the urban landscape, the work place, or our foods, are influenced by our culture, social structure, and relationships. And these in turn influence our bodies.

THE SOCIAL CONSTRUCTION OF IDEAS ABOUT THE BODY

Ideas too are constructions. Every society has many levels of shared ideas about bodies: What is defined as healthy and beautiful in one society might be considered unhealthily fat and ugly in another; what is seen as thin and lean in one group might be defined as sickly in another. Aging may also be defined as something to be either conquered, feared, accepted, or revered. Likewise, some societies picture the body as working like a machine, whereas others see it as a spiritual vessel.

Health Beliefs and Practices

Because they are social constructions, one's ideas of the body and its health and illness are influenced by both one's culture and one's social position, such as class or gender. Both cultural and social structural factors are important in understanding people's behavior and health. People act as they do not only because of their beliefs about health (the cultural aspects) but also because of structural aspects, such as how power is distributed and relationships are organized. Thus although we conceptually distinguish cultural and social structural aspects in actuality they overlap.

Culture is the beliefs, values, actions, and material objects shared by a people. Culture includes such elements as language, beliefs about the universe and the nature of good and evil, ideals such as justice or freedom, and more mundane considerations such as what constitutes appropriate food, dress, and manners. Culture also encompasses objects that a people produce and share. Cooking utensils, films, cemeteries, blueprints, crucifixes, musical scores, and flags are among the items that represent cultural values and notions.

How do our cultural conceptions of a person's physical abilities affect those abilities? In our society, we used to believe that women were unable to carry heavy objects. While biology contributes somewhat to women's physical abilities, so do cultural ideas. In a patriarchal society, women's expectations that they will be weak, together with the experience of being treated as weak because of their social status, have a self-fulfilling result: Women do not become strong.

Social structure (or social organization) is the relatively stable, ongoing pattern of social interaction. In a particular society, there are recognizable patterns of interaction that are appropriate to different social positions and relationships, such as parent-child, supervisor-employee, teacher-student, and friend-friend. Behavior in these relationships is regulated through a number of mechanisms, including social control and shared cultural values. Various persons in social relationships occupy different social statuses. These relationships are often part of larger social organizational contexts; for example, the supervisor and employee positions may be part of a business corporation.

Social status is an individual's position in any system of social ranking. People can be stratified or ranked according to such dimensions as class, ethnicity, age, and gender. Social class (often measured by income or occupation or both) is one important indicator of social location; it influences how much power individuals have to manage their bodies and their external environment.

Class is not the only determinant of power. The particular position of power we occupy in our family (e.g., child or parent) and our gender, race, and ethnicity are also all important factors. Even health status (being chronically ill, for instance) will determine the stressors we are exposed to and the coping resources that are available to us. Our position in institutional arrangements (such as being a hospital patient) can also affect our health (Volicer, 1977, 1978).

In understanding health and illness, cultural aspects to be considered might include people's eating and hygienic habits, and their ideas about health, illness and healing. By contrast, structural elements might include a person's position and relationships in the work place, family, and medical settings as well as such social status indicators as gender, race, age, and class.

Both scientific and nonscientific ideas about health, illness, and the body are the result of social construction, as are the facts that we assemble as evidence for our ideas about the world. *All* descriptions, including medical descriptions, are constructions in that they include some information and exclude other information. Similarly, definitions of health are social constructions. For example, the *International Dictionary of Medicine and Biology* defines "health" as "a state of well-being of an organism or part of one, characterized by normal function and unattended by disease" (Becker, 1986: v. 2, 1276). This definition delineates well-being only in terms of bodily functioning and the absence of disease. But are we necessarily healthy if we simply lack disease? And are all diseases necessarily unhealthy? Is it healthy to function under all (however miserable) conditions? Why should functioning be such an important criterion? Is it because our society places so much cultural emphasis upon certain forms of functioning?

The Medical Model

Our culture derives many of its ideas about the body from the Western biomedical model. A sociological perspective on health and illness, however, does not take this model as "truth." Rather, medical ideas of the body and its diseases are also seen as socially constructed realities that are subject to social biases and limitations. Biomedical ideas are based upon a number of historical assumptions about the body and ways of knowing about the body; the following are some of these historically created assumptions that have become embedded in the Western medical model. Chapter Nine develops these concepts in more detail.

One biomedical assumption is *mind-body dualism*. The medical model assumes a clear dichotomy between the mind and the body; physical diseases are presumed to be located solely within the body. As a result, biomedicine tries to understand and treat the body in isolation from other aspects of the person inhabiting it. The history of Western medical science suggests several of the sources of this image of the body as separate from mind or spirit (some are described in Chapter Nine).

Not only does the medical model dichotomize body and mind, but also it assumes that illness can be reduced to disordered bodily (biochemical or neurophysiological) functions. This *physical reductionism* excludes social, psychological, and behavioral dimensions of illness. One result is that medicine "sees" disease as localized in the *individual* body. Such conceptions prevent the medical model from conceiving of the *social* body or how aspects of the individual's social or emotional life might affect physical health. Thus, medicine generally ignores social conditions contributing to illness or promoting healing.

A related assumption of the biomedical model is what Dubos (1959) called the *"doctrine of specific etiology."* This belief holds that each disease is caused by a specific, potentially identifiable agent. The history of Western medicine shows both the fruitfulness and the limitations of this assumption. Dubos noted that while the doctrine of specific etiology has led to important theoretical and practical achievements, it has rarely provided a complete account of the causation of disease. An adequate understanding of illness etiology must include broader factors, such as nutrition, stress, and metabolic states, which affect the individual's susceptibility to infection. As noted in Chapter 2, the search for specific illness-producing agents worked relatively well in dealing with infectious diseases but is too simplistic to explain the causes of complex chronic illnesses. Also, as Dubos observed, this approach often results in a quest for the "magic bullet" to "shoot and kill" the disease, producing an over-reliance on pharmaceuticals in the "armamentarium" (stock of "weapons") of the modern physician.

The Machine Metaphor is another implicit assumption in the medical model. Accordingly, the body is a complex biochemical machine, and disease is the malfunctioning of some constituent mechanism (e.g., a "breakdown" of the heart). Other cultures use other metaphors; for example, ancient Egyptian societies used the image of a river, and Chinese tradition refers to the balance of elemental forces (yin and yang) of the earth (Osherson and AmaraSingham, 1981). In combination with the assumption of mind-body dualism, the machine metaphor further encouraged an instrumentalist approach to the body; the physician could "repair" one part in isolation from the rest (Berliner, 1975).

Partly as a product of the machine metaphor and the quest for mastery, the Western medical model also conceptualizes the body as the proper *object of regimen and control*, again emphasizing the responsibility of the individual to exercise this control in order to maintain or restore health. This assumption meshes with other values, resulting in the medical and social emphases upon such standardized body disciplines as diets, exercise programs, routines of hygiene, and even sexual activity (Turner, 1984: 157–203).

THE CENTRALITY OF POWER IN THE SOCIOLOGY OF HEALTH AND ILLNESS

One of the unifying themes of this text is the social construction of both ideas about the body and the body itself. In this process power and control play an important role. In the most general sense, **power** is the ability to get what one wants and to get things done.

Power is a ubiquitous factor in our daily lives. It both enables us to accomplish tasks (such as to get enough food) and constrains the number and types of possibilities open to us. This text emphasizes the relationship between health and power, such as the power of workers over their work pace; the power of people to control the quality of their physical environments; the power of various groups or societies to shape health policy or to deliver what they consider healing; the power of people of different statuses to control, receive, and understand information vital to their well-being; and the power of the mass media to shape ideas about food and fitness. In addition these objective manifestations of power, we also subjectively experience power. A person's sense of empowerment—a feeling that one can handle stressful situations, for instance—is important to health and well-being, and is strongly related to one's ability to manage one's environment and to feel safe and secure in it. The power of individuals is not simply personal but also usually has a social basis.

The concept of social power in particular implies that the will of one individual or group can prevail over that of others. One's statuses (e.g., age and social class) in society determine the resources available for the exercise of power. For example, if I own a business and control its resources, I can decide how they will be used; generally, I have power in my work place and have more resources to enforce my will than do the workers in my business.

Often our experiences deal not with overt power or control but relative, implicit power. For example, if I feel in control of my family life, I thus feel able to resist others' attempts to wrest control, whether by direct confrontation or by subtle manipulation. For this reason, power is typically enhanced when its exercise is accepted as legitimate. Likewise, when people do not recognize that power is being exercised, they may submit to control unwillingly and unknowingly. Thus concepts like "social status" and "social control" are significant in understanding the relationship between power and the body. **Control** refers to the exercise of power in a particular situation. Like a sense of empowerment, control is related to one's ability to manage one's environment and to feel safe and secure in it.

Social control may be defined as those ways in which a society assures itself of its members' proper and respectable behavior, appearances, productivity, and contributions. Social control assures the relatively smooth functioning of the social order and the maintenance of hierarchical relationships such as class.

This control may rely on violence, force, persuasion, and/or manipulation. Internalized forms of control, such as individual conscience, are far more subtle and effective means of assuring uniformity. The standards by which persons learn to measure themselves are another way in which society uses the social self as a means of control. Social organizations also use their control of information to maintain power. For example, the regulation that workers have to punch a time clock is a device for assuring work attendance. Social control measures also affect those who are in power, as when they become their own "slave drivers."

THE PERSPECTIVE OF THIS TEXT

While our focus is sociological, we have drawn from many other disciplines and subdisciplines, such as medical sociology, medical anthropology, socio- and psychophysiology, medical economics, sociology of health and illness, social psychology, history, philosophy of the body, and ethics. Each has its

separate focus, and persons contributing to one discipline are often unaware of related work in other fields. We emphasize synthesizing work
from several disciplines to achieve a more holistic appreciation of health
and illness that views healing and prevention in the broadest sense: The
body is not treated as a self-enclosed machine, and health and illness are
understood in their social, cultural, and historical contexts.

A holistic perspective is necessary but difficult, because it requires us
to go beyond the rigid separations of concepts about the body, mind, and
society. As Scheper-Hughes and Lock (1986: 137) wrote:

> We are without a language with which to address mind-body-society interac-
> tions, and so are left hanging in mid-air, suspended in hyphens that testify to
> the radical disconnectedness of our thoughts. We resort to such fragmented
> concepts as the biosocial, the psychosomatic, the psychosocial, the somato-
> social, as feeble ways of expressing the complex and myriad ways that our
> minds speak to us through our bodies, and the ways in which society is in-
> scribed on the expectant canvas of our flesh and bones, blood and guts.

We stress the interactions of mind, body, and society, and the importance of symbols and subjective experience in understanding health and illness. The narrow focus and unifactorial models of disease characterizing
much of modern medicine and some of the sociology of health and illness
deflect attention from the social issues implied by persisting inequalities in
health status within most modern societies (Comaroff, 1982: 61), as well as
the yet greater gaps of inequality between "developed" and less-developed
nations.

SUMMARY

This text on the sociology of health and illness deals with the social construction of bodies, with an emphasis on how power shapes this construction.
How cultural and social structural factors and central power relationships
influence us physically and how we perceive, care for, maintain, and "repair" our bodies constitute the major questions to be addressed. The perspective of this book is a holistic one, emphasizing the interpenetration of
mind, body, and society.

The first part, Chapters Two through Five, deals primarily with the
ways in which society and culture affect physical functioning, and the material environments in which people exist. The second part, Chapters Six
through Nine, emphasizes people's experience of their own and others'
bodies, especially social aspects of the illness experience. The last part,
Chapters Ten through Twelve, examines social and cultural factors in the
medical systems' treatment of sick persons, and the political economy of
health care in the United States.

Chapter Two

Who Becomes Sick, Injured, or Dies?

Sickness does not just "happen." Rather, there are discernible patterns in the distribution and frequency of sickness, injury, and death in human populations. **Social epidemiology** is the study of these patterns and the social factors that shape them (Mausner and Bahn, 1985).

Noticing relationships between specific illnesses and people's social situation is hardly a new phenomenon: Early Greek and Egyptian writers made such connections (Sigerist, 1960). Popular lore also includes awareness of the linkage between, for example, an occupation and a sickness. *Alice in Wonderland*'s Mad Hatter was a plausible "madman" because people had recognized a connection between the occupation of hat-making and bizarre behavior long before the relationship was traced to the effects of the mercury with which hat-makers regularly worked (Stellman and Daum, 1971: 255). Similarly, long before medicine identified the problem, villagers living by the Niger River in Africa recognized that their proximity to the river was related to the prevalence of a horrible sickness characterized by intense itching and eventual blindness. Often they would move away, abandoning valuable farmlands, when the sickness had affected too large a proportion of the community (Eckholm, 1989).

During the late eighteenth and early nineteenth centuries, the historical process of industrialization set the stage for the development of the disciplines of both sociology and epidemiology (Spruit and Kromhout, 1987). The changes that accompanied industrial capitalism created radically different conditions for health and illness:

> The rates of smallpox, typhus, typhoid fever, diphtheria and scarlet fever all increased: two cholera epidemics had swept through the warrens of the Great Towns, a third was on its way. . . . The reordering of the circumstances of everyday life . . . ensued. Industrial capitalism gave rise to novel physical arrangements for work and dwelling (the factory, the company town), created new patterns of economic exploitation (mass displacements from land, urban migration in unprecedented numbers, wage labor). . . . Hazardous and fatiguing work, damp cold and stifling living quarters, cheap gin and adulterated foods, demoralization—the legacy of disease bequeathed by early capitalism stems from such an environment (Susser et al., 1985: 4).

Epidemiology, as a discipline, evolved from early studies of epidemics among people living in such environments. Like sleuths tracing the path of a suspected criminal, epidemiologists examined clues to the path of a suspected source of infection. For example, in 1854 a cholera epidemic broke out in London. Sir John Snow pinpointed known cases of the disease on city maps, thus narrowing the search to certain neighborhoods. He then interviewed survivors and neighbors of cholera victims about everyday behavior, such as what the victims had eaten, where they had played, and so on. Snow discovered that all of the victims had obtained their water from the same pump. He concluded that there was a relationship between this source of water and cholera infection, and he had the pump shut down, thereby ending the epidemic (Snow, 1855).

While modern epidemiologists have far more sophisticated tools such as computers and complex bacteriology laboratories, their underlying method remains much the same as Snow's: They search for patterns linking the types and incidence of sickness of a people with their way of life. Thus epidemiological studies often highlight the political and social contexts of health and illness. The famous nineteenth-century epidemiologist Rudolf Virchow declared, " 'Medicine is a social science, and politics nothing but medicine on a grand scale' " (quoted in Susser et al., 1985: 6). Political and social factors are readily evident in studies showing certain diseases to be characteristic mainly of the rich, while others occur almost exclusively among the poor. Political implications also follow, for instance, from epidemiological studies demonstrating certain occupations to be the causes or major contributing factors in certain illnesses and death. Epidemiology is only one of many approaches to understanding the connections between social arrangements and sickness or death, but epidemiological data receive special attention from policymakers because they describe large-scale differences that are applicable to entire industries or nations.

Because the connections between a group's lifestyle and its disease are often remote and not readily apparent, epidemiological research can reveal unexpected and/or indirect consequences of human activities. At the turn of this century, for instance, there was an outbreak in Asia of the Manchurian plague, which was transmitted by wild rodents, such as the furry marmot, which were sickened when they got the disease. The plague was preceded by a change in Europe, as marmot furs became exceptionally fashionable. In response to the dramatically heightened demand for the Manchurian marmot, hunters began to violate traditional taboos against hunting and trapping sick animals. Infected hunters then spread the disease to each other and eventually to the population at large. Thus a change in women's fashions in Europe indirectly contributed to the outbreak of a deadly plague in Manchuria (Dubos, 1968).

COMPLEX WEBS OF CAUSAL FACTORS

Epidemiology examines the interaction of complex disease-producing factors: a "web of causation" (MacMahon and Pugh, 1970: Chapter 2). This web is composed of three main, intertwining aspects: agent, host, and environment. The *agent* is the source of a disease, such as a virus in an infection or asbestos in asbestosis. The agent is a necessary-but-not-sufficient cause of disease; disease does not occur without an agent, but the agent alone is not sufficient to produce the disease (Mausner and Bahn, 1985).

The site within which an agent creates a disease is called the host. The host and agent interact within a biosocial environment, which includes the external conditions linking the agent to the host (such as unsanitary living conditions); the vector, or the means through which the agent is carried (such as diseased marmots or contaminated drinking water); and the condition of the internal environment of the host (such as relative immunity). To cause disease effectively, an agent must be able to survive in the environment and find a susceptible, fertile host. For example, a human body (host) may harbor tubercular bacilli (agent), but if the body's resistance (environment) is high, this disease agent cannot produce infection. Thus disease is not the outcome of just one factor; rather, many factors contribute to the complex "web of causation." Epidemiology is a generally holistic approach to health and illness.

As the name implies, epidemiology arose from the study of widespread infectious diseases, or epidemics. The maturing field has more recently begun to include study of the distribution, spread, and cause of noninfectious diseases, such as heart disease. The epidemiology of these sicknesses is, however, more difficult, because they develop more slowly, often over decades. The causal factors are thus obscured by time. A sixty-year-old victim of a heart attack is not likely to be able to recall accurately relevant information about his life as much as forty or fifty years earlier.

Noninfectious diseases also often involve multiple contributing factors rather than a single infectious agent. Thus it is difficult to identify all possible factors and determine their relative weight. For example, the hormones in birth control pills have been implicated in the development, many years after their use, of breast cancer. It is difficult, however, to determine just how significant a factor they may be for several reasons. The disease does not develop in clinically observable forms immediately upon use of "the pill." Other factors (such as the age of the onset of menstruation) are also involved and, in combination, greatly increase probability of developing the disease. It is extremely difficult to determine the relative importance of these various other factors (such as the woman's leanness, her age at the birth of her first baby, and whether she breastfed her babies) or even whether some possible factors are not being considered. It is difficult to determine, many years after the fact, exactly how much or which type of hormones women received; formulations for early contraceptive pills contained much higher dosages of hormones and in different combinations than more recent formulations. If a woman is now forty-eight, she may have taken several different formulations for many periods of varying length since the age of eighteen (cf. Kolata, 1989).

Early epidemiological studies examined relatively crude social factors, such as occupation or social class. Increasingly, social epidemiology is trying to tease out more refined categories of social influences on morbidity and mortality. For example, rather than look only at broad categories of occupation, research might examine the health impact of characteristic patterns of work-place time pressures or supervisor-worker relationships. Subsequent chapters describe some of these studies.

METHODOLOGICAL ISSUES

Epidemiology proceeds by observing statistical correlations between two or more variables pertaining to health, sickness, or death. The data for these statistical procedures are often drawn from records that are kept for other institutional purposes; researchers must therefore contend with discrepancies or errors created by the original records.

Statistical Associations

The existence of a statistical correlation between two variables is not sufficient evidence of a causal link between them. Many statistical relationships are spurious. For example, a ninteenth-century observer noted that the incidence of cholera was inversely correlated with the altitude of a community; low-lying places had higher rates of the disease than did those at higher altitudes. This correlation confirmed a prevalent notion that stagnant air (miasma) caused cholera; accordingly, because their air was "fresher," communities at higher altitudes had less miasma and thus less cholera. Later epidemiological discoveries showed that impure water was actually the vector (means of spreading the agent) for cholera. Because low-lying places were more likely to have both stagnant air and impure water, investigators were led to a spurious correlation between the disease and miasma (Mausner and Bahn, 1985).

It is often difficult to determine whether a statistical correlation is the product of an indirect relationship actually explained by intervening variables. For example, epidemiological data from the rural southern regions of the United States may show a statistical correlation between low birth weight and childhood deaths from diarrhea.[1] Does that mean that low birth weight causes subsequent death from diarrheal dehydration? This is a plausible interpretation, since birth weight may affect the child's susceptibility to illness, but birth weight may be only a by-product of some other causal

[1] Diarrhea is a major killer of children in the Third World; an estimated 4.5 million children die from it each year. In the United States, about 200,000 children under the age of five are hospitalized each year because of diarrhea, and several hundred a year die from it. While vaccines against the virus that is the disease's primary agent are not yet available, the treat of oral rehydration therapy is simple, safe, and inexpensive. The epidemiology of diarrhea shows that in America these preventable deaths occur disproportionately among poor black children in the rural South; social policies addressed to alleviating poverty, improving sanitation, and increasing access to health care and health care education could thus eliminate an entire category of infant mortality (Stevens, 1988).

factors. One clue to these other factors is to ask a somewhat oversimplified question: What kind of children are likely to experience both low birth weight and diarrhea? The profile of children with these conditions suggests several related features: They are likely to be from poor families in which the mother was young and received little or no prenatal care (Stevens, 1988). To establish a direct causal link between low birth weight and death due to diarrhea, it would be necessary to identify and hold constant all other factors. Any causal analysis must take into account multiple factors that may operate at several levels in the web of causality.

Data Bases

Many records upon which epidemiological studies are based are seriously flawed. Some statistics come from the records of schools, industries, insurance companies, hospitals, and public health departments. Since these data are kept for various other institutional reasons, they are often of limited accuracy for epidemiological purposes. For example, industrial accident statistics can be distorted by an industry's attempt to give the impression of a low accident rate.

Likewise, death certificates are very inaccurate and unreliable sources of information about the causes of death (Hill and Anderson, 1988). A Connecticut study found that 29 percent of death certificates inaccurately stated the cause of death, based upon autopsy reports and patients' medical records (Kircher et al., 1985). In a further 26 percent of the cases, the autopsy and death certificate gave the same general disease category but attributed death to different specific diseases. Thus more than half of the certificates provided seriously flawed data about the cause of death. Similar conclusions about the inaccuracy of death certificates were found in a Scottish study of postmortems (Cameron and McGoogan, 1981).

The usefulness of data from both medical records and death certificates may also be diminished by judgments made by the medical personnel who keep the records. Deliberate misrepresentations often occur when the cause of death is a stigmatizing sickness, such as alcoholism or AIDS. Such reporting problems make it difficult to assess the scope and actual impact of these important health problems. Not only the concern over stigma but also political, economic, and ideological considerations often figure into the deliberate underreporting of the incidence of AIDS. Data have been flawed, for example, by racist attitudes, fears of hurting tourism, and the assumption that AIDS affects only stigmatized minorities (Bolton, 1989: 93–94).

Death certificates also often state only a final cause of death, rather than the initial or contributing causes. For example, a person who dies of a gunshot wound may be listed as having died of internal bleeding. Although the bleeding is a fact in the case, the gunshot wound does not appear in the mortality statistics. Certain causes of death, such as adverse reactions to prescribed medications, are also systematically underreported (Altman, 1988b).

The *International Statistical Classification of Diseases, Injuries and Causes of Death*, revised about every ten years by the National Center for Health Statistics of the U.S., specifies standards to be used by attending doctors, coroners, and others in an attempt to produce internationally comparable data. Changes in these guidelines for classification, however, yield different rates of morbidity and mortality. One revision of the manual required coders to disregard medically induced (iatrogenic) causes of death, such as postsurgical bleeding or drug reaction, and instead to record the medical condition that first necessitated the treatment (Bloor et al., 1987). The proposed new form of death certificates in the United States asks for the immediate cause of death and a sequential listing of *all* underlying causes. It is likely that these new data will result in the "discovery" of comparatively high rates of medically induced conditions leading to death.

Despite recent efforts to change the format of U.S. death certificates to allow for more complex and thorough reporting, the data entered upon them remain problematic. Most death certificates are based upon doctors' clinical judgments about the cause or causes of death; autopsies are expensive and performed for decreasing numbers of cases. Even when an autopsy subsequently contradicts the certificate or adds significant new information, physicians often do not amend it (Altman, 1988b).

Even if autopsy findings are included on death certificates, these data may be slanted by the criteria used to select cases for autopsy. Women are less likely to be autopsied than men. In some states, nonwhite deaths are less likely to be investigated than those of whites (Bloor et al., 1987). Social status and/or the perceived social worth of the victim may also influence the thoroughness with which a death is investigated (cf. Sudnow, 1967). Thus the cases autopsied are not a representative sample of all deaths.

"Errors" or variations in diagnosis are not random; they are often socially produced. For example, medical personnel's judgments may vary according to the perceived social class of the dead person. In earlier medical reporting, the cause of a professional person's death from heart disease was likely to be labeled as "angina," whereas the cause of death of a working-class person with the same condition was usually classified as something else (Marmot et al., 1987). Similarly, diagnoses (and thus morbidity statistics) are influenced by doctors' attitudes toward patients' social characteristics, such as gender, social class, or occupation, as discussed further in Chapters Nine and Ten. For example, earlier data indicated that the rate of deaths due to alcoholism in Scotland were about twice those in England and Wales; these data are now in question, because studies show that doctors in England and Wales are much less likely than those in Scotland to attribute death to alcohol-related diseases such as cirrhosis (see Altman, 1988b).

Cultural differences in medical practice, even among Western industrial nations and among doctors trained in modern biomedicine, account for some variations in diagnoses. For example, blood pressure readings considered hypertensive in the United States would be considered normal in England (Payer, 1988). Doctor characteristics may also affect the diagnosis or reported cause of death. Because of differences in their training, younger British doctors were less likely than older ones to report stomach cancer as a diagnosis (Bloor et al., 1987). Thus a falling rate of mortality due to stomach cancer may be at least in part an artifact of differences in doctors' education.

These examples show that many health statistics may be artifactual, or produced by the social arrangements by which the statistics themselves are gathered and processed. Such artifactual evidence is misleading and often altogether incorrect. With these limitations in mind, let us examine some results of epidemiological investigation. The cautious use of epidemiological information can give us a broad "picture of health."

CHANGES IN LIFE EXPECTANCY IN THE TWENTIETH CENTURY

American males born in 1920 could expect to live 53.6 years and females, 54.6 years. By 1980 the life expectancy for both sexes had increased, but so had the gap between male and female rates. Males born in 1980 could expect to live 69.8 years, while females born that same year could live on the average to the age of 77.5 years. Figure 2.1 shows the dramatic increase in life span in the United States from 1900 to 1983. It also demonstrates the general decline of infant mortality and the increasing difference in life expectancy between men and women that began to emerge around 1920. There are also dramatic differences between blacks and whites in both general life expectancy and infant mortality.

Along with life expectancy changes, there have also been changes in the causes of death in Western industrial societies. Despite the recent development of some infectious diseases such as AIDS, there has been a general decline in death rates due to infectious diseases and an increase in death rates due to chronic degenerative diseases (McKinlay et al., 1989). Figure 2.2 illustrates this important change.

Table 2.1 shows the changing causes of death in order of their frequency. In 1900 acute infectious diseases (pneumonia, influenza, and tuberculosis) were the foremost causes of death in the United States. Chronic diseases (heart disease and cancer) were the major killers in 1985. Since the 1950s, the death rate from coronary heart disease in the United States has been decreasing. This is perhaps due to changes in diet, exercise patterns, and smoking habits. Rates of death from cancer have increased during the same time (Pear, 1984).

The increased incidence of chronic degenerative diseases cannot be

Stretching the life span
Life expectancy at birth

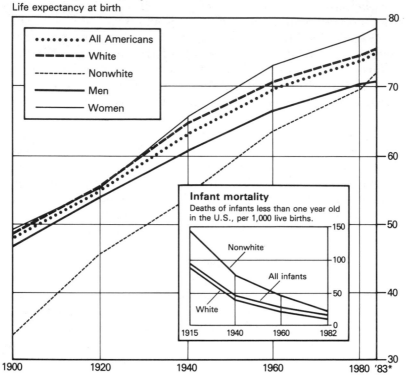

FIGURE 2.1   Changes in U.S. Life Expectancy and Infant Mortality, 1900–1983. (*Source:* "Stretching The Life Span" *New York Times,* February 17, 1985:E5. Copyright © 1985 by The New York Times Company. Reprinted by permission.)

attributed simply to the fact that people are living longer. It is true that the longer people live, the more likely they are to develop a chronic disease; however, increased longevity does not account for the fact that, beginning in the 1950s, even *younger* age groups have shown an increased incidence of these afflictions (Eyer and Sterling, 1977). This premature development of degenerative sickness may be the result of contemporary dietary, environmental, and social factors. Evidence that the social, biochemical, and physical environment of industrialized societies create new health problems, such as increased rates of cancer, comes from a comparison with "preindustrial" societies, which have lower incidence of these problems. Aspects of the way of life in industrialized societies are implicated, because the rates of chronic degenerative diseases increase among groups that migrate from agricultural to industrial communities (Doyal and Pennell, 1981; Janes, 1986).

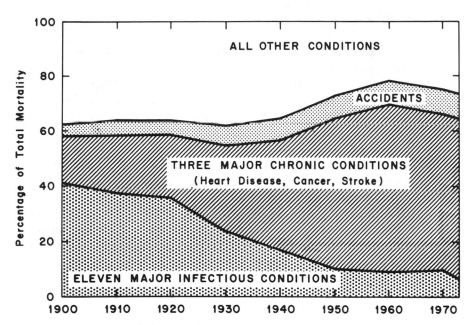

FIGURE 2.2   Proportion of Chronic and Infectious Disease Contributing to U.S. Mortality, 1900–
1973. (*Source:* John B. McKinlay and Sonja M. McKinlay, "The questionable effect
of medical measures on the decline of mortality in the United States in the twentieth century," *Milbank Memorial Fund Quarterly* 55, 1977: 416. Reprinted by
permission.)

TABLE 2.1   Causes of Death in the United States, 1900 and 1985

	1900		1985	
CAUSES OF DEATH	DEATH RATE (PER 100,000)		CAUSES OF DEATH	DEATH RATE (PER 100,000)
All causes	1,719.0		All causes	876.6
Pneumonia and influenza	202.2		Diseases of the heart	324.2
Tuberculosis	194.4		Malignancies	193.2
Diarrhea, enteritis, and ulceration of the intestine	142.7		Cerebrovascular disease	64.3
			Accidents	38.3
Diseases of the heart	137.4		Influenza and pneumonia	27.8
Senility, ill-defined or unknown	117.5		Suicide and homicide	19.8
Intracranial lesions of vascular origin	106.9		Diabetes mellitus	15.8
Nephritis	88.6		Cirrhosis of the liver	11.3
All accidents	72.3		Arteriosclerosis	10.0
Cancer and other malignant tumors	64.0		Bronchitis, emphysema, and asthma	9.1
Diphtheria	40.3		Certain diseases of early infancy	7.9

Source: U.S. Department of Health and Human Services, National Center for Health Statistics, "Births,
marriages, divorces, and deaths for 1985," *Monthly Vital Statistics Report* 34(12), 1986: 5.

THE MYTH OF MEDICAL PROGRESS

Many people believe that "miracles" of medical progress have been responsible for the improved health and longevity in Western industrial countries since the turn of the century. Media imagery often contributes to the notion, but much evidence suggests the contribution of medical intervention to increased life expectancy has been rather limited. McKeown (1979) argues that improved nutrition and population control, the control of predators, and improvements in urban dwelling conditions and hygiene have played a much greater role in extending life expectancy than did medical technology. The impact of these various factors on health can be documented through epidemiological studies.

A study of mortality rates in the United States shows that that medical intervention (such as innoculations) accounts for only a small percentage of the decline in mortality from infectious diseases during the early part of the twentieth century. Figure 2.3 shows that, of nine common infectious diseases, only poliomyelitis began to decline significantly *after* the introduction of the vaccine. All the other major infectious diseases had declined dramatically *prior* to the introduction of a vaccine or antibiotic (McKinlay and McKinlay, 1977). The decline of tuberculosis likewise preceded the introduction of chemical therapies (Friedman, 1987). Nonmedical factors, such as improved nutrition, clean water, garbage and sewage disposal, and other public health measures, may account for the primary decline in mortality due to many infectious diseases.

The precise contribution of medicine to increased life expectancy, to the reduction of morbidity, and to the quality of life is difficult—if not impossible—to assess. Some have argued that the iatrogenic (i.e., medically induced) health risks of modern medicine and its institutions outweigh its benefits (Illich, 1975). This position probably overstates the harmful effects of modern medicine. Nevertheless, any evaluation of the contribution of medical intervention must take into account its iatrogenic consequences, such as unneeded surgery, over- and misprescription of drugs, the negative "side effects" of medication, and infections transmitted in medical settings.

There is no doubt that medicine has made significant contributions to human health. It is effective in treating many acute diseases. Emergency medicine has saved many lives, and technological innovations in medicine since World War I have made it possible for many to survive previously mortal health crises. Medicine has also played a major role in the virtual eradication of some infectious diseases, such as smallpox and polio. The ability of medicine to treat or prevent chronic, degenerative diseases is, however, more limited. Furthermore, the benefits from medical progress must be distinguished from social-environmental changes and public health measures that have played a major part in improving people's health. The contributions of public health measures are often devalued by modern medi-

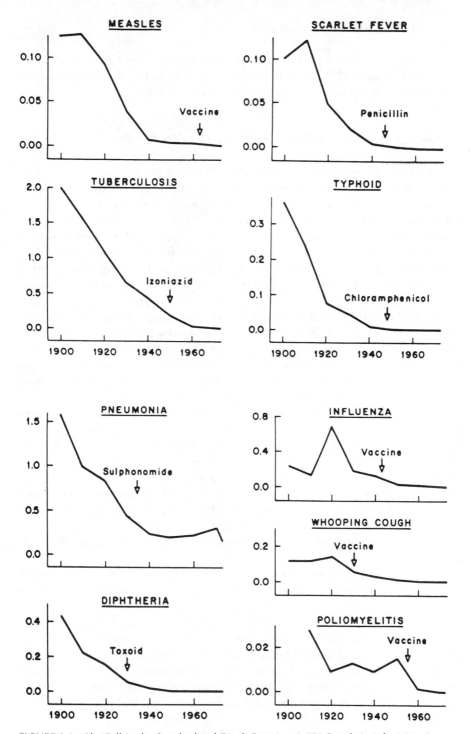

FIGURE 2.3 The Fall in the Standardized Death Rate (per 1,000 Population) for Nine Common Infectious Diseases in Relation to Specific Medical Measures in the United States, 1900–1973. (*Source:* John B. McKinlay and Sonja M. McKinlay. "The questionable effect of medical measures on the decline of mortality in the United States in the twentieth century," *Milbank Memorial Fund Quarterly* 55, 1977: 422–423.)

cine, resulting in social policies that allocate the vast majority of health care expenditures to medical research and treatments rather than to preventive programs such as maternal nutrition or work-place safety).

MORBIDITY AND MORTALITY IN THIRD WORLD COUNTRIES

The pattern of high rates of mortality due to infectious diseases seen in industrialized societies at the turn of the century still characterizes the health situation of many Third World societies. In Sweden, Japan, and the Netherlands, the average person born in 1987 can expect to live about seventy-seven years; in the United States and Canada, that person will live seventy-six years. By contrast, life expectancy for those born in 1987 in Ethiopia is forty-five; in Bangladesh, fifty-one; in India, fifty-six; and in Haiti, fifty-four (World Bank, 1987). Average life expectancies are somewhat misleading, however, because they do not reflect the variations between subgroups (e.g., class, gender, and rural-urban differences) within each society. In Third World countries, as in nineteenth-century Europe and America, such factors as inadequate diet and unsanitary conditions contribute greatly to the high mortality rate and prevalence of infectious diseases. Childhood diseases such as measles are much more likely to result in death where nutrition and sanitation are poor.

Many Westerners consider Third World countries to be inherently disease-ridden, eagerly awaiting the benefits of modern civilization. In the nineteenth century, Africa was viewed as a "white man's grave," a disease-filled "dark continent." Many diseases, however, such as smallpox, syphilis, measles, influenza, cholera, and tuberculosis, were introduced to Africa from Europe and Asia, devastating native populations, which had no immunity to diseases to which they had never been exposed. At the same time, sailors, explorers, colonists, and merchants were exposed to diseases, such as malaria, that were new to them. Since they had no immunity, they too were hard hit.

The colonization of Africa and the slave trade created massive sociocultural dislocations and altered patterns of land use. Migration to the cities and the attendant overcrowding, as well the ecological disruption of the land, generated conditions that bred and spread certain infectious diseases. In epidemiological terms, alterations in the environment made for a changed relationship among host, agent, and environment. For instance, in western Africa the development of logging, commercial agriculture, roads, railways, and other changes in the landscape created sites (infection reservoirs) for breeding mosquitoes and thus for spreading malaria (Epstein and Packard, 1987).

Similarly, the transmission of the AIDS virus depends on the geosocial context in which it is spread. In North and South America, Western Europe, Australia, and New Zealand, AIDS affects mainly males. The mode of transmission often involves anal intercourse, whereas the rate from transmission by vaginal intercourse appears to be relatively low. In these countries, AIDS is concentrated primarily among homosexual men, contributing to the myth that it is essentially a "gay plague." Intravenous drug users are the second largest risk group; transmission occurs by sharing unsterile needles. The epidemiological profile of AIDS in countries like the United States, however, may be changing. More people in racial and ethnic minorities—men, women, and increasingly children—are becoming AIDS victims. In New York City, more than one-half of AIDS cases are among blacks and Hispanics (Shulman and Mantell, 1988). Among Hispanics, the rates are highest among Puerto Ricans, whereas the rates among Mexican-Americans are similar to those of non-Hispanic whites (Selik et al., 1989). The rate of new cases in the gay community may be leveling off because of dramatic changes in sexual practices (Fauci, 1988). AIDS is also becoming more geographically widespread in the United States, with one-half of new cases occurring outside of major urban centers. This development may be even more dramatic than it appears, because AIDS may be particularly underreported in regions like the Midwest and among persons of higher socioeconomic standing (Laumann et al., 1989).

In central Africa, the patterns of transmission to hosts and course of infection are quite different. One-third to one-half of all those with AIDS are women, with a large concentration of cases among prostitutes. This suggests that in Africa heterosexual intercourse is a more common means of transmitting AIDS than homosexual contact and intravenous drug use. By mid-1988, there were an estimated 250,000 AIDS cases worldwide, with about 100,000 cases in Africa (Mann et al., 1988). At the same time, the United States had about 66,000 cases (Heyward and Curran, 1988).

In countries such as South Africa, radically different pictures of health exist side-by-side in the same society. As a whole, South Africa has a highly "developed" economy. Nevertheless, the policy of apartheid produces the social and economic domination of a white minority over a nonwhite majority by radical segregation of housing, education, occupations, and legal status. This social arrangement results in very different living conditions for whites and nonwhites, and hence in different patterns of morbidity and mortality. The infant mortality for blacks in South Africa is at least six times higher than that of whites. One-quarter of black children under fourteen years of age are chronically malnourished or undernourished. By contrast, there is hardly any malnutrition or undernutrition among whites, and whites generally die of "diseases of affluence," which are linked with affluent lifestyles such as high-calorie diets and sedentary occupations. Blacks, on the other hand, are more likely to die of infectious diseases, such as typhoid, cholera, tuberculosis, and measles (a disease that is rarely fatal in "affluent" societies). Thus in one nation, two very different ways of life produce different health profiles. These differences are a dramatic illustration of how social-structural arrangements (i.e., apartheid) can produce different patterns of health, illness, and death (Frankel, 1986; Susser et al., 1985).

Not only are diseases themselves spatially and socially segregated, but various forms of segregation also reduce people's ability to know and understand others' way of life. Probably most members of the white minority in South Africa do not fully perceive the physical consequences of apartheid. The ability of the affluent to see the world of the hungry and poor is blocked by their spatial and social segregation from each other. Similarly, a reporter in Ethiopia noted that many members of the urban middle and upper classes did not have any knowledge of the famine in their *own* country until foreign correspondents wrote about it (May, 1985). A censored press, as in Ethiopia and South Africa, can thus mute social conscience. In many cities in the United States, economically comfortable middle-class persons may likewise live only blocks from squalor and never be truly aware of it.

VARIATIONS IN MORTALITY AND MORBIDITY

The wide range of mortality and morbidity within societies is distributed along basic sociological variables such as region, age, gender, ethnicity, and class. Variations in health and death are linked to people's different locations in social space and structure. The following discussion examines major variables in mortality and morbidity for the United States.

Age

As expected, death rates increase with age. In the United States, until the age of forty, death rates increase gradually. After forty, they virtually double for each decade of age (Mausner and Bahn, 1985: 120). Figure 2.4 shows population pyramids for the United States, which indicate, for a given year, the relative numbers of males and females in each age bracket. The data for 1910 take the shape of a conventional pyramid because the birth rates are balanced by death rates, for both sexes, in a somewhat even pattern. The 1980 pyramid, however, is less conventionally shaped because of decreased birth rates and lower death rates, a pattern that characterizes industrialized nations. This trend, in which fewer people are born and more live past the age of fifty, has been called the "graying" of society, because ever larger proportions of the population survive into old age.

Although chronic degenerative diseases have been increasing in all age groups, their rates increase most dramatically for older people. In 1965, one out of five Americans under fifty had chronic diseases; among

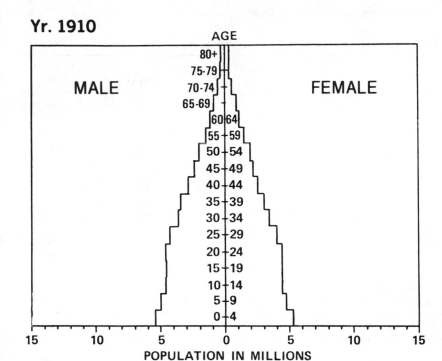

Yr. 1910

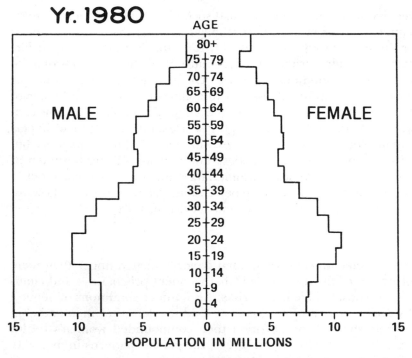

Yr. 1980

FIGURE 2.4 Age Composition of U.S. Population, 1910 and 1980. (*Source:* Population Reference Bureau, Population Bulletin 37(2), 1982: 30, 31.)

TABLE 2.2   Percentages of Deaths, by Cause, at Various Ages in the United States, 1980

	UNDER 50	50 TO 64	65 AND OVER
All causes	14.5	20.1	65.4
Heart disease	4.3	17.1	78.6
Cancer	9.7	30.3	60.0
Pneumonia	10.8	11.4	77.8
Diabetes	7.4	21.1	71.5
Cirrhosis of liver	27.4	44.7	27.9
Emphysema	2.7	22.3	75.0
Nephritis and nephrosis	11.2	20.3	68.5
Septicemia	24.7	17.0	58.3
Tuberculosis	15.7	27.2	57.1
Suicide	61.8	21.6	16.6
Homicide	81.3	12.8	5.9
Motor vehicle accident	76.4	12.0	11.6
All other accidents	49.6	16.2	34.2

Source: U.S. Congress, House Select Committee on Aging, 1980 Census of Population, Vol. 2, Subject Reports. Washington, DC: Government Printing Office, 1980.

those over sixty-five, four out of five had such disorders, with heart disease most frequent (Susser et al., 1985). Table 2.2 shows the major causes of death for three age groups in 1980. Only rates for death due to homicide, accidents, and suicide decline with age; rates of death due to chronic illnesses and disabling conditions increase. The increased number of people in our society with chronic illness and disabilities has raised a number of sociopolitical issues, discussed further in Chapter Eight. Many chronic conditions are not a "natural" result of aging. For example, the rate of hypertension (high blood pressure) increases with age in American society but not in hunting and gathering societies. The nomadic !Kung bushmen of the Kalahari Desert in Africa consume large quantities of dietary salt, a factor that some have linked to hypertension, yet they do not show increased blood pressure with age (Schnall and Kern, 1981).

Gender

In the nineteenth century, women typically died younger than men. One explanation of the difference is that frequent pregnancies and childbirth involved considerable health risks. Also, under conditions of general material scarcity, women often got what food was left after men and children ate their share. Poor nutrition then compounded women's health difficulties (Shorter, 1982). By the 1920s, the gender patterns in mortality rates had changed, and women generally were living longer than men. By 1983, the life expectancy at birth for U.S. males was 70.9 years; for females, 78.2. Similar differences between men and women exist in most Western industrialized countries (Sagan, 1987).

Biological factors may partially account for the higher mortality rates of males. Higher fetal mortality rates have been reported for males (Waldron, 1976). Because the male-female mortality rate difference occurs cross-culturally, it cannot readily be explained by social factors. There is evidence that female life expectancy is also higher among many other animal species (Sagan, 1987). This biological advantage for women may come from hormonal differences, although these differences may also produce in women higher rates of some sicknesses, such as gallstones (Friedman, 1987).

Men die earlier and have more life-threatening illnesses, but in general women become ill more frequently (Cleary, 1987: 55). Chronic illnesses are more prevalent among women than men, but they are less severe and life threatening than those of men (Cleary, 1987: 55; Verbrugge and Wingard, 1987). Women also report more episodes of illness and more contact with physicians (Susser et al., 1985: 71). Women's higher rates of sickness and doctor visits can be partly explained by gynecological or reproductive problems, which men would not have, but the incidence of these problems is not great enough to account for the difference in morbidity rates between men and women. Perhaps women are more willing than men to admit they are sick and/or to visit physicians. If this is true, then lower morbidity rates for men are deceptive, since they are a function of the underreporting of sickness rather than differences in rates of actual disease (see Waldron, 1976). It has been suggested that women learn more effective coping skills and ways of caring for themselves (such as seeking care and calling in sick), but there is no firm evidence for this hypothesis (Verbrugge, 1985).

Men are more likely than women to engage in high-risk behavior, such as smoking or driving fast, and risks associated with work roles may be higher for men (Verbrugge, 1985). Furthermore, there may be some differences in personal styles. Women are perhaps less likely to exhibit Type A ("coronary-prone") behavior, described in Chapter Five. The mortality gap between men and women may be narrowing in recent years. As women adopt more high-risk behaviors (e.g., smoking) and enter into work places with job stressors and other risks, and as men, by contrast, improve their health behaviors, the gap may narrow further (Cleary, 1987; Verbrugge and Wingard, 1987). While biological factors such as hormonal differences play some role, sociocultural factors linked with differences between men's and women's roles probably account for much of the sex-linked variations in mortality and morbidity rates.

Race and Ethnicity

Patterns of morbidity and mortality also vary among ethnic and racial groups in a society. Some differences may be explained by hereditary factors that are disproportionately characteristic of certain groups. Genetically transmitted sicknesses include sickle cell anemia (among blacks and some other groups) and Tay-Sachs syndrome (among persons of Eastern European Jewish descent).

Hereditary factors also combine with sociocultural factors to produce ethnic differences in morbidity and mortality. For example, Mexican-Americans are more likely to have inherent lactose intolerance than Anglo-Americans; lactose intolerance combined with social factors (e.g., higher rates of poverty) produces serious nutritional deficiencies (Schreiber and Homiak, 1981: 283). Similarly, genetic tendencies may be a component factor that, together with stressful living and working arrangements, leads to disproportionately high rates of diabetes among Mexican-American migrant workers (Angel, 1989; Scheder, 1988).

Patterns of variation are linked indirectly to ethnicity through other factors: nutrition, housing and sanitary living conditions, employment and types of occupation, family patterns, and lifestyle. Epidemiological data reflect these variables, but cannot always separate them neatly to show just how much variance is explained by any one variable. Other connections are more obvious. For example, a study of the incidence of childhood lead poisoning showing a large number of the victims to be inner-city black preschoolers could determine rather easily whether the causal connection was in fact that disproportionate numbers of urban blacks live in substandard, older housing where the crumbling lead paint may be ingested by young children. The following discussion gives some of the highlights of U.S. data about racial and ethnic variation in morbidity and mortality.

Black Americans constitute by far the largest racial/ethnic minority in the United States. Epidemiological data referring to "nonwhites" are thus mainly describing blacks. The pattern of health of black people is very different from that of whites. In 1980 black life expectancy was 69.6 years compared to 74.3 years for whites. Thus white males born in 1980 are predicted to live, on average, 8 percent longer than black males; white females born the same year are predicted to live 5.5 percent longer than black females (Hacker, 1983). These rates represent a dramatic improvement since 1920, when life expectancy was 45.3 years for blacks and 54.9 years for whites.

One major factor in the lower life expectancy for blacks is their high rate of infant mortality. Table 2.3 shows differences in infant mortality between white and nonwhite Americans for selected years between 1940 and 1985. Even though infant mortality has been steadily declining for both groups, the nonwhite rate has generally been about twice that of

TABLE 2.3   U.S. Infant Mortality Rates by Race for Selected Years, 1940–85

| | INFANT MORTALITY RATE[a] | | |
YEAR	ALL RACES	WHITES	NONWHITES
1940	47.0	43.2	73.8
1950	29.2	26.8	44.5
1960	26.0	22.9	43.2
1965	24.7	21.5	40.3
1970	20.0	17.8	30.9
1972	18.5	16.4	27.7
1975	16.1	14.4	22.9
1982	11.5	10.1	18.9
1985	10.6	9.3	18.2

[a]Infant mortality rate is the number of deaths of infants under one-year of age, per 1,000 live births.
Source: U.S. Department of Health and Human Services, Health, United States, 1986. Hyattsville, MD: National Center for Health Statistics, 1987.

whites. Infant mortality is especially high among newborns with low birth weight or very young mothers or both. The rate of live births of babies with low birth weight (less than 2,500 grams) was 12 percent for blacks compared with 6 percent for whites; 38 percent of black mothers did not receive prenatal care until after the first trimester of pregnancy, compared to 20 percent of white mothers (Anderson et al., 1987). These factors are clearly linked with socioeconomic factors. Low birth weight is often the direct result of poor maternal nutrition and inadequate prenatal care. Compared to other industrialized countries, the U.S. infant mortality rate is frighteningly high, largely due to this country's failure to address the problems of poverty, especially nutrition and health care. Indeed, since 1980 cutbacks in federal spending resulted in reduced or inadequate prenatal care for poor mothers (cf. Physicians' Task Force on Hunger in America, 1985).

The proportionately higher rates of hypertension and hypertensive heart disease among blacks compared with whites illustrate the complexities of causal factors with which epidemiological studies must contend. Factors accounting for these differences include genetic factors in susceptibility, greater stress due to racism, lower socioeconomic status, less access to good medical care, and a higher rate of obesity among blacks (Friedman, 1987). The genetic susceptibility explanation seems doubtful, because cross-cultural studies found no such patterns among genetically comparable peoples of Africa. Whereas American blacks show a rapid increase in blood pressure after the age of about twenty-four, African blacks living in tribal communities do not have increased blood pressure as they age. Migration to industrialized, urban settings, however, does promote increased blood pressure (Janes, 1986). The lower socioeconomic status of many blacks probably accounts for some of the differences in hypertension and other problems. Even after one takes social class into consideration, however, some small yet significant differences remain (Navarro, 1989). Such factors as stress produced by racism may explain some of these remaining "racial" differences.

Some American ethnic groups comprise individuals whose families came to the United States in different waves of immigration. Thus comparative studies have the potential of identifying which factors in sickness and death are due to the particular living situation and lifestyle of a group in the United States compared with the country of origin. For example, while the rate of tuberculosis among Chinese-Americans is higher than among the general population, it is nevertheless lower than in the "old country." Similarly, both first- and second-generation Chinese-Americans have more coronary heart disease than Asian Chinese; diet and stress are both implicated (Gould-Martin and Ngin, 1981).

Patterns of morbidity and mortality among Native Americans reveal another set of factors. American Indians are among the most disadvantaged ethnic groups in the United States; their death rate is about 30 percent higher than that of the general U.S population (Weeks, 1986). Like many peoples of developing nations, Native Americans are experiencing a demographic and epidemiological transition over a relatively short period of time.

Demographic transition refers to the changes populations undergo (usually in the course of so-called modernization) as they move from a situation of high mortality and fertility to a stage in which mortality has declined but fertility is still high. The third phase is characterized by low fertility and mortality (Omran, 1971). Native American groups have experienced more decline in mortality than in fertility, and the decline in mortality is largely due to the reduction of epidemic infectious diseases. The resulting rates of morbidity and mortality, at this stage of transition, reflect a shift in causes of death. For example, among Navahos overall mortality has declined, especially mortality due to influenza, pneumonia, gastritis, and certain diseases of early infancy; at the same time, there is increased mortality due to accidents and alcohol-related diseases (Kunitz and Levy, 1981).

There thus appears to be considerable racial and ethnic diversity in the United States in rates of mortality and morbidity, but precise figures are not available since national epidemiological data do not differentiate among white ethnic groups or nonwhite ethnic groups (for critical summaries of various studies on urban black Americans, Chinese-Americans, Haitian-Americans, Italian-Americans, Mexican-Americans, Navajos, and mainland Puerto Ricans, see Harwood, 1981a). Most differences, however, appear to be largely due to social-structural factors, especially class. Cultural factors also influence diet, health-related behavior (e.g., smoking and drinking), reproduction, and the like.

Social Class

Social class is probably one of the most useful shorthand indicators of a person's power. Class is usually measured by income, education, occupation, or a combination of these factors. Generally, there is a consistently significant relationship between class and health (Dutton, 1986). The lower the social class, the higher the rates of morbidity and mortality. This relationship is not surprising, considering the important part that social class plays in the quality of our everyday lives (Mausner and Bahn, 1985). Infant mortality and social class are also clearly linked. While infant mortality has declined for the population as a whole in the past century, class differences are still quite large and have remained constant over the years (Wilkinson, 1986a).

The relationship between social class and rates of mortality has been documented for England, Wales, Denmark, Finland, France, Japan, New Zealand, and the United States (Marmot et al., 1987). Table 2.4 shows some relationships between social class (measured by occupational classifications) and morbidity, mortality, and health behavior in England and Wales. Lower-class persons had consistently higher rates of perinatal (infant) mortality, maternal mortality (the mother's death from pregnancy- or birth-related problems), and mortality from all causes. Class differences are also linked to rates of coronary heart disease and diseases of the respiratory system. Morbidity rates (measured by respondents' reports of long-standing illness and the number of restricted activity days per year) show a regular correlation with social class. Class differences are particularly pronounced between the highest class (professionals) and lowest class (unskilled manual workers).

These data illustrate that differences that at first appear to be individual are often actually social variations. While smoking is an individual behavior, for example, those in the lowest socioeconomic positions are almost three times as likely to smoke as those in the highest positions (Marmot et al., 1987), which may partially explain the higher rates of respiratory diseases among the lower classes. Similarly, alcohol consumption is highest among the lower classes, as is the incidence of obesity (Dutton, 1986).

The Black Report, a famous British study on the relationship between class and health, concluded that lack of personal control over one's life was an important factor linking low social status with poor health (Black, 1980; see also Gray, 1982). Syme and Berkman (1976) have argued that this lack of control and other adverse features of lower-class life create a "generalized susceptibility" to disease. The issues of generalized susceptibility, control, and health will be discussed further in the next three chapters.

The conditions of lower-class life include living and working in more polluted and crowded environments, exposure to higher noise levels and risks of accidents, and inadequate housing and transportation. Medical care for the poor is less accessible and of lower quality than that for higher social

TABLE 2.4   Birth Weight and Mortality in England and Wales by Social Class.[a] Morbidity and Health Behavior in Great Britain by Socioeconomic Group.[b]

		SOCIAL CLASS[a]				
	I	II	IIIN	IIIM	IV	V
Birthweight ≤ 2500 g, 1980 (%)	5.3	5.3	5.8	6.6	7.3	8.1
Mortality						
Perinatal mortality/1,000, 1978–1979	11.2	12.0	13.3	14.7	16.9	19.4
Mortality 1–14, 1970–1972 M	74	79	95	98	112	162
F	89	84	93	93	120	156
Maternal mortality, 1970–1972 (standardized maternal mortality rate)	79	63	86	99	147	144
All cause mortality 15–64, 1970–1972 (SMR) Men	77	81	99	106	114	137
Married women	82	87	92	115	119	135
Single women	(110)	79	92	108	114	138
Coronary heart disease, men 15–64, 1970–1972 (SMR)	88	91	114	107	108	111
Diseases of respiratory system, men 65–74 (PMR)	60	74	82	105	108	123

		SOCIOECONOMIC GROUP[b]				
	1	2	3	4	5	6
Morbidity (age 45–64)						
% Reporting long-standing illness M	35	31	41	42	47	52
F	32	36	40	41	49	46
Average number of restricted activity days M	4	14	30	31	27	38
per person per year F	22	23	28	27	33	39
Health Behavior						
Prevalence of cigarette smoking, 1984 M	17	29	30	40	45	49
F	15	29	28	37	37	36
Participation in active outdoor sports (%), M	42		34	23	17	15
1977 F	30		27	17	14	11

[a]Registrar-General's Social Class: I, Professional etc; II, Intermediate; IIIN, Skilled occupations (nonmanual); IIIM, Skilled occupations (manual); IV, Partly skilled; V, Unskilled.
[b]Socioeconomic group: 1, Professional; 2, Employers and managers; 3, Intermediate and junior nonmanual; 4, Skilled manual and own account nonprofessional; 5, Semiskilled manual and personal service; 6, Unskilled manual.

Source: M. G. Marmot, M. Kogevinas and M. A. Elston, "Social/economic status and disease," Annual Review of Public Health 8, 1987: 113. Reproduced, with permission, from the Annual Review of Public Health, Volumn 8, © 1987 by Annual Reviews, Inc.

classes. Furthermore, health problems of the poor are typically more serious, complex, and difficult to treat (Dutton, 1986).

Measuring social class variables is difficult. Occupation is one frequently used indicator of social class, but occupational categories are often broad and not neatly tied with a single social stratum. For example, the category "teacher" might include a nursery school teacher and a professor at a prestigious university. How would the classification scheme distinguish between a farmer who owns fifty acres and cultivates them for family subsistence, and a "farmer" who owns four thousand acres and hires numerous workers to cultivate them (Susser et al., 1985)?

Despite such definitional problems, studies of many societies document a consistent relationship between social class and health. Rates of mortality and social class are clearly linked, but the relationship between class and specific causes of death is not so consistent, and may change over time. Rates of coronary heart disease in England and Wales, for example, first began to increase in the 1930s among men of the upper classes. By 1950 the disease was more common among the lower classes. A similar downward shift in the incidence of coronary heart disease took place in the United States (Susser et al., 1985). A possible explanation of the variation is that the upper classes were initially more susceptible to coronary heart disease as a "disease of affluence" (for example, they may have eaten much more meat and enjoyed more sedentary leisure time). All lifestyles changed, however, concern with dieting and exercise became values for many middle- and upper-class persons, and coronary heart disease declined. The lower classes did not adopt such lifestyle changes, and thus their rates of coronary heart disease remained high (Marmot et al., 1987; Susser et al., 1985).

The epidemiology of poliomyelitis also illustrates how the relationship between class and mortality from specific diseases may change over time. In lower-class areas, characterized by overcrowding and poor sanitation, children often developed antibodies and hence immunity to polio after being exposed to the virus early in life. Thus the poor had lower risk of paralysis and death than the more "sheltered" middle and upper classes. When the polio vaccine was introduced in the mid-1950s, however, this relationship between class and vulnerability to the disease changed. Those upper- and middle-class children who were first vaccinated were the first to benefit. An education campaign eventually resulted in the widespread acceptance of immunization, but pockets of underimmunized persons still exist in the United States, particularly among lower-class minority groups (Susser et al., 1985: 229–231).

These examples show that the relationship between specific kinds of morbidity or causes of mortality may not follow the usual relationship with social class and may shift over time. On the whole, however, the lower classes bear higher burdens of mortality and morbidity. The general incidence of morbidity and mortality decreases as one moves up the social ladder.

Even when data show a strong correlation between two variables, such as social class and health status, the direction of causality is sometimes difficult to determine. Does variable *A* produce variable *B*; does variable *B* produce *A*; or are they related in even more complex ways, mutually influencing each other or indirectly influencing each other through some third (intervening) variable. For example, do lower social status and the poor living conditions that accompany it produce poor health, or does poor health lead to downward mobility and lower income, or do both situations interact (Dutton, 1986)? The explanation that poor health results in downward mobility has been called the "drift hypothesis," which suggests that those who acquire disabling diseases "drift" down the social ladder in the course of their lives (Lawrence, 1958).

Some evidence hints that serious illness in childhood is related to downward mobility in later life. Boys who were seriously ill are more likely than those who were healthy to gravitate to a social position below that of their fathers (Wilkinson, 1986b). Downward drift may be linked only to specific "diseases" such as schizophrenia (Marmot et al., 1987), so the drift hypothesis does not satisfactorily explain the entire relationship between social morbidity and mortality. The hypothesis does appear to hold more for chronic illness than for acute illness. The two explanatory models may, however, be complementary: Chronic illness may lead to lower socioeconomic status, the conditions of which may increase the likelihood the person will suffer acute diseases, thus producing a vicious downward circle for the disadvantaged (Wolinksy and Wolinsky, 1981).

Some of the relationship between social inequality and specific kinds of morbidity and mortality may be more artifactual—a product of the way the variables are measured—than real. An extensive critique of the Black Report argues that the correlation between social class and mortality due to chronic degenerative diseases is essentially artifactual (Bloor et al., 1987). For example, the perceived social class of the decreased person influences whether the cause of death was classified as heart disease. The significance of such artifacts in the correlations between social class and health is not clear. Other reviews (compare Marmot et al., 1987) consider artifacts to be relatively unimportant in explaining the social class differences in health. They observe that a large number and variety of studies, done in several societies, indicate a strong relationship among class, health, and death.

SUMMARY

There are observable patterns to the frequency and incidence of human sickness and death. As opposed to the clinical-medical model, which focuses on individual bodies and a limited number of causal factors in disease, the epidemiological approach looks at social patterns of morbidity and mortality and the complex "web of causation." Epidemiological studies show that many patterns of morbidity and mortality are connected with social variables, such as the kind of society, race, ethnicity, age, social class, and gender. These epidemiological variables are also rough indicators of the social distribution of power and of the different power relationships people experience. With its broad generalizations, social epidemiology sets the stage for a more refined analysis of the ways a society produces, defines, experiences, and treats sickness and death.

RECOMMENDED READINGS

Article

John McKinlay and Sonja McKinlay, "The questionable contribution of medical measures to the decline of mortality in the United States in the twentieth century," *Milbank Memorial Fund Quarterly* 55, 1977: 405–428.

Books

Gary D. Friedman, *Primer of Epidemiology* (third edition). New York: McGraw-Hill, 1987. A clearly written introduction to epidemiological concepts.

Alan Harwood, ed., *Ethnicity and Medical Care*. Cambridge, Mass.: Harvard University Press, 1981. A well-integrated set of articles comparing U.S. ethnic groups on demographic and epidemiological characteristics, concepts of disease and illness, illness patterns, native and ethnic healing practices, encounters with mainstream medical practitioners, and adherence to biomedical treatment regimens.

Sol Levine and Abraham Lilienfeld, eds., *Epidemiology and Health Policy*. New York: Tavistock, 1987. An excellent collection of articles dealing with problems such as nutrition, coronary heart disease, cancer, injuries, and occupational health.

Mervyn Susser, William Watson, and Kim Hopper, *Sociology in Medicine*. New York: Oxford University Press, 1985. An interesting interpretation of the sociology of health and illness from an epidemiological perspective.

Chapter Three

The Material Foundations of Health and Illness

Certain social practices contribute to the production of a healthy body; others lead to its destruction. The very condition of our bodies—whether we are healthy or sick, whether we live or die—depends not on luck but on social circumstances.

In Chapter 2 we discussed some of the patterns of distribution of sickness and death according to social variables like socioeconomic status, ethnicity, race, and gender. In this chapter we shall examine certain social environments and practices that produce physical conditions contributing to these differences in health and illness. Basic health requirements—a satisfactory diet and a safe, clean physical environment—are very much influenced by many cultural and social-structural arrangements.

Much in our social activities endangers our health. How we organize production, and what and how we produce and consume are central to creating our way of life as well as to producing health or illness. This discussion begins by examining material (i.e., physical) sources of health and illness, and how they are shaped by social factors, especially the power of different groups to control physical resources such as food and the quality of the physical environment.

FOOD

World Hunger

Every few years the news media alerts the public in economically "developed" nations to widespread starvation in parts of the world such as Ethiopia or Bangladesh. The public conscience is mobilized, and money and food are collected. The furor then dies down, and for a while the public forgets the routine starvation that plagues much of the world. At the same time, the World Food Council of the United Nations estimates that 40,000 children die each day of hunger-related causes (Lewis, 1987). Another estimate suggests that approximately 10 to 20 million people die each year from hunger-related causes (Robinson, 1983). More than 1 billion people of the world's population of approximately 4.9 billion (Brown et al., 1987) are chronically hungry (Bennett and George 1987).

More common than outright malnutrition is undernutrition, or a diet that lacks certain basic nutrients (i.e., enough protein or vitamins). Approximately 6 million people suffer from blindness due to vitamin A deficiency. Another 750,000 die from this deficiency, which also lowers resistance to disease. There are 350 million people (mostly women between the ages of eighteen and forty-five) who suffer from iron-deficiency anemia (Latham, 1987: 330), which results in symptoms of constant fatigue. The mortality rate in Mexico from measles is 180 times that of the United States; in Ecuador it is 480 times as high. Differences in vulnerability to an infectious disease such as measles (which kills few people in the United States), tuber-culosis, and even diarrhea are partly due to nutritional factors (Eckholm, 1977: 48). While not starving, many people in the world suffer from stunted physical development, a greater vulnerability to disease, and a low-ered quality of life brought on by undernutrition.

An adequate diet is characterized partly by the quality of food con-sumed and by a certain amount of various vitamins, protein, fiber, and other components. An adequate diet also requires the consumption of a sufficient number of calories to support the body's activity. (A calorie is a measure of how much energy is generated by food eaten.) Table 3.1 shows variations in per capita calorie consumption in selected countries. We can see from this table that the figure for some nations, such as Ethiopia in 1985, was a little more than half that of countries such as the United States. Per capita figures, however, do not show how these calories are distributed within the population. Thus in Ethiopia some are well-fed, whereas others consume far *less* than their minimum daily caloric requirement.

There is a certain irony to the fact that although undernutrition and malnutrition are more common in Third World countries, they are also features of well-to-do countries such as the United States, where an entire industry is devoted to producing foods that taste like the "real" thing but lack caloric substance, and where some use jogging and other exercises to cope with the tendency to overconsume and overeat. In the 1960s, however, studies such as *Hunger U.S.A.* (1968) showed the extent of undernutrition in America. The introduction of food stamps, increased health care and wel-

TABLE 3.1   Nutrition of Nations, 1965 and 1985

NATION	DAILY CALORIE SUPPLY PER CAPITA	
	1965	1985
China and India	2,061	2,428
Other low-income economies (e.g., Ethiopa, Mali)	1,997	2,073
Lower-middle economies (e.g., Bolivia, Indonesia)	2,115	2,514
Middle-income economies (e.g., Chile, Jordan)	2,357	2,731
High-income oil exporters (e.g., Kuwait, Libya)	1,969	3,265
Industrial market economies		
All (reporting)	3,114	3,417
Ireland	3,530	3,831
United Kingdom	3,346	3,131
Canada	3,289	3,432
United States	3,292	3,663
Soviet Union	3,231	3,440

Source: World Bank, *World Bank Development Report, 1987.* New York: Oxford University Press, 1987: 260–261. Reprinted by permission.

fare benefits, school lunches, and other "poverty" programs since that time has helped to decrease the incidence of hunger. Some evidence suggests that cutbacks in these programs under the Reagan administration in the 1980s have led to the increased incidence of hunger. The recent report of the Physicians' Task Force on Hunger in America (1985) estimates that approximately 20 million Americans are hungry and that about 500,000 children are undernourished. Recent economic crises in the farming sector have ironically increased hunger among the families of the nation's food producers (Schneider, 1987).

Overpopulation and Scarcity.   One common theory explains world hunger as a matter of overpopulation combined with lack of natural resources, such as arable land and favorable climate. Accordingly, poor people exceed their ability to feed themselves by reproducing too fast. This is often called a "Malthusian" explanation, after Thomas Malthus, a nineteenth-century British economist whose theories of population growth still have influence (Hess, 1987). Malthus ([1798] 1965) argued that the growth of the world's food supply would not be able to keep pace with the growing population unless it were reduced by "natural" forces such as war or famine, or by poor people's abstinence from sex. Innovations in agricultural productivity, which were already apparent in Malthus's time, cast doubt on his theory. His interpretations nonetheless influenced many social scientists and policy-makers, particularly the nineteenth-century social Darwinists, who argued that social life and survival could be explained using the principles of evolution and that evolution favored the "survival of the fittest." Malthus's predictions were correctly characterized as "dismal" and led some (including the social Darwinists) to believe that while food aid and improved sanitary measures might help the poor in the short run, they would simply encourage them to breed more, thus creating more long-term suffering (Hess, 1987).

The Malthusian notion of an absolute scarcity of food and thus the need for poorer nations to control population growth still prevails. While there is some truth to this position, advocates often exclude policy measures, such as land reform, that would more equitably redistribute the resources needed to grow food (Moore-Lappé and Collins, 1986).

Malthus, of course, could not fully grasp the potential of modern technology to stimulate the food supply. It is estimated that, with existing levels of technology, it is possible to feed a much greater number of people than the world's current population (George, 1982; Moore-Lappé and Collins, 1986; Ross, 1975). However, in many countries hunger seems to have increased just as the world food surplus has grown. In fact, many poor countries in which undernutrition and malnutrition prevail are *exporting* large quantities of food. During a 1984 drought, for example, Zimbabwe was exporting a record harvest of tobacco, soybeans, and cotton, and Kenya was exporting asparagus and strawberries (Bennett and George, 1987). During a famine in Mali, there were likewise increased exports of cotton and peanut cake, which is fed to European cattle (Moore-Lappé and Collins, 1986).

After the communist revolution, life expectancy in China increased dramatically, from the age of twenty-four in 1929–31 to sixty-five in 1982; infant mortality also sharply declined. Except for periods of famine in some areas caused by natural disasters, China has been able to feed its people not simply by increasing food production but also by more equitably distributing food (Warnock, 1987; Lardy, 1983; George, 1982).

The improved standard of living brought population growth to China. Agricultural practices and land use for urban areas and industry have subsequently decreased the available arable land, which, relative to other countries, was already minimal (Warnock, 1987). To increase its living standards and diversify people's diet further, China may have to import food. If the nation continues to increase its use of energy-intensive agricultural methods to increase crop yields, it will become dependent on oil imports.

Nevertheless China—an extreme example of the Malthusian problem of many people and few resources—managed to bring about dramatic decreases in hunger through political changes. Population growth will be a significant factor in the long-term standard of living, but population is not the only factor, nor can the mechanisms that affect population growth be considered independently of sociopolitical and economic factors.

Emphasis on population control as the primary solution to hunger problems often places the burden of solutions on poor people whose attitudes toward birth control appear irrational to outsiders. High birth rates in developing countries may, however, be very rational to the people themselves, who believe they need more babies (in the face of high infant mortality) to care for them in old age and to provide a family labor force. Population growth is thus not simply the *cause* of poverty. Large families are a way of coping with impoverished conditions, and hence a *result* of poverty (George, 1982).

The scarcity argument also holds that many countries lack sufficient natural resources such as arable land. Only about 44 percent of the world's cultivatable land is being used, to grow food. Much lies unused for investment purposes (i.e., the owners are waiting for its value to increase). How land is used and who determines this use are thus important considerations. Colombia, for example, uses arable land for such export crops as carnations, which bring the large landowners more profit than subsistence crops. In Brazil, land that had once been used to grow food beans for local consumption is now cultivated in soybeans for export. Due to a diversion of land use for export crop production, bean prices tripled. At the same time Brazil's GNP (gross national product) increased, as did its supply of foreign currency. Brazil industrialized and its rich prospered, while hunger grew among the poor (George, 1982). Moore-Lappé and Collins (1977) have argued that every country has enough land to feed itself, and that hunger is often the result of patterns of land use and ownership that are shaped by the social distribution of power in these societies.

While overpopulation and geography contribute to world hunger, more important reasons involve sociopolitical and economic factors as well as technology and knowledge.

Technology and Knowledge.   There is no doubt that modern technologies, such as farm machinery, allow people to work the land more effectively and often to increase food production. Indeed, some improvements in health in the Western world were the consequence of advances in agricultural production. Yet these technologies must be viewed in their sociopolitical and economic contexts.

Modern technologies are expensive; people living at bare subsistence levels lack resources to purchase them. To get a loan from the Agricultural Development Bank, for example, a Pakistani farmer must own at least 12.5 acres, a regulation that excludes 80 percent of the nation's farmers (Moore-Lappé and Collins, 1977).

Toxic substances are often a part of modern agricultural technologies, but developing countries do not have effective regulatory controls (Norris, 1982). About one-half of the world's countries have no effective legislation to control toxic chemicals (Gelber, 1981: 53). Many pesticides such as DDT and DBCP, which have been banned in the United States, continue to be sold and used in the Third World. Beyond their widespread and deadly effects on farmers who often do not know of their risks, these toxic chemicals often come back to our dining room as residues on vegetables and fruits, thus completing a "circle of poison" (Weir and Shapiro, 1981). Industrialized nations export substances that are banned in their own countries but that subsequently are imported back into their own food supply.

The high yield these agricultural technologies produce has other negative consequences. They are typically energy intensive, requiring considerable quantities of oil to build and fuel machinery, and to make pesticides and fertilizers. Thus a great deal of nonrenewable resources, like oil, is required to produce relatively little food energy. The need to import such resources for energy and for agricultural technology increases the foreign debts of many Third World countries, which means that more land must be devoted to producing export crops to pay those debts. Should the market price of a major export crop drop, the problem becomes more acute. When coffee prices dropped in 1981, for example, El Salvador had to spend 70 percent of its coffee earnings on oil imports (Everett, 1984).

Energy-intensive technology is a mixed blessing for many people. Small farmers cannot afford it, and its uncontrolled use may deplete the land and cause extensive pollution. Technological solutions alone are thus of little use to many developing nations. Many farmers would benefit from less energy-intensive ways of growing food, but such possible options are not likely to be developed by the companies that profit from existing technologies. In short, technologies do not develop in sociopolitical and economic vacuums.

Some critics attack many of the agricultural practices and consumption patterns of the Third World poor as irrational factors contributing to their hunger. On the surface, nothing appears more ironic than starving Hindus in India who will not eat their cattle. Harris (1985), however, has argued that many of these seemingly "irrational" practices make ecological sense, given local conditions. Cows can be used to plow land and produce milk, their blood (which can be drained without killing them) is a source of protein; and their manure provides fuel and fertilizers. In the context of Indian culture, large-scale meat production may actually be "ecologically impractical," since it takes about twenty pounds of grain to produce one pound of beef (George, 1982). In fact much of the world's grain is used for animal feed. The major barriers to subsistence are thus not the lack of technology, overpopulation, or a scarcity of land but rather economic, political, and social considerations that relate to land use, distribution, and control.

Land as a Resource: Use and Distribution.   In South America, 90 percent of the land is controlled by 17 percent of the landowners (George, 1982). In Honduras, one of the poorest countries in Central America, 4 percent of the people control 65 percent of the arable land (Wijkman and Timberlake, 1984: 74). In El Salvador, another extremely poor Central American country, 81 percent of the arable land is used to grow coffee and is owned by 3 percent of the population (Kotzsch, 1985). This pattern of land ownership and use is typical of many Third World countries. In Africa, three-quarters of the population has access to only 4 percent of the land.

Bangladesh is an example of how patterns of land control are significant in explaining world hunger. In that country, the per capita calorie consumption is considerably less than the necessary nutritional minimum, yet Bangladesh actually produces enough food to be able to feed its hungry. In fact it exports large amounts of food. The wealthiest 16 percent of the rural population controls two-thirds of the land, however, while almost 60 percent of the poor have less than one acre (Crittenden, 1981). Those who own less than .2 hectares of land or who own *no* land consume an average of 1,924 calories per day. People owning 1.2 hectares or more consume 2,375 calories per day, and consume 28 percent more protein than those with less land (Brown et al., 1987: 31). In short, farmers' access to land and their ability to grow what their family needs are prerequisites to subsistence. Land reform that would make this subsistence possible is very difficult to institute, however, since the parliament is dominated by landowners (Crittenden, 1981).

Hungry Bodies Are Socially Produced.   A basic requirement for health is a good diet. At first glance, it would seem that the problem of hunger in many parts of the world revolves around issues of scarce resources, a lack of technology, and overpopulation. These undoubtedly *are* factors, but technology depends on who controls it, whether it is available to all, and whether it is geographically and culturally appropriate. Most countries have the resources to feed even very large populations, but the key factors in determining whether they do so appear to be political considerations as well as corporate control of technologies and often, of large amounts of land used to grow export crops.

Many have criticized food aid on the grounds that it is used as a political tool: Countries may withhold needed food aid from governments with policies of which they disapprove (Doyal, 1981; Kinley et al., 1981). A more serious problem, however, is that much aid never reaches those who need it because of local power arrangements. A World Bank study of Bangladesh discovered that about one-third of the food aid went to police, military personnel, and civil servants; that about one-third went to the urban middle class; and that only one-third reached the rural poor, who constitute the vast majority of the hungry. A similar pattern prevails in other countries (Parker, 1981; Kinley et al., 1981).

Hunger in poor countries is affected by their relationship with rich nations. Many Third World countries must contend with the impact of colonialism on their society, physical environment, and system of food production. Furthermore, rich nations' models of industrial food production may be inappropriate for less developed countries, and their pressure to adopt "advanced" food production methods often hinders the development of culturally and ecologically viable alternatives. Many Third World countries also serve rich nations as a source of markets, raw materials, and export crops. Fluctuations in global food prices are furthermore affected by the capitalist world market in which rich nations are a dominant force (Warnock, 1987).

The basic requirement of health, a good diet, therefore is linked to the distribution of power. It is easier to blame nature, scarcity, a lack of technology, or individual reproductive practices than it is to indict social systems. Yet it is the social systems and the way that power is distributed within them that shape the material world in which we live and hence the condition of our bodies.

The Sociocultural Dimensions of Eating Habits: "You Are What You Eat"

A society's habits of food consumption also play a role in nutritional problems. These eating habits are in turn influenced by sociocultural factors and issues of power. So-called affluent societies, with their diets high in animal fat, salt, and sugar, are often characterized by poor eating habits. At the end of the eighteenth century, sugar consumption in Europe (13 pounds per person per year) was already relatively high compared to previous times. With time sugar found even more and more uses as a flavor enhancer and preservative. By the middle of the twentieth century, sugar consumption in the United States was over 120 pounds per person per year (Mintz, 1979). In some respects our diets have become healthier (e.g., increased consumption of protein); however, in other ways (e.g., significantly increased consumption of food additives, sugar, animal fat, and salt), they have become unhealthier. We tend to view eating habits as a matter of individual free choice. While this is partly true, they also reflect sociocultural preferences, and the way we eat is shaped by sociopolitical and economic factors. In this section, the interrelationships among society, power, and food will be examined from that perspective.

We do not eat merely to survive or because food provides us with sensuous pleasure. For humans, food takes on symbolic meanings, and activities related to the consumption of food have social functions and dimensions. Sharing food reflects social bonds. A family dinner is an occasion to communicate, affirm social ties, and remind members of their respective social statuses. There are food taboos in virtually every society. For instance, Moslems and Jews prohibit the consumption of pork. A breach of such a taboo can affect one physiologically. A person who knowingly eats a proscribed food may get sick or even die. For example, when the Ponape, a people of the South Pacific, ate a forbidden fish, they would break out in hives (Farb and Armelagos, 1980).

Culturally rooted aversions to particular foods are not restricted to religious groups or "preliterate" societies. A priest in San Francisco once suggested that, since Asian refugees in the area liked to eat dogs and cats, the humane society could supply them with stray animals (which unless adopted, would be killed anyway) to use as food; his proposal was met with a great deal of opposition. Many Americans would get physically ill if they discovered that they had just eaten "puppy parmigiana," yet in some parts of the world dogs are a normal source of meat protein and are even considered a delicacy. Americans enjoy cheese, but most Chinese people find it disgusting. Cultural factors thus shape our food preferences, our reactions to food, and our very appetites (i.e., when we feel hungry).

The diets of specific cultures are often well suited to the physical environments and biological constitution of the people who inhabit them. A genetic intolerance of lactose, a prime component of milk, is not uncommon among *most* peoples of the world (Harris, 1985; Overfield, 1985). Such physical intolerance, common among the Chinese, may partially explain their aversion to cheese, for example. Biological variations are not the only reason some foods are defined as unpleasant or preferred. Cultures also adopt certain food habits for practical benefits, as exemplified by the

Hindu prohibition against eating cows (Harris, 1985). Some foods may be too costly in their demand on land, human, and fuel resources. The Chinese custom, for example, of rapidly cooking food in a wok over high flame developed because of fuel scarcity (Farb and Armelagos, 1980).

Sociocultural Change, Eating Habits, and Multinational Corporations.   When external forces alter the eating habits or way of life of a culture, new nutritional problems can ensue. In many societies, dental cavities were rare until Western influences introduced large amounts of refined sugar into the diet (McElroy and Townsend, 1985). Several decades ago the Zuni Indians of the American Southwest had a very low incidence of diabetes. As farmers and hunters, their bodies had developed a capacity to store fat efficiently to survive periods of food shortage. Their cultural values defined being fat as healthy. As they "modernized," their lifestyle became more sedentary, and they replaced their traditional diet with the low-income food culture of fast food that was high in salt, and sugar. Their biological capacity to store fat then became a liability, as they burned less energy and consumed more food. The incidence of diabetes subsequently increased (Peterson, 1986).

In recent years, multinational corporations have found new markets for their food products in the Third World. Often these products are promoted and introduced into sociocultural environments in which their widespread use may be inappropriate and unhealthy. Soft drinks and white bread, for example, have been aggressively promoted in countries like Mexico. Advertising campaigns and the fact that these products are seen as coming from a "high status" culture make them prestigious, and they may come to symbolize modernity and social status. Given the limited cash income of Mexican peasants, however, such products consume disproportionate amounts of the family budget and provide little nutritional return. A Mexican family may sell chicken and eggs (rich in protein) to get money for Coca-Cola (Barnet and Mueller, 1974). In a marginally nourished population, this exchange is a poor trade.

In the 1960s and 1970s, several companies such as Nestlé promoted commercial baby formula in Third World countries. Their advertising presented bottle feeding as modern and healthy for babies. Bottle feeding, however, required much of the family cash income (from 15 to 85 percent, depending on the country), and many mothers diluted the milk to stretch supplies, thus unintentionally starving their babies. The lack of the clean water, fuel, and sanitary conditions needed for formula preparation and storage also prevented the product's safe use. Even a marginally nourished mother can usually produce breast milk, which also transmits to the infant her natural antibodies that fight infection. As bottle-feeding practices were adopted in such places as Kenya, infant malnutrition increased. Doctors gave this form of commercially encouraged malnutrition a medical label: "bottle-baby syndrome." In recent years, because of a boycott and other pressures, the transnational companies were persuaded to stop many of their practices promoting this inappropriate product in Third World countries (Barnet and Mueller, 1974; Eckholm, 1977; Norris, 1982).

The world's eating habits are increasingly influenced by global corporate interests, which not only control much food production but also influence the information disseminated through advertising. One author concluded, "Backed by such powerful advertising, the standardization of food values at a global level at the expense of the local specificities has divorced people's eating habits from their history and culture" (Mansour, 1987: 16). Large corporations have not only more and more control over the growing and processing of food, but also access to powerful means of disseminating information about their products (e.g., advertising). These factors increasingly shape the food habits of the world.

Nutritional and Commercial Practices in Industrialized Countries. Commercial messages that promote foods are often directed at such vulnerable targets as children. A considerable portion of Saturday morning television commercials, for example, promote sugar-laden cereals and snack food. With the exception of a few token public service nutrition ads, most commercials imply that such food is consumed by the viewer's heroes, and that eating it will result in personal pleasure and status among one's peers (Gussow, 1978: 229; Barnouw, 1978: 91–92). One study indicated that children influenced by these commercials may exert significant control over their mothers' shopping habits (Barnouw, 1978: 92–93).

Not only do individual advertising messages affect eating habits, but their cumulative tone also suggests a cultural attitude toward food. The more implicit messages often have a greater effect. Bottled drinks, such as beer and soft drinks, are heavily advertised. The implicit message is less a matter of which product one drinks, but rather that one should want a commercial drink instead of water or a home-produced beverage to satisfy thirst. Advertising has thus sold a behavior, not just a product (Gussow, 1978: 222). Some ads suggest that when people are hungry and do not have time to eat, they should deaden hunger pangs by consuming a candy bar, which produces a sugar "high." Other ads urge the audience to eat or drink more, even after the hunger or thirst is satisfied; expanded appetites are thus created. To sell products, commercials often urge people to override their bodies' signals by either deadening them or overconsuming. Their messages are often contradictory: "Be thin," "control your eating," "eat, drink, and be merry," and "gorge, gorge, gorge."

Affluent societies often consume overly rich diets with too much sugar, fat, and salt, and too little fiber. Absence of fiber in a diet has been linked to the high incidence of colon cancer (Burkitt, 1973). Food processing enables modern societies to preserve, store, and transport a wide variety of foods, increasing their availability throughout the year in regions far from their origins. Processing also increases the convenience of preparation of many foods. By its very nature, however, processing causes the loss of many nutrients (Farb and Armelagos, 1980: 211). It also frequently takes away some of the natural flavors; to compensate for lost flavor, manufacturers then add sugar, salt, or artificial flavoring (Silverstein, 1984).

The diet of our modern society is more varied, interesting, and in many ways more nutritious than that of our medieval ancestors, who, prior to the fifteenth or sixteenth centuries, subsisted on a plain fare mainly consisting of grains and vegetables with few spices (Braudel, 1973). Increased trade, the availability of new foods and seasonings, and advance in agricultural technology and food processing have made an improved diet possible. The growth of capitalism helped to stimulate trade and technology to the benefit of many. Food processing, however, is also used to increase profit. Technologies have been developed to store foods longer, to increase yield of products (e.g., hormones make chickens grow faster and fatter), to enhance flavor in place of using expensive ingredients, and to disguise products with artificial colors, scents, and shapes (Center for Study of Responsive Law, 1982). Yet rather than reducing food prices, processing often increases costs (Silverstein, 1984). Corporate control over food production and distribution also affects the choices available. Relatively few people have access to and can afford to buy unprocessed foods, which are now sold as part of a growing health food industry. In many places, supermarket fare is the only option.

Dieting and Fitness. An estimated 10 to 20 percent of all children and 35 to 50 percent of middle-aged people in the United States are overweight (Eckholm, 1977). The excessive consumption of salt, sugar, and animal fats have been linked to many "diseases of affluence," such as hypertension, diabetes, and coronary heart disease (*Economist*, August 31, 1985). Since the mid-1970s, there has been a slight decrease in the number of deaths from heart disease in the United States. Some of this decrease has been linked to changes in habits of eating and exercise (*New York Times*, November 18, 1984). Stress, other psychosocial factors, and environmental factors like pollution have also played a role.

The motivation and opportunity to consume a healthy diet and to exercise are socially distributed. Several studies show a relationship between social status and obesity (Sagan, 1987). One study indicated that 30 percent of lower-class women, 16 percent of middle-class women, and 5 percent of upper-class women are obese (Goldblatt et al., 1965). Some of this variation is explained by differences in availability of adequate nutrition (i.e., starchy food satisfies hunger and is cheaper). Another factor is that people overeat to manage stress; also, different classes assign different social meanings to obesity. Obesity is not as heavily stigmatized in the lower class. Dieting and fitness rituals are primarily a middle- and upper-class phenomenon, not motivated simply by a concern for better health. In some cultures fat is a sign of prosperity; in middle-class American culture, however, fat symbolizes loss of self-control. Such differences lead some anthropologists to consider obesity to be a culture-bound syndrome, or a condition that "makes sense" as an illness only in certain cultural contexts (Ritenbaugh, 1982). In recent years, there has been an increasing concern with thinness. The pressures to be thin are greater for women than for men.

What constitutes being overweight, and how much excess weight is unhealthy? Questions of overweight and overnutrition are difficult to calculate with precision. While "objective" scientific facts bear upon the definition of "normal" weight, the facts change, and various groups challenge particular standards of evaluation. Table 3.2 shows the changes between 1960 and 1983 in the standards for normal weight as established by actuarial tables (statistical calculations, especially of factors related to life expectancy). Critics argue that these tables are based on samples unrepresentative of the general population (Cahnman, 1968), and groups like Weight Watchers, the American Cancer Society, and American Heart Association do not accept these changed standards as valid. In short, there is no tidy, universal standard for how much one should weigh (Schwartz, 1986; Attie and Brooks-Gunn, 1987).

Our cultural obsession with dieting and fitness reflects a concern not merely with health but also with self-control and physical appearances. In our society, looking good and feeling well tend to be confused. In all societies, health is judged to some degree on the basis of appearances, but in our society, a person's image is especially important, partly due to mass media influence.

Concern about weight and fat is one expression of a generalized societal anxiety about physical appearances. Since the 1880s, societal tolerance for high weight may have narrowed, and the criteria for acceptable weight have become more demanding (Schwartz, 1986). Eating disorders are on the increase (Sagan, 1987: 55, Attie and Brooks-Gunn, 1987), while cultural

TABLE 3.2   Metropolitan Life Insurance Actuarial Tables, 1960 and 1983

SUBJECT	YEAR	SMALL FRAME (POUNDS)	MEDIUM FRAME (POUNDS)	LARGE FRAME (POUNDS)
Woman, 5'4"	1960	108–116	113–126	121–138
	1983	114–127	124–138	134–151
Man, 5'9"	1960	136–145	142–156	151–170
	1983	142–151	148–160	155–176

Source: Society of Actuaries and Association of Life Insurance Medical Directors of America, *1979 Build Study* New York: Metropolitan Life Insurance Company, 1983. Reprinted by permission.

standards for women's bodies have shifted from fat to thin. In recent decades, the number of articles and books about diets have increased (Hatfield and Sprecher, 1986). In 1986 25 million people (mostly women) attended Weight Watchers meetings; 700,000 attended regularly, and $10 billion were spent on weight reduction drugs alone (Kleinfield, 1986). Women's and increasingly men's anxiety about weight and fat constitutes a major source of profit. A 1985 survey found that, in comparison to 1972 data, respondents (both male and female) showed more dissatisfaction with their body image. While the proportion of women expressing such dissatisfaction was still higher than in 1985, the differences in the level of dissatisfaction between the sexes had narrowed. Weight was the one physical feature that evoked the most anxiety among these males (Cash et al., 1986). A small 1981 survey found that 40 percent of the respondents considered "getting fat" to be a major personal fear (Schwartz, 1986: 246).

Such fears are not totally without foundation. Obesity is strongly stigmatized in our culture, particularly among the middle and upper classes (Attie and Brooks-Gunn, 1987). Negative attitudes toward obese people tend to be learned at an early age. One study showed ten- and eleven-year-olds pictures of a "normal" child, one with an amputated limb, one with facial disfigurement, one in a wheelchair, one with crutches and a wheelchair, and an obese child. When the children were asked to rank the pictures in terms of their preference for a friend, the majority made the obese child their *last* choice (Richardson et al., 1963).

Obesity *does* contribute to physical problems such as high blood pressure. While obesity functions to raise blood pressure because of the physical strain it puts on the body, other factors may also be involved. Perhaps the social meanings of obesity affect the body as well (Attie and Brooks-Gunn, 1987). Since obesity is perceived as a negative attribute, it may affect an individual's self-esteem. Anxieties about one's body may also contribute to increased blood pressure (Lynch, 1985).

Society's stigmatization of those who are overweight is related to the social norm of control, but there is a question of whether obesity is a metabolic disorder beyond some people's control (Brody, 1983). If this is the case, to focus on the individual's responsibility is cruel and futile. The regulation of appetites is not merely biological, however; there are important social factors too. To regulate our appetites, we need to know whether we are hungry. It is possible that obese people are more vulnerable to social forces that short circuit hunger signals from their bodies. One study found that "normals" were more oriented to internal cues as signals as to when to eat, while obese people relied on external cues such as the appearance, taste, and smell of food and the time of day, In one variation of the experiment, a wall clock had been moved forward a few hours, displaying the wrong time. Subjects of normal weight did not eat the available food, even though the clock falsely signaled meal time, whereas the obese subjects ate (Schachter, 1968).

Some have observed that this culture encourages people to rely on external signals for eating. Snack ads urge us to deaden hunger signals; meal schedules encourages us to look to the clock for signs of hunger. In a culture that encourages high levels of consumption, physiological hunger and nutritional considerations may be eclipsed by advertising messages designed to create demand (Silverstein, 1984). If there are "natural" limits to human appetites (and this is debatable), the economic system's impetus to sell must overcome them. This factor does not explain individual differences in responding to social pressures, but it does suggest that cultural pressures may affect the way people perceive their bodies, and hence how they control their eating.

All societies value some degree of self-control, but in modern societies such a concern is pervasive. Turner (1984: 112) observes:

> We jog, slim and sleep not for their intrinsic enjoyment, but to improve our chances at sex, work and longevity. The new asceticism of competitive social relations exists to create desire—desire which is subordinated to the rationalization of the body as the final triumph of capitalist development. Obesity has become irrational.

The contemporary emphasis on fitness, especially among the middle class, is not simply a matter of health but of conformity to the norms of an eternally youthful, lean body. Moreover, fitness activities may be a way of displaying control over one's body and hence over one's self in a culture in which control is valued and yet powerlessness seems to be a pervasive experience (Glassner, 1989).

A study of workers in California's "Silicon Valley" suggests that their almost compulsive tendency to exercise and diet (along with compulsive shopping and extensive drug abuse) represents a way of coping with the powerlessness, alienation, stress, and loneliness of much of their lives (Hayes, 1989). As with dieting, a vast industry has arisen to meet fitness "needs," producing endless streams of commodities and specialized technologies, from electronic rowing machines to digital pulse meters. Commercialized diet and fitness thus transform simple needs into marketable commodities (Glassner, 1989).

In modern society, appearances are very important in achieving success in work, play, and sexual relationships. A competitive society makes such successes important to the individual's sense of self. To achieve them, a rational mastery over the body and appearances becomes a central concern in life. By these norms, then, obesity reflects an irrational inability to control oneself, and fitness activities (beyond their contribution to health) promote a sense of self-mastery.

Gender, Power, and Eating Disorders.   Much concern about weight is a concern about appearances. The standards for physical appearances or somatic (body) norms vary from time to time and place to place. The importance of conforming to such standards also varies. Our society tends to evaluate women by their appearances and men by their performance (such as occupational, athletic, and sexual). Despite some shift in attitudes, men are generally more anxious about functioning and women about appearances (Melamed, 1983; Lakoff and Scherr, 1984). Furthermore, the responsibility for whether one is successful in one's area of competence rests with the individual:

> Ours is a culture of personal responsibility; we are told to captain our own souls and "take responsibility" for our successes and failures. Traditionally, men have been able to demonstrate success through their achievements in work, but it has mainly been through what a woman does with her appearance that she has been able to exhibit her mastery and achievement to others and to herself (Millman, 1980: 155).

While this "double standard" is changing somewhat, it still prevails. A heavy man can be seen as solid and powerful. Think of media heroes like "Cannon" and "Ironsides." Heavy women television stars, however are unlikely to have heroic roles (Silverstein, 1984: 107); they are typically portrayed as sloppy, weak willed, or comic.

Women are more likely than men to believe that they are overweight when in fact they are not, if judged by "objective" standards (which themselves are not so objective). A 1980 survey of college women found that 70 percent believed they were overweight, while only 30 percent actually fit insurance chart definitions of being overweight. Women's anxieties about weight are thus out of proportion to the facts. Fears about one's body and appearances are fueled by the mass media, which reminds audiences how inadequate their bodies are. One woman observes:

> The mass media tells us all day and all evening that we are inadequate, mindless, ugly, disgusting in ourselves. We must try to resemble perfect plastic objects, so that no one will notice what we really are. In ourselves we smell bad, shed dandruff, our breath has an odor, our hair stands up or falls out, we sag or stick out where we shouldn't. We can only rook people into liking us by using magic products that make us products too (quoted in Hatfield and Sprecher, 1986: 291).

Concerns about weight are a source of chronic stress for many women (Attie and Brooks-Gunn, 1987). Pressures on women to look thin may contribute to eating disorders like anorexia and bulimia (Fallon and Rozin, 1985), which are much more common among women than men. Anorexics lose the desire to eat and starve themselves. Bulimics binge, consuming vast amounts of food, and then purge themselves by vomiting or using laxatives.

Our culture gives members seriously conflicting messages about eating. On the one hand, people are urged to control their appetites and to diet in order to be sexy and desirable. At the same time, there is a conflicting message to enjoy life, to consume, to indulge ourselves and our appetites. The cultural contradiction of our times lies in the conflict between one set of messages, which emphasizes the importance of discipline as producers (i.e., the work ethic), and another, which stresses our role as pleasure-seeking consumers (Turner, 1984: 200). We are thus asked to be both ascetic (disciplined and in control of our flesh) *and* hedonistic (pleasure seeking and indulgent) at the same time. This dual expectation compounds problems for women, whose traditional role as nurturers and food providers places them in frequent contact with food (Charles and Kerr, 1986).

Anorexia can be interpreted as a woman's body discipline carried to an extreme. Families of anorexics often stress perfection and success. The anorexic woman takes the mandate to use diet to control appearance a step further than most would. The bulimic person perhaps responds to the contradictory messages of the culture by "both having her cake and eating it." The purge-and-binge cycle characterizing bulimics enables them to overindulge their appetites yet remain thin. Eating disorders are extreme, self-destructive ways of responding to cultural conflicts that affect most women to some degree.

Advertising for a variety of products may promote the bulimic solution in a seemingly benign way. One "lite beer" commercial promises, "Oh, you can have it all!," trumpeting both a message of the good life and the promise of a beer that tastes like it has substance but in fact has little actual substance. A vast array of diet foods offer a "banquet without food," which promises all the pleasures of eating without its unwanted consequences (Schwartz, 1986).

Eating disorders are not really problems of appetite for food but rather self-destructive responses to cultural constraints and contradictions. Somatic norms of femininity limit female appetites (not only for food but also for public power, independence, and sexual gratification). Gender role norms expect women to feed and nurture others, and not the self. And the culture subtly promotes the expectation that women be circumscribed in their access to and amount of public space (Bordo, 1989).

Similarly, overeating is sometimes a means of asserting control. Millman (1980) found that some of the obese women she interviewed experienced eating as the one area of a controlled life where they felt able to "let go," while others used eating as a way of protecting themselves against parental domination. One respondent reported that she ate and gorged herself as a defiant response to her mother, who was always harassing her about her appearance. Millman (ibid., p. 73) observed:

This woman (like several others I interviewed) has throughout her life used food and weight to assert and feel control in her relationships and her place in the world. And when these assertions run against the wishes of parents or husbands, eating and weight become associated with a refusal to bow to social control.

Others have argued that fat may represent a form of "armor" by which some women can protect themselves from unwanted sexual advances. Eating may also help to alleviate the anxieties about identity and devalued sense of self that our society engenders in women (Chernin, 1981). The double standards of physical appearances, together with the strong link that our culture encourages between women's looks and their sense of self, has led some writers to declare that "fat is a feminist issue" (Ohrbach, 1981). This approach suggests that eating disorders are not simply a loss of control but may reflect an attempt to *assert* control (albeit in ultimately self-destructive ways). It is simplistic to view eating disorders as a sign of personal weakness or as a purely individual matter, independent of social factors.

THE PHYSICAL ENVIRONMENT AND HEALTH

The physical environment is another crucial factor in health and illness that is profoundly shaped by sociocultural forces. The notion that clean air and healthy spaces are essential ingredients for well-being is by no means new. In the fifth century B.C. the Greek physician Hippocrates wrote about the importance of such factors. As described in Chapter 2, infectious diseases are more likely to develop and spread among poorly nourished, weakened "hosts." Even the earliest epidemiologists knew that environmental conditions, such as unclean water supply or poor sewage disposal, spread infectious diseases.

Development and Environment

Famine in parts of Africa has been blamed on unfavorable geography and climate. Some research suggests that colonialism disrupted traditional African farming practices that were adapted to the local environment. The best land was appropriated to grow export crops like peanuts. Brush and trees were cleared, thus hastening erosion and desertification (Danaher, 1985a; Franke and Chasin, 1981; Warnock, 1987). In the West African Sahel,

> while French science developed improved varieties of peanuts and the French vegetable oil business prospered, African farmers were being coerced through taxation and physical brutality into peanut mono-cropping that depleted the

soil, overuse of fallow areas, seasonal labor migrations that interfered with millet production and a breakdown of mutually beneficial grain milk exchanges with pastoralists from the Sahara desert fringe, whose animals had also manured the farmer's fields (Franke, 1987: 462).

In Central America, Nicaragua's landscape has been damaged by the stripping away of its rain forest, pesticide pollution, and industrial contaminants. Deforestation and pollution were a legacy left by the dictator Anastasio Somoza, the small local landholding elite that supported him, and U.S.-based corporations that invested there. Expansion of cotton plantations and cattle ranches forced poor farmers away from the fertile lands into the forests that they cleared. U.S. lumber companies also deforested vast regions. Cotton growers used large quantities of toxic pesticides, which polluted the soil and poisoned local people in epidemic proportions (Karliner and Faber, 1988).

The Sandinista regime came into power in Nicaragua in 1979 and tried to rehabilitate the land, impose environmental regulation, reforest, and find less toxic ways of controlling pests. Their ongoing war with the "Contras," however, hampered these efforts by diverting government funds for environmental protection into the war effort. "Contra" targets also included environmental workers and reforestation projects. Similar ecological destruction as the result of political and social conditions similar to those that prevailed in Nicaragua under Somoza can be found in other Central American countries like Honduras and Guatemala (Karliner and Faber, 1988). In many developing countries, the poorer inhabitants face the hazards of unregulated development but share in few of its benefits (Eckholm, 1977).

The transformation of the land through unregulated development may result in unforeseen epidemiological consequences. Massive deforestation in South India, for example, facilitated the spread of Kyasanur forest disease, an influenzalike viral infection spread by ticks. With deforestation, formerly tree-dwelling monkeys began to spend more time on the ground, thereby coming into contact with ticks. Cattle grazed on the cleared forest edge and were also exposed to the ticks. Human contact with monkeys and cattle that carried the ticks created an epidemic of this disease among people. Agricultural workers, who had the most contact with the cleared land between forest and pasture, were the most vulnerable (Nichter, 1987).

As we manage to control and pacify various external threats, ironically it is many of our own activities that cause many modern health problems. Even so-called natural disasters, such as floods, famine, and drought, are themselves affected by human activity. Human practices exacerbate the effects of flooding (Wikjman and Timberlake, 1984). For example, deforestation destroys natural barriers against flooding and fosters mudslides. Some agricultural practices that destroy the soil's ability to absorb water may also aggravate flooding. Deforestation often speeds up erosion and the growth of deserts. In short, even "natural" disasters often have social and political dimensions.

The Social Organization of Space and Motion

Our fitness, health, and physical comfort depend in part upon the quality of the physical space we inhabit and our options for movement within it, which in turn depend greatly on the social organization of that space and on the opportunities or constraints that social forces place on our movement. The social organization of space and motion is affected by the distribution of power in any given society. Some people have more influence in shaping their physical surroundings than others; some have more freedom of movement. The following examples of the work place and transportation illustrate how powerfully various social forces shape our physical space and motion with significant implications for our well-being.

Space, Motion, and Occupational Health.   The design of physical environments reflects social status. One indicator of social status is the amount and quality of an individual's space. Large private offices with windows, for example, are reserved for executives (Lindheim, 1985). Certain physical arrangements of the work place would appear to be essential for health, yet many low-status workers do not have access even to toilets or facilities to wash their hands. A 1984 study (Weinstein, 1985) showed that over one-third of U.S. farm workers did not have access to toilets and that one-fifth did not have access to drinking water. OSHA (Occupational Safety and Health Administration) has only recently passed regulations requiring employers to provide such necessities, the lack of which can spread infection. Because many farm workers work with toxic substances such as pesticides, the absence of washrooms is not just an inconvenience but also a health hazard.

Uncomfortable work environments are also problematic for the large proportion of employees who work in offices. The vast majority of jobs in the expanding information service sector are low-level positions in which workers have little control over their environment, which is designed to maximize cost effectiveness and worker control. The following arrangement is characteristic of white-collar offices:

> Of the people surveyed in one large modern office building by our Columbia University research team, 34 percent could not decorate or personalize their work areas in any way. They couldn't even hang a picture or keep a plant. Ninety percent could not control the number of people passing by their desk area, and 69 percent had no say over whether others could come directly up to their desk at any time without permission. Eighty-four percent of the office workers reported that they were always in the view of someone else and had

no way to avoid this contact; 80 percent also reported that they had no control over whether their work or conversations were overheard. The overwhelming majority of office workers could not alter the ventilation (88 percent), open the windows (96 percent), adjust the lighting (83 percent), rearrange the furniture or equipment (75 percent), or change the temperature (75 percent) (Stellman and Henifin, 1983: 112).

How the work place regulates our movements may literally shape or misshape our bodies. Friedrich Engels ([1845] 1973: 282–283), writing over 145 years ago, describes the crippling effects of their work on the bodies of women and children coal carriers:

The first result of such over-exertion is the diversion of vitality to the one-sided development of the muscles, so that those especially of the arms, legs, and the back, of the shoulders and chest, which are commonly called into activity in pushing and pulling, attain an uncommonly vigorous development, while all the rest of the body suffers and is atrophied from want of nourishment. More than all else the stature suffers, being stunted and retarded.

A 1978 analysis of injuries among office workers reported that two-thirds of the claims filed were for musculoskeletal disorders, and it is estimated that 76,000 such injuries occur annually. A study of VDT (video display terminal) operators found that 14 percent suffered backaches, that 25 percent had shoulder pains, and that 19 percent had wrist pains (Stellman and Henifin, 1983: 15). People whose occupations require the use of their arm, wrists, or fingers in quick, repetitive motions, such as cashiers, packers, mail sorters, and typists, may suffer from inflamation of their tendons (tendonitis) or from compression of their nerves (carpal tunnel syndrome or tenosynovitis). Reported cases of "repetitive strain" injury have risen in the United States in recent years (Tuller, 1989). Certain work movements may cause disproportionate wear and tear on certain parts of the body. While some of these problems are inherent in the type of activity involved in an occupation, they can be reduced by frequent breaks, job rotation, and opportunities to stretch as well as by the proper ergonomic design of equipment and work space.

Ergonomics is the study of the relationship between the workers, their movements, and the physical features of their work environment. For example, is the chair designed to minimize backaches after long hours of sitting? Is the control panel easily readable and within comfortable reach? Ergonomic studies have tended to emphasize designing machines and work places that will enhance productivity; however, less attention has been directed toward worker health or comfort (Goldsmith and Kerr, 1982). Furthermore, ergonomists design work places with the "average" person in mind, with little provision for those whose bodies are not average.

In many work places, even basic ergonomic considerations are often ignored to enhance productivity and profits. Workers may be forced to work in cramped, uncomfortable positions. For instance, one welder comments:

> I got moved to a new job spot-welding where I had to stand on my toes with my head all the way against my back and my arms stretched out all day long. I told my boss that we had to disassemble the piece in order for me to do the job without injuring myself, and he insisted that I could do it the way it was. Well, I did it until finally I hurt my back so bad that I was out for 5 months (quoted in Back, 1981: 24–25).

Until a few decades ago, farm laborers were forced to use short-handled hoes, which raised productivity by increasing traction but also caused serious back pains. It was only after pressure from unions and workers that the farm owners finally allowed workers to use long-handled hoes. Healthy movements are thus related not just to the nature of the activity, but also to the design of the tools and environment.

Varying the position of the body frequently during the workday is important for orthopedic health and psychological well-being. Some workers come to experience themselves and their bodies as "spirit" or disoriented when their work involves uncomfortable, uninterrupted, repetitive motions:

> I sit in one place all day facing a wall. My fingers are moving all the time, my eyes are staring into a machine that is placed so I have to hold my neck stiff to see the words clearly. Everyone is typing or using machines so there is a lot of noise. It's impossible to talk or even to turn around and look at someone else. My job is basically to copy numbers and letters all day, but most of the time I'm not even aware of them. *It's like my hands and my eyes are alive and my mind and my body are dead* (quoted in Back, 1981: 41–42 [emphasis added]).

People can adapt to unhealthy environments, but often at a cost. A significant portion of time in our everyday lives is spent on such unnoticed forms of body activities as walking up and down, pacing, stretching our limbs, tapping our feet, drumming our fingers, smoothing our hair, and hugging our body. These kinds of activities are integral to our self-image and contribute to stress reduction and to fitness (Csikszentmihalyi, 1978: 297). They may also foster a sense of self-control and physical-emotional satisfaction. The social arrangements of many work places affect workers' ability to engage in these natural activities.

The work place illustrates the relationship between the organization of space and the regulation of motion, and workers' psychophysical well-being. Disempowering spaces force people's bodies into standard forms or the motions of a machine. Workers need to vary their movements and to distribute more evenly the stressors that cause bodily wear and tear. The ability to control movements and to adapt work spaces to one's own well-being in turn depends on various political and economic factors.

Space, Motion, and Transportation.   Another arena in which space and motion affect health is the automobile. In many parts of the United States, someone with no automobile transportation has severely curtailed access to medical care, shopping, leisure activities, friends, and work. It has been estimated that more than 57 percent of U.S. households with incomes under the poverty level do not possess a car. About 45 percent of elderly households lack a car. Similarly, most youths and persons with disabilities are unable to transport themselves (Myers, 1972). In American society access to transportation is thus unequally distributed, based on race, income, age, and class (Yago, 1985). The system of transportation dominated by the individual passenger car was created not merely by individual consumer choices but also by political and corporate interests. The major portion of public funds spent on transportation in the United States goes for highways as opposed to mass transit (Snell, 1982).

Reliance on automobile transportation is related to various problems of physical fitness. Difficulties in commuting can increase stress; for example, the heart rate of a train passenger is lower than that of a passenger in a private car (Lundberg, 1976). Driving causes increased levels of stress hormones, blood sugar, and cholesterol (Robinson, 1988), and can create problems like "motorist's spine" and "driver's thigh" (Homola, 1968). Persons who drive a car for twenty miles or more a day are at special risk for lumbar disk herniation (lower back injury). Truck drivers suffer a high rate of back injuries (National Institute on Disability, 1987).

The shape of modern transportation networks is the result not merely of society's love affair with the automobile but also of concrete economic and political decisions that affect the location of corporation offices, shopping malls, industrial parks, and restaurants. These decisions thrust individuals into reliance on private automobiles, whether they love or hate them. Advertising campaigns of automobile companies, furthermore, have imbued the car with symbolic meanings of masculinity, freedom, and social status; reliance on cars is thus not simply a matter of preference. Through their various interventions in the marketplace, manufacturers have shaped social space to the needs of automobile transportation. According to Snell (1982), from the 1930s to the 1950s the automobile industry (specifically General Motors) promoted the homogenization of the urban landscape by dismantling alternate transportation networks (e.g., trains and trolleys) and replacing them with inefficient, polluting trucks, buses, and automobiles. Once other modes of transportation had declined, the automobile become a virtual necessity rather than a luxury.

Accidents: An Individual or Social Problem?

Following heart disease, cancer, and stroke, accidents are among the foremost causes of death in American society. Automobile accidents constitute a large percentage of total accidents; work-related injuries are another important component. Accidents result from the interplay among an unsafe environment, unsafe equipment and tools, and the behavior of the individuals involved. Accidents are usually treated as the results of individual fault, but often social and environmental problems also play a significant causal role. The very definition of events as "accidents"—as opposed to socially produced, preventable incidents—has political and social policy implications.

Auto Accidents.   While the death rate due to auto accidents in the United States is by no means the highest among industrialized countries, some 43,000 to 53,000 Americans die each year in such accidents, producing a death rate of over 26 deaths per 100,000 population (National Safety Council, 1986). Worldwide, some 200,000 people died in traffic accidents in 1985 (Renner, 1988). There are approximately 4 to 5 million injuries related to motor vehicles each year in the United States. Of these, 500,000 people require hospitalization (averaging a stay of nine days). More deaths occur from automobile accidents than from any other injury-producing event. Motor vehicle accidents are the largest single trauma-induced cause of paraplegia and quadriplegia, and a major cause of epilepsy and head injuries (Claybrook et al., 1984); each year about 20,000 Americans develop epilepsy as a result of auto accidents (Schneider and Conrad, 1983). Auto accidents are a leading cause of death for young people between the ages of five and twenty-four; young males between the ages of fourteen and twenty-four are at highest risk (Baker et al., 1987). Per passenger mile, cars are more dangerous than trains, buses, or planes.

Why the automobile exacts such a high health risk is a complex question. Much public attention focuses on drunk driving; some estimate that it is connected to about half of all of traffic fatalities. These estimates are somewhat misleading, however, since they include all traffic deaths in which any of the parties involved consumed alcohol, even if the person who was drinking was not at fault. Other estimates place the figure of alcohol-related deaths at 25 percent (Ross and Hughes, 1986). Many alcohol-related traffic fatalities, furthermore, involve cofactors such as fatigue, inexperience, poorly designed or inadequately lit roads, and unsafe cars (Gusfield, 1981). Such devices as air bags have been shown to significantly reduce fatalities, yet the automobile industry lobby has regularly worked to prevent the implementation of regulations to require air bags in cars (Baker et al., 1987).

Although individual drivers have a responsibility to drive safely, focusing merely on individual behavior neglects the social, cultural and environmental dimensions of auto accidents. Some roads are designed without barriers between oncoming cars; cars lack protective devices like air bags, and drivers use vehicles capable of killing speed (Schrank, 1977: 77). When New Jersey residents were given the option of free and readily available public transportation on New Year's Eve, the accident rate declined. In many parts of this country, the automobile is the only available means of transportation, pressuring drunken drivers and other impaired persons (e.g., those with vision problems) into driving (Syme and Guralnik, 1987). Such factors in traffic fatalities are the result of social policies.

Policy responses to traffic accidents emphasize raising the *drinking* age, but few legislators would consider raising the *driving* age, because in many parts of the country to be without a car is to be helpless, especially given an atrophied public transportation system. Social factors also explain why males are at particularly high risk. Many young males are socialized into taking lots of risks and into feeling or appearing invulnerable; media messages glorify speed and risk-taking; many car-chase scenes convey a relatively carnage-free image of fast or reckless driving; advertisements glamorize cars as images of masculinity, speed, power, and excitement; and young men often view the use of seat belts as not "macho" (Horton, 1985b).

Economic pressures may also contribute to vehicular accidents by promoting reckless behavior on the road. Truck drivers have a high rate of drug consumption (especially stimulants). Economic considerations lead them to drive longer hours with unsafe equipment and larger payloads. Thus social-structural forces contribute to trucking accidents (Sherrill, 1977).

In addressing the problem of automobile accidents, most policy focuses on changing individual behavior through education or various sanctions (Gusfield, 1981). However, individuals are hard to reach, influence, and control; traffic penalties are not consistently and rapidly imposed on violators; and to monitor and educate all drivers is difficult and not very cost effective. By contrast, an **ecological approach** to the problem emphasizes changing the social and physical environment (e.g., building safer highways), producing safer cars, and making many alternative ways of traveling available to drivers (Syme and Guralnik, 1987). These kinds of preventive measures have, however, been consistently constrained by the marketplace. The political and economic power of the automobile industry, in consideration of the cost of designing safer vehicles and highways, seriously limits the government's power or willingness to choose and implement solutions to prevent auto accidents (MacLennan, 1988).

Work-Place Accidents: Unsafe Behavior, Unsafe Conditions?

Work-place *accidents* (some prefer the term "injury," since an accident implies a random occurrence) differ from occupational *diseases* in that in the former the exposure to the source is sudden, and the damage as well as its cause is readily apparent (Baker et al., 1987: 177). By contrast, the cause of work-related diseases is not always apparent, and the effect may be gradual. Accidents are thus discrete, clearly identifiable events that happen suddenly.

Work-place accidents alone cause some 5 million reported injuries, of which 2.2 million are disabling and 13,000 result in death (Hills, 1987). Like other health problems, their incidence and severity tend to be socially distributed. Lower-status jobs generally involve more accidents (Dutton, 1986). Because black males tend to work in high-risk occupations (e.g., coke-oven stokers) with little control over their work environment, they have 37 percent greater likelihood than whites of suffering occupational injuries or illnesses (Goldsmith and Kerr, 1982). The rate of injuries, particularly fatal ones, have generally declined somewhat in the past fifty years (Baker et al., 1987). The legislation of safety regulations, such as the 1969 Federal Mine Safety and Health Act, seems to have helped reduce injuries.

Data on work-place safety are highly problematic. Job injury rates are sometimes calculated in terms of the number of workdays lost per week, month, or year due to injury. However, employers often keep injured workers on the job or temporarily move them to easier jobs to keep injury down (Goldsmith and Kerr, 1982). Some companies simply do not report all injuries. In 1986 the Chrysler Corporation was fined a substantial sum for failing to report 182 injuries at one work site alone (Noble, 1986). Since official government data are based on company self-reports, these figures also tend to underestimate injuries. In 1985 the U.S. Bureau of Statistics reported that 3,750 workers died on the job, whereas the National Safety Council (an independent agency) reported 11,600 worker deaths (Noble, 1986). Part of this discrepancy is due to the fact that the government does not count injuries in private businesses employing fewer than eleven people. Because the current administration of OSHA uses injury rates to decide whether to inspect a work place, this undercounting of injuries has serious policy and regulatory implications.

Until recent decades, much research focused on work-place accidents rather than diseases, partly because the source of the damage is easier to identify. It is also easier to emphasize the individual's role in an accident. For example, textbooks on occupational health argue that changing the work environment reduces occupational diseases, but treat occupational accidents as essentially a problem of individual attitude and safety awareness (Baker et al., 1987: 197).

The concept of "accident proneness," first coined in 1926, became the focus for whole generations of industrial psychologists who searched for specifiable characteristics causing some individuals to be especially likely to have accidents. In a chapter on "industrial and occupational" psychiatry, the 1966 *American Handbook of Psychiatry* described the "accident syndrome" as involving an "impulsive character" and "reaction of anxiety." The handbook does not suggest, however, that the psychiatrist should take into account the characteristics of the work place in which the "accident prone" behavior occurs (Berman, 1978: 23–24). Empirical research has been unable to isolate any personality traits, independent of specific situations, that could be categorized as "accident proneness" (Members of the Working Party, 1973).

Environmental factors also contribute to accidents. Work-place accidents involve "accident prone" tools and environments, as well as social pressures that encourage risky behavior. As for automobile accidents, the ecological model appears more useful than the individual behavior model for understanding work-place accidents. At one steel plant, for example, the higher the rate of production grew, the higher the monthly injury rate rose (Hills, 1987). Similarly, in the past decade or so the meat-packing industry has been under increased competitive pressure. Wages have decreased, but productivity pressures in this shrinking industry have grown, simultaneously increasing the rate of on-the-job injuries (Glaberson, 1987). Especially when linked with other factors such as increased job alienation, situational pressures enhance the likelihood of accidents (Back, 1981).

Design of equipment itself is sometimes the source of accidents. Although machines can be built in an ergonomically sound fashion to reduce accidents, more often they are designed mainly to enhance productivity (Goldsmith and Kerr, 1981). The burden of accident prevention in these environments is thus on the individual worker. An assembly-line worker commented:

> When there are accidents they always blamed us for not using safety equipment. Six of us had to work with an acid solution and we were all given plastic goggles. But no one could wear them because they didn't fit and you couldn't see very well with them on. This was a piece work job and there was no way we were going to make our bonus if we wore our glasses. I always felt caught between being worried about my health and being worried about not making production. You know it could've been fairly easy to put a shield over the whole operation so we wouldn't have to worry about it (quoted in Back, 1981: 15).

Engineering controls that alter the environment, such as putting a protective "shield over the whole operation," are typically more expensive than giving workers individual safety equipment, such as respirators to prevent breathing dust. So-called passive safety approaches, which rely on safe equipment and environment more than on behavior, are more effective but also more expensive (Baker et al., 1987). While respirators are cheaper for corporations, they create problems for workers. Respirators are physically uncomfortable, especially if worn the whole day under conditions of high temperature and noise. They may also be ineffective or create such side effects as breathing difficulty or heart strain. Work-place physical stressors, such as high noise levels and toxins, may also affect workers' perception, alertness, and reflexes, thereby producing "accident proneness" (Doyal, 1981).

Some social scientists consider accidents to be related to the social structure of the work place. In many work situations, there is a split between those who plan and organize work and those who execute it. As described in Chapter 6, this division may influence the perception and treatment of occupational health problems (Navarro, 1981). Experts who study accidents and occupational health problems are often far removed from the day-to-day routine of the work places they analyze. Furthermore, management concerns with productivity and cost effectiveness are not always compatible with workers' needs for safe work places. Human error (e.g., due to drug use) and carelessness *are* important factors in work-place injuries. It is also important, however, to focus on how such variables as styles of managerial control also contribute to work-place health problems (Members of the Working Party, 1973: 74–75). One basic issue in occupational injuries is the conflict between, on the one hand, managerial pressures to enhance productivity, control, and profit margins, and, on the other hand, the needs of workers to work in the safest technologically feasible working environment. Box 3.1 illustrates some structural ways of reducing work-place injuries.

BOX 3.1   Swedish Road to Better Conditions

The Swedish approach to health and safety has four main features.

First, Swedish workers have won real power at the local level to prevent hazards. Sweden's OSHA—the National Board of Occupational Safety and Health—sets standards and inspects work places, but unions view its role as secondary to their own efforts.
Second, Swedish workers have the information and training to enable them to use that power.
Third, unions have a major voice in safety and health research and research is often geared to finding practical solutions to hazards.
Fourth, Swedish unions are concerned about the total work environment, not just safety and health as narrowly defined in the U.S. They consider physical safety hazards, chemical and noise exposures, heat and cold, speed-up, boredom, and stress as related problems. The Swedish unions are concerned not only about injuries and illnesses but also discomfort, an unpleasant work place and lack of job satisfaction.

They believe that workers are entitled to a humane work environment and control over their jobs.

Source: In These Times, January 18–21, 1986: 17. Reprinted by permission.

ENVIRONMENTAL POLLUTION

The concept of pollution usually carries the connotation of the fouling of the environment by humans, but volcanoes pollute the air and various nonhuman species pollute the environments with their excreta. In fact, most atmospheric pollution is not of human origin. Only 9 percent of the carbon monoxide in the air comes from human sources, such as automobile use. Of all particulates (i.e., bits of metal and the like) emitted into the air, only 11 percent comes from human activity (e.g., cars and industrial pollution). Various industrial processes account for 16 percent of the hydrocarbons in the atmosphere. About 45 percent of the sulfur dioxide in the atmosphere comes from human activity (Botkin and Keller, 1982: 172–173).

Table 3.3 shows the quantities and sources of major pollutants emitted in the United States. There was a significant decrease of lead emissions between 1975 and 1980, coinciding with an approximately 50 percent decline in the use of leaded gasoline. Motor vehicles are a major source of carbon monoxide, a gas that interferes with the blood's ability to carry oxygen. Sulfur dioxides and nitrous oxides come from fuel combustion used to heat dwellings, generate electricity, and power motor vehicles (Renner, 1988). These emissions are important components of acid rain, which has a destructive impact on forests and the life in lakes and rivers, contributes to the erosion of building surfaces, and may contribute to human respiratory problems. Because acid rain often falls in regions distant from where the pollution originates, the economic activity in one region damages the environment in another, causing political strains between regions and nations, such as the United States and Canada.

While humans are not the only sources of global pollution, their

TABLE 3.3   Air Pollution in the United States in 1984 (Calculated Emissions Estimates)

TYPE OF POLLUTANT	ALL SOURCES	TRANSPOR- TATION	STATIONARY FUEL COMBUSTION	INDUSTRIAL PROCESSES	SOLID WASTE	OTHER
Particulate matter[a]	7.0	1.3	2.0	2.5	0.3	0.9
Sulfur oxides[a]	21.4	0.9	17.4	3.1	(1)	(1)
Nitrogen oxides[a]	19.7	8.7	10.1	0.6	0.1	0.2
Carbon monoxide[a]	69.9	48.5	8.3	4.9	1.9	6.3
Lead[b]	40.1	34.7	0.5	2.3	2.3	(2)

[a]Emissions in 10^6 metric tons per year
[b]Emissions in 10^3 metric tons per year
(1) Emissions of less than 50,000 metric tons per year
(2) No emissions calculated

Source: U.S. Department of Health and Human Services, Health, United States, 1986, Hyattsville, MD: National Center for Health Statistics, 1987:134.

activities have increasingly produced ecological changes in climate, atmosphere, and the very shape of the earth's surface. Our social institutions may not be able to effectively regulate the impact (Shabecoff, 1987b: A6). This impact of humans on the "spaceship earth" is not merely the result of technology or "progress" but is also linked to the failure of political, economic, and social policy to regulate the use of technology or to create "healthier" technologies.

Discussions of pollution often pronounce that "we" (referring to humans in general) pollute. This expression, however, masks the sociopolitical dimension of environmental health by equating the individual "litterbug" with the corporate polluter whose impact on the environment is more far-reaching and potentially dangerous than that of the individual (Bookchin, 1962). Not all of "us" pollute equally, nor are we all equally affected by pollution.

"Don't Let the Smoke Get in Your Lungs":
The Individual as Polluter

While tobacco smokers do not contribute significantly to atmospheric pollution, their habits do have a significant impact on health (U.S. Department of Health, Education, and Welfare, 1972). They obviously pollute their own air, and are at increased risk of coronary heart disease, emphysema, bronchitis, and lung, bladder, and esophagal cancer (U.S. Department of Health and Human Services, 1987: 50). An estimated one-quarter of the U.S. population smokes tobacco, and one-sixth (37 million) will die prematurely from their smoking habit (Blair, 1979). In Britain, an estimated 100,000 people each year die prematurely from smoking (Doyal, 1981: 80). Some experts argue that smoking is as serious an addiction as heroin and, in the long run, perhaps even more damaging to the body (Weil and Rosen, 1983).

Individuals who smoke also affect the quality of air shared by others in the enclosed spaces of offices, homes, and restaurants. Passive smoking (the inhaling of someone else's cigarette smoke) has been linked to a variety of health risks. Parents' smoking has an impact on the respiratory health of their children, and a smoker's spouse may have increased risk of lung cancer (Fielding and Phenow, 1988; Sandler et al., 1988). The effect of the smokers' habit on nonsmokers raises fundamental issues regarding individual rights as opposed to collective rights:

> Air pollution makes us take seriously the fact that we exist, not as isolated entities secure behind our fences, but as fellow creatures in a shared and threatened environment. While in some settings—when looking at second-hand smoke or workplace hazards—we can insist that individual consent remains fundamental, in others we may have to look beyond consent to auton-

omy and beyond the individual to a deeper sense of community. If anything is our birthright, it is the air that we breathe (Center for Philosophy and Public Policy, 1985:5).

Some research suggests that there may be a synergistic (i.e., mutually enhancing) relationship between smoking and air pollution from other sources. For example, smokers in urban areas of high air pollution are at a greater risk of lung cancer than their rural counterparts who smoke (Epstein, 1978).

Movements to restrict smoking in public places are becoming widespread in the United States (Cummings, 1984). One company told workers that they would either quit smoking or lose their jobs (*New York Times*, January 25, 1986). The courts subsequently overturned the company's efforts to control its workers' private lives (i.e., smoking outside of work). This company manufactures accoustical tiles and insulation containing various fibers that may contribute to respiratory problems and lung cancer. Union officials saw the company's emphasis on smoking as an attempt to evade the more costly issue of clearing the work-place air of these dangerous fibers. Smoking is often a way of dealing with the stress induced by the work place (see Chapter 6). Are the employers who wish their workers to stop smoking willing to give them more breaks, alternative means of stress reduction, more relaxing work conditions, and a slower pace of work? The tendency to focus only on smoking may distract from issues of other sources of environmental pollution that are often heavily concentrated in work places (Fettner, 1987).

The tobacco producers form a major industry in the United States. On one hand, pronouncements and public service messages from the Surgeon General and Department of Health and Human Services condemn smoking; on the other hand, the Department of Agriculture continues to subsidize tobacco growers heavily. Taxes on tobacco sales are also a source of revenue for the government, so there may be some conflict of interest on the issue. The threats of job losses and of the death of a large industry are also involved (Doyal, 1981: 82–83; Milio, 1985). Rather than deal with such massive economic and political issues, however, policymakers find it easier to focus on changing individuals' habits (Milio, 1985). While smoking is an individual behavior and only the individual can decide to stop, the practice of smoking is firmly rooted in a sociocultural context. Advertising has glamorized smoking, associating it with vigor, sexiness, and sophistication. Other social factors supporting the habit include peer pressure among teenagers, and the use of smoking for sociability and for stress reduction. Smoke cessation programs, some argue, have little impact, because their focus is on changing individual behavior rather than addressing its sociocultural sources (Syme and Guralnik, 1987). As with accidents, an ecological method that considers individuals *and* their relationships to their social and cultural environment is a fruitful approach to supposedly "personal" addictions like smoking.

Pollution in the Work Place

Approximately 100,000 Americans die each year of occupational diseases (*not* including occupational accidents). About 390,000 new cases of disabling occupational diseases are diagnosed each year (Elling, 1986). These estimates vary according to criteria for the category of "occupational diseases." Many respiratory problems experienced by coal miners, for example, were not immediately classified as black lung. They were so designated only after years of political conflict between mine owners, workers, unions, and various health professionals (Smith, 1981). The same symptoms were previously diagnosed as bronchitis, emphysema, or health problems resulting from workers' personal habits. In fact, occupational diseases are often hard to distinguish from "ordinary," nonwork-related problems (Elling, 1986: 18). To a physician untrained in diagnosing occupational diseases, lung cancer caused by asbestos looks like cancer due to smoking. Many cases of brown lung (a disease caused by inhaling cotton fibers) among textile workers go unrecorded, since the symptoms may be misinterpreted as emphysema (Guarasci, 1987). Stress-related diseases (discussed in Chapter 5) are also not included in occupational disease statistics.

Obtaining sound statistics on occupational disease is a complicated process, because they vary depending upon who decides which health problems are job related. Company doctors, for example, are less likely to view symptoms as work related than union-affiliated doctors. One doctor working for the textile industry claimed that brown lung is

> best described as a 'symptom complex' rather than a disease in the usual sense. We feel that this term may be preferable, first in order not to unduly alarm workers, as we attempt to protect their health and secondly, to help avoid unfair designations of cotton as an unduly hazardous material for use in the textile industry, raising the fear that the engineering control of it may be costly, and that it may be better, therefore, to switch to some less costly material (quoted in Berman, 1978: 93).

Industry has focused on individuals and their "susceptibility" to occupational diseases. For years, instead of cleaning the air of cotton dust, the textile industry tried to identify hypersusceptible workers or "reactors" (Green, 1983). Employers' concern with workers' health is often inextricably tied to economic interests that influence what is or is not perceived and treated as occupational disease. As with accident prevention, management favors individual devices rather than "passive" engineering controls for the prevention of occupational disease. The issue of having the worker adapt to the work place rather than adapting the work place to the worker is thus not merely an economic one. Nelkin and Brown (1984: 70) observe that

> the dispute over precautions extends beyond the question of immediate cost. Personal protective equipment places responsibility for protecting health on the workers themselves. Ill health can then be blamed on their failure to comply. Conversely, engineering controls place responsibility on management, shifting both the burden and the blame. To insist on personal precautions is to reinforce the belief that individuals are responsible for their own health and safety. To accept engineering controls is to accept the notion of corporate responsibility.

Because the people who study or make policy decisions about occupational health are often remote from the work place, workers' reports of symptoms are often ignored or invalidated, despite the fact that workers are often the first to recognize occupational health hazards. A Labor Department study found workers' self-reporting of health hazards to be highly reliable, except that workers tended to underestimate the effects of chronic diseases caused by occupational exposure (Nelkin and Brown, 1984: 31). Coal miners have, for generations, known of "miner's asthma" and black lung; their awareness is documented in song and popular writings. Such knowledge was, however, dismissed as unscientific or as excuses for malingering. While workers' reports are not based on scientific observation, ignoring their observations delays effective responses to occupational health hazards.

Workers do not always report work-related health problems, however; some may not complain out of fear of repercussions. Many others do not make the connection between low-level, long-term exposure to hazards and diseases that developed slowly or gradually. For example, the symptoms of asbestosis appear twenty to forty years after asbestos exposure. Most private physicians have little training in occupational medicine and may not recognize patients' symptoms. A 1985 survey of 111 U.S. medical schools found that only 66 percent offered courses on occupational health, and only 54 percent of the schools required any course on the topic (*Science For the People,* 1985). Many doctors do not record a patient's occupational and work history, and often they fail to connect symptoms to work conditions.

Tens of thousands of different chemicals are used in commercial production processes, and the list grows at the rate of about a thousand a year. Of the 2 million known chemicals, only a few thousand have been tested for their dangerous properties, and only a few hundred of these have been thoroughly tested. Production processes often use several chemicals in conjunction with each other, but very little is known about health hazards created when these chemicals (which individually may be harmless) interact with each other (Eckholm, 1977: 108; Nelkin and Brown, 1984). Regulatory standards are typically set only after a problem has been identified among workers. In this sense, workers often function as human guinea pigs.

Regulatory agencies such as the Environmental Protection Agency (EPA) or OSHA must rely heavily on company data about various chemicals. However, the very companies with an economic interest in producing the chemicals are often the ones that test them. Cutbacks in funding to regulatory agencies, such as those in the 1980s, further limit effective research to determine regulatory standards. In many cases, OSHA has not set standards even for those chemicals known to be carcinogenic (i.e., cancer causing).

Many dusts and particles inhaled by workers produce serious health problems. It is estimated that about 10 percent of active miners have black lung disease (pneumoconiosis). The inhalation of various fibers (such as cotton dust) affects about 85,000 U.S. textile workers, 35,000 of whom are disabled by brown lung (byssinosis) and other respiratory problems (Hills, 1987). Tunnel workers' asthma (silicosis) comes from inhaling particles of sand. Table 3.4 shows the number of male deaths due to exposure to some of these substances. Exposure to chemicals used in many manufacturing processes has also been linked to cancer and various other serious diseases.

Pollution in the work place is not confined to blue-collar or industrial jobs. For example, the computer industry, which seems "high tech" and clean, exposes workers to solvents, chemicals, and gases that may be toxic. Adequate health and safety standards have not been established for this relatively new industry (Hayes, 1989; Howard, 1985). Supposedly "clean" office work sometimes involves inhaling ozone, a gas that can aggravate respiratory problems, from photocopiers or chemical copier fluids (Stellman and Henifin, 1983). Several studies document "office sickness" due to the high pollutant content of modern office buildings that are often airtight and rely on centralized air sources (Sterling et al., 1983). Persons who do housework may also be exposed to a variety of chemicals and air pollutants, such as fungal spores and bacteria (Chavkin, 1984).

Work-place pollution spreads beyond the confines of workplace.

TABLE 3.4 Death from Selected Occupational Diseases for U.S. Males, 1970–84

CAUSE OF DEATH	1970	1975	1980	1984
Malignant neoplasm of peritoneum and pleura	602	591	552	584
Pneumoconiosis	1,155	973	977	923
Asbestosis	25	43	96	131
Silicosis	351	243	202	160

Source: U.S. Department of Health and Human Services, Health, United States 1986, Hyattsville, MD: National Center for Health Statistics, 1987:118.

Some wives of asbestos workers developed asbestosis from dust brought home on their husbands' clothes (Doyal, 1981). Factory pollution also tends to spread into the immediate vicinity. A high percentage of urban dwellers have some asbestos fibers in their lungs, even though they have not worked with asbestos. Atmospheric pollution from asbestos plants, construction sites, and even from auto brake linings spreads asbestos fibers into public spaces. An estimated 10 to 15 percent of lung cancer deaths is due to asbestos (Moss, 1980: 237).

Just as the fruits of production are not equally distributed, so too are the costs of production, such as pollution, unequally shared. People living in urban poverty areas are exposed to larger quantities of chemical and air pollution than their middle-class suburban counterparts (Dutton, 1986). Likewise, developing countries experience increasing pollution and industrial hazards, even while already industrialized countries are achieving greater environmental and work-place health and safety regulation. Many developing countries want to attract industry, but they lack technical information to evaluate processes, resources for testing products, effective power to set enforce standards, and worker organizations to voice concerns (Navarro and Berman, 1981).

In the United States, the Occupational Safety and Health Act of 1970 was passed to "assure as far as possible every working man and woman in the United States, safe and healthy working conditions." This assurance has not been realized, however, in large part due to political abuses and to underfunding of the vast task of researching and enforcing standards (see Berman, 1978; Elling, 1986; Howard, 1985; Simon, 1983; Szasz, 1986). Compared to Sweden, Finland, East Germany, West Germany, and the United Kingdom, the United States ranked last, or tied for last place, on five out of six criteria for effective occupational safety and health: a strong national policy mandate for occupational health and safety; the provision and organization of services related to occupational health; workers' ability to control their work environment; the level of financing for occupational health activities; worker education; and the information about the work place available to workers and experts. Sweden and East Germany ranked highest on all six criteria (Elling, 1986).

Comparative data on actual levels of occupational health and safety in each of these countries are scant and difficult to evaluate, because countries use different methods of collecting and categorizing information. Elling (1986) argues that those countries with the most protection have the lowest rates of occupational disease and injury. Calculating admittedly crude work-related death rates, he finds that the United States has the highest rate, with 50 such deaths per 100,000 workers; the United Kingdom has 2.5 per 100,000, and Sweden has 3.6 per 100,000. Comparing rates of occupational disease and injury, Sweden and East Germany have the lowest; Finland and the United Kingdom fall in the middle; West Germany is next, and the United States has the worst (Elling, 1986: 22). The other countries appear to have stronger regulations and generally safer working conditions than the United States (Goldsmith and Kerr, 1982). For instance, Swedish workers have the right to veto plans for new machines, work processes, or construction on health and safety grounds. They are also trained in health and safety (including ergonomics) at the employers' expense. In one SAAB automobile plant, the accident rate decreased 33 to 50 percent after some of these policies were implemented (Engler, 1986). Since an estimated 25 percent of disease and disability in the United States is work related (American Public Health Association Chartbook, 1975), issues of regulation and the politics of regulation become important health considerations.

SUMMARY

Sociopolitical factors and culture "construct" our physical environments and hence our bodies. Cultural meanings, shaped by social status as well as corporate and other political interests, influence physicial activities: working, eating, and fitness. Social factors determine people's opportunities for a healthy material environment and lifestyle. Thus human activity produces important factors in bodily health and life, or illness and death.

RECOMMENDED READINGS

Articles

Nicke Charles and Marion Kerr, "Food for feminist thought," *The Sociological Review* 34(3), 1987: 537–572.

Carol A. MacLennan, "From accident to crash: The auto industry and the politics of injury," *Medical Anthropology Quarterly* 2(3), 1988: 233–250.

David Michaels, "Waiting for the body count: Corporate decision-making and bladder cancer in the U.S. dye industry," *Medical Anthropology Quarterly* 2(3), 1988: 215–232.

Mark Nichter, "Kyasanur forest disease: An ethnography of a disease of development," *Medical Anthropology Quarterly* 1(4), 1987: 406–423.

Barbara Ellen Smith, "Black lung: The social production of disease," *International Journal of Health Services* 11(3), 1981: 343–359.

Books

Joseph R. Gusfield, *The Culture of Public Problems: Drinking-Driving and the Symbolic Order*. Chicago: University of Chicago Press, 1981. A sociological study of ideologies about drinking and driving.

Marcia Millman, *Such a Pretty Face: Being Fat in America*. New York: W. W. Norton, 1980. An excellent, highly readable empirical study of dieting, "fat camps," the social meanings of obesity, and the relationship of such issues to gender.

Jeanne Stellman and Mary Sue Henifin, *Office Work Can Be Dangerous to Your Health.* New York: Random House, 1983. A well-written handbook for workers about the hazards of office work.

John W. Warnock, *The Politics of Hunger: The Global Food System.* Toronto: Methuen, 1987. A comprehensive discussion of world food problems, with an emphasis upon both political and ecological aspects of the situation.

Chapter Four

Mind, Body, and Society

We have briefly reviewed some of the ways in which social and political factors affect the quality of and our use of our material environment. In previous chapters, we looked at physical determinants of health and at their social contexts. Here we shall examine other ways in which our bodies are affected less visibly, but perhaps more directly, by social relationships and structures. In this chapter and the next, we focus on the issue of sociopsychological stress and health. Stress and related concepts provide the basis for a holistic perspective in which individual minds and bodies are integrally interrelated with social environments.

"STICKS AND STONES MAY BREAK MY BONES, AND NAMES CAN ALSO HURT ME"

In everyday life, we are sometimes aware that sociopsychological factors affect our health. We might say, "I always get a cold after a tough exam."[1] Conversations contain various psychosomatic references such as, "You're a pain in the neck!" "She'll be the death of me yet!" "Grandma died of a broken heart!" These references show a commonsense awareness of the connections among the mind, body, and society. Particularly among middle-class persons, there appears to be a recent increase in self-consciousness about bodies and stress.

Despite this recent interest in mind-body relationships, psychological and social factors are not perceived to be truly important in determining health, because they are not "real," that is, countable and tangible. Viruses, radiation, chemicals, and smoking are physical factors whose effects on the body can be measured and observed. Because medical science has viewed mind and body as separate entities to be studied and treated separately, doctors often do not assign these factors much reality or tangibility. Thus while we may intuit the reality of psychosomatic connections, we also believe that "sticks and stones may break my bones, but words will never hurt me" (at least not physically!). Yet is this adage really true?

Some evidence suggests that a conversation with another person (even a nonthreatening one) will automatically raise our blood pressure; a conversation with our boss, even more so (Lynch, 1985). What are we to make of accounts of "voodoo death," when a chieftain utters a death curse at a woman who violates a tribal taboo, and the woman, who believes her death to be inevitable, soon dies of no clear physical causes (Cannon, 1942)?[2]

---

[1] In fact, studies do show that immunity to disease among medical students is lower than usual during finals (Suter, 1986).

[2] There may well be other mechanisms involved in voodoo death besides being scared to death. For example, other people, such as relatives, friends, and neighbors, withdraw their emotional support from the victim. Funeral rites may be carried out while the person is still alive thus symbolically defining the individual as dead. (This has been called social death.)

Modern equivalents of voodoo death occur in such cases as sudden death after retirement or widowhood. Engel (1971) argues that such phenomena are due to intense emotional arousal, which interrupts the regular rhythm of the heart; in other words, it causes a cardiac arrhythmia that can be deadly. We do not wish to overstate the case that words can kill, but do want to make the point, developed further below, that human physiology is responsive to its social environment and that symbolic meanings can physi cally affect us.

Placebos: A Case of Mind or Body?

Research on placebos provides some suggestive linkages between mind and body. A placebo is a chemically inert or inactive substance (e.g., a sugar pill) that looks like real medication. It is a sham treatment that is supposed to have no actual physical effects. The Latin word "placebo" means "I will please." Doctors sometimes give placebos to patients who want and expect treatment yet seem to have no physical, organic basis to their complaints. Placebos are also used in tests of drugs and treatments to determine how much of a drug's effectiveness is due to its specific physical properties and how much is due to subjective or psychological factors. The placebo is used as a standard (or a control) against which a drug being tested can be compared.

While chemically inert, placebo "pain medication" can actually reduce pain in as much as 35 percent of patients (Beecher, 1959). In the late 1950s, there was even a controversial experiment with placebo surgery. (Recent tighter rules for experiments with human subjects prohibit such experiments.) It was found that an early version of coronary by-pass surgery (called mammary artery ligating surgery) was no more effective than sham surgery, in which patients were put to sleep and had an incision made, although no actual surgery was performed on the heart arteries (Cobb et al., 1959). Some observers have suggested that current coronary by-pass surgery may likewise derive part of its success from a placebo effect. Many by-pass patients experience considerable relief, even though their surgery produced *no* functioning, patent grafts (i.e., it did not improve ventricular function). The operation's symbolic and metaphorical effects may thus account for much of the patients' relief from angina pain (Moerman, 1983). Since patients usually

---

However, there may also be a withdrawal of material support, such as refusing the victim water. The literature on voodoo death differs on how the process works. Some argue that dehydration (loss of body fluids) is a vital factor. Relatives may withhold water, and the victim believing he is doomed, loses the desire to drink or obtain water (Eastwell, 1982). Thus according to some, voodoo death has mainly physical causes (e.g., dehydration), with psychological causes being secondary. Others argue that while physical causes are important, psychologically giving up on life produces lethal physical consequences (such as cardiac arrhythmia). There is some laboratory evidence that animals who give up die because their physiological systems have been depressed to a point of death (McElroy and Townsend, 1985).

hope that treatment will work, almost all treatments involve an element of the placebo effect. Medical settings—with their impressive equipment, diplomas and certificates on doctors' office walls, white uniforms, clipboards and stethoscopes—contribute to this "faith" or expectancy.

Some researchers view the placebo effect as being all in the mind and having no physical basis. Others suggest that placebos actually induce internal physical changes in the body (Sternbach, 1964; Weil, 1983; Bakal, 1979). Placebos may in fact stimulate the body's production of natural opiates, called endorphins (Levine et al., 1978; Davis, 1984). If this is true, it may be an oversimplification to consider the pain-relieving properties of a placebo merely psychological. Doctors' "bedside manner" or communication may likewise have concrete physical effects, such as reducing pain or speeding recovery. As one physician notes,

> But what if it is demonstrated in the future that reassurance provided by a health professional is capable of releasing endogenous morphine-like substances within a patient's brain? Without doubt, the phrase "laying on of hands" will acquire a new meaning (Bakal, 1979: 251).

The Western assumption of a division between mind and body is not shared by all cultures. In many cultures being sick or being healed is neither all biological nor all psychological but a psychophysiological process (Grossinger, 1980; Weil, 1983; Kleinman, 1978). We shall examine this issue in later chapters. For our present purpose, research on placebos illustrates that they may have a psychophysiological effect and that biomedicine's assumption of a mind-body split may not be supportable. A growing body of evidence suggests that the assumption of such a mind-body dualism limits medicine's ability to understand health and illness.[3] Furthermore, mind and body exist in a social environment with which they also interact. Thus social meanings, pressures, and relationships have at least *some* impact on us. The following sections sketch some of the possible pathways through which social pressures (or stressors) can become the source of psychophysical troubles.

[3]There is not always definite evidence, and much of the research is controversial, yet it is very suggestive. The research comes from a host of newly developing disciplines with a bewildering array of names, including psychological medicine (Bakal, 1979), psychosomatic medicine, psychophysiology (Suter, 1986), health psychology (Millon et al., 1982), sociophysiology (Barchas and Mendoza, 1984a, 1984b; Waid, 1984) and recently psychoneuroimmunology, (Locke et al., 1985). These names become less intimidating if we break them down into smaller units of meaning. In the case of psychoneuroimmunology, *psycho* refers to the mind, *neuro* to the nervous system, and *immuno* to immunity. The ending-*ology* generally means *study of.* Thus psychoneuroimmunology is the study of the interactions among the mind, the nervous system, and the immune system. A central theory that underlies much research in this area is that the immune system may be the connecting point between psychosocial experiences and diseases (Solomon, 1985). For instance, such factors as social stress may have an impact on immunity, which in turn lowers a person's resistance to disease.

The value of placebos is sometimes misconstrued as a simplistic mind-over-matter argument, which leads to the trap of another form of mind-body dualism: the mind ruling the body. Mind and body must be seen as interacting and not as separate elements. Diseases clearly have biological components, but they also have a psychosocial dimension. Psychosocial factors, however, do not magically transform bodies. Psychosocial pressures generally take years to exact their toll; for instance, social stress does not generate coronary heart disease or hypertension overnight. Some health problems experienced in adulthood may have begun much earlier in the person's life, even early childhood, when the organism is not yet fixed in its patterns of physical responses. Physical damages brought on by long-term stress, for example, may not be easily reversible. The fact that a health problem is affected by social factors, however, does not make it any less real.

The Open Quality of Human Bodies: Dogs Don't Brood

All creatures interact intimately with their environments; they have an impact on their environmental conditions and in turn are affected by them. When studying organisms and their surroundings, we have a tendency to make a sharp distinction between the environment and the creatures inhabiting it (Levins and Lewontin, 1985), but this distinction is misleading. We speak of animals adapting to their environments, but creatures also transform the world they live in, often modifying it to their needs and in turn being shaped by the world they have shaped. Humans, more than other creatures, can transform their social and physical environments, but they are also more liable to being affected mentally and physically by the world they create.

Creatures are shaped not only by physical surroundings but also by their social relationships and expectations. Social relationships affect physical responses. The social position of animals, for instance, affects their behavioral responses to amphetamines. Given amphetamines, both dominant and submissive monkeys increased dominant and submissive behaviors "appropriate" to their status. When a monkey changed its social position, so did its response to the drug. Thus, under amphetamines a monkey with increased status changed its behavior from being submissive to being more threatening and making more dominant displays (Haber and Barchas, 1984).

In a similar experiment with humans, four subjects were told that they would be given a sleeping pill, but one of the four was actually given a stimulant. All *four* subjects became drowsy and quiet (including the one who had unknowingly been given the stimulant). This study shows the importance of social expectations, the influence of the experimenter, and the behavior of one's peers (in this case the other three subjects) for one's physical response. Psychosocial factors were thus as important as the drug's biochemical properties in influencing people's behavior (Bakal, 1979: 180).

Becker (1967) argued that culture and social learning affect how the individual experiences the effects of drugs. The ability of the hallucinogen LSD, for example to produce a psychotic episode does not depend merely upon the chemistry of the drug but also on the sociocultural setting in which it is experienced.

Human physical functioning is more responsive than that of other animals to its environment (Berger and Luckmann, 1967: 47–50). This is true for a number of reasons:

1. Human beings leave the womb more unfinished than other creatures and exist in an extrauterine social womb of dependence on others. Social learning begins before we are biologically complete (e.g., our central nervous system is not fully developed) for an extended period after birth. Since human young are more open and malleable, early social learning has a deeper impact on them both physically and mentally. Although rats are far more "closed" than humans, studies show that activity and social stimulation can modify the brain of infant (and even adult) rats (Diamond, 1988). The role of early stimulation in constructing human physiology is much greater. Because human interconnectedness and dependence on others are thus partly a result of biology, human physiological functioning is more deeply affected by social surroundings (Birke, 1986: 85).

2. Humans communicate through the use of symbols, which allows them—unlike other creatures—to reflect on themselves and their bodies, and to attach meanings to events (Berger and Luckmann, 1967). Symbols allow humans to remember experiences in a way that other creatures cannot. Humans reflect on their past and anticipate their future, but dogs cannot brood about old grudges. This is not to say dogs do not remember past pain or wait in anticipation, but relative to humans, they tend to be more grounded in the here and now. Such a capacity to reflect on the meaning of events may generate a chronic, low level of stress, since our brooding can contribute to a constant degree of psychophysical arousal. The capacity to symbolize widens the range of events to which humans respond as psychologically and physically stressful. A human can respond to the fear of being humiliated in the same way that an animal responds to physical threat. Unlike animals, however, humans do not generally respond to threats motorially (i.e., by running or fighting) but by mulling them over in our minds. This response has an impact on our health, because the wider range of anxiety and guilt about our past, present, and future that may result can affect us physically.

3. Research shows ways in which seemingly involuntary physical processes, such as blood pressure, digestion, and the functioning of the immune system, can be changed in "lower" animals by conditioning (i.e., reward and punishment) and in humans by learning (such as learning through biofeedback). People are capable of a great deal of voluntary self-

regulation and, as yogic practitioners demonstrate, can initiate the regulation of even "involuntary" aspects of physical functioning (Pelletier, 1977).
While one can *condition* an animal to lower its blood pressure, humans can
place themselves into states of mind that will alter their blood pressure. This
means that the regulation of blood pressure and other supposedly involuntary physical functions are not closed systems that simply operate automatically, but rather that are responsive to the psychosocial environments of
which the person is a part. Human sexual responses are modulated by
"higher" cognitive functions. Fantasies may amplify or diminish excitement
(Cohen and Taylor, 1976). All organisms are capable of *self*-organizing their
physical functioning; in humans this capacity seems greater. This capacity
may be affected by moods, emotions, and feelings about ourselves that are
in turn connected to our social existence (Buytendijk, 1974).

In sum, one might loosely characterize human physiology, relative to
that of other creatures, as more responsive to its environment and more
capable of self-regulation. Humans have more open and more controllable
bodies; hence, we are more "makeable." Our bodies have greater access to
the outer physical and social world because humans are free from fixed
instinctual patterns and have greater capacity for self-regulation. One human aspect of our bodily nature is this particular openness to the world.
"Our body in its relative independence has an opening to a formed outer
world" (Buytendijk, 1974: 19).

Through these mind-body "thoroughfares," our movements are
shaped by the physical constrains of our world, and our internal environment fluctuates to some extent with our experiences in the social and
physical world. The way in which conversation can raise blood pressure
serves as an example. Our way of life in a society and how we experience
this way of life are linked to the functioning of our bodies through muscular, neurohormonal, cardiovascular, respiratory, and other systems. Due to
our developed self-consciousness and capacity to reflect, the self can
dampen or incite the physical systems and in turn be affected by them.

The ability to communicate symbolically (which is intrinsically tied
with this open quality) makes us susceptible to a wider range of stressors
than other forms of life experience. Humans respond physically to both
physical and socially symbolic threats. Most psychosomatic illnesses are
therefore peculiarly human. Humans also possess a greater ability to modify stressors' impact by the way we interpret them.

Body and society can intersect in many ways. We have reviewed some
obvious connections, such as the impact that cultural and social factors have
on our diet and hence on our physical condition. Other interrelationships
between body and society are more subtle, such as ways our biochemistry
may be influenced by the temporal rhythms of social environments or
relationships. Some body-society influences involve surface modifications

of our muscular-skeletal structure, including our posture, movements, and the shape of our bodies. Others may penetrate our body by changing blood pressure or the responsiveness of our nervous system. While showing relative internal stability, our bodily systems are "never completely withdrawn from a relationship to a way of existence" that is constantly changing and affecting these bodily systems (Buytendijk, 1978: 29).

Respiratory functioning, which is both voluntary and involuntary, exemplifies such body-society connections. We breathe automatically, yet can hold our breath (Suter, 1986: 56). How we breathe may be affected by our mood. Anxious people breathe more shallowly. Anxiety in turn may be produced by social settings. What we have here is a kind of society-mind-body bridge. Similarly, blood pressure, blood sugar, and immunity are affected by patterns of neuroendocrinological arousal (Gruchow, 1979), which are themselves linked to the way we live and respond to our life experiences. The early empirical and theoretical foundations for such linkages can be found in the pioneering works of W. B. Cannon (1929) and his student who became the father of contemporary stress research, Hans Selye (1956).

The Neurohormonal Connection: Stressor and Stress Response

Of all the bridges that connect the body to the mind and to the "outside" world, the best known and explored is the neurohormonal connection. A **stressor**, or a stress situation (Suter, 1986), refers to stimuli, or environmental conditions or events, that elicit stress. We include here those stimuli that come from our minds, such as recalling a frightening event. The threat of a dog's bite is a stressor, and our body's response to that stressor is called the **stress response** or **fight-or-flight response**. The stress response is the body's way of getting ready to deal with the stressor by mobilizing itself to either fight or to flee. This "fight-or-flight reflex," as Cannon (1929) called it, involves neurohormonal changes in the body (Suter, 1986: 73), which elicit a particular pattern of arousal or excitation in the nervous system and release of certain hormones. One function of these hormones is to "stimulate and coordinate distant organs" (Selye, 1975: 148).

Hormones are released by the endocrine glands directly into the body, and they stimulate or depress various physical functions. These hormones act as the body's chemical messengers, telling it to step up or to slow down its activities. Adrenaline (also known as epinephrine) and noradrenalin (norepinephrine) are examples of a class of stress hormones known as catecholamines. The stress response involves changes in the central nervous system (CNS; the brain and nerves in the spinal cord) and the release of some of these hormonal substances. The response goes through a series of stages that Selye called the **General Adaptation Syndrome** (GAS) (Selye, 1956).

The fight-or-flight response is a general physiological response that involves a number of systems throughout the body and can be evoked by any number of nonspecific stimuli (stressors) in the environment. Selye noted that his medical training encouraged a blind spot for the idea of nonspecific factors. In the course of his medical education, specific diseases and their causes "assumed an ever increasing importance and pushed the syndrome of just being sick, the question 'what is disease in general?' out of my consciousness into that hazy category of the purely abstract arguments that are not worth bothering about" (Selye, 1956: 17).

As shown in Chapter 1, most biomedicine emphasizes specific diseases and causes. Selye's research, however, did not merely focus on specific physical reactions to specific stimuli but rather on general physical responses that might be evoked by a whole range of environmental factors. It is only recently that medicine has begun to investigate such ideas as nonspecific disease factors.

The fight-or-flight behavior described by Cannon is an adaptive response to environmental stressors, because the body is mobilized for action either to flee or to flight the threat. For this reason Selye (1956) later called stress-related disorders "diseases of adaptation." Many physical problems do not come so much from outside factors as an invading bacteria or an injury, but from the body's attempt to protect itself. When a wound is infected, the sore and resulting inflammation come from the body's reaction to invading bacteria.

The fight-or-flight response involves various hormones and the CNS, which is divided into autonomic (i.e., involuntary) and voluntary components. The voluntary part of the CNS controls conscious movements, such as walking and talking; the involuntary part controls such functions as blood pressure, respiration, and heartbeat. The complex nature of human physical functioning necessitates operating on "automatic" to a great extent. We could not survive if we constantly had to remind our heart to beat or our lungs to breathe. Animals can be conditioned to control various autonomic physical functions; humans also can learn such control (Suter, 1986).

The autonomic (involuntary) nervous system in turn is divided into sympathetic and parasympathetic parts. These two branches often have opposing effects on an organ. Sympathetic excitation or arousal may speed up a function, while parasympathetic activity in the nervous system may slow down a function. During the stress response, the sympathetic nervous system is activated by messages from the hypothalamus, a small part of the midbrain that receives messages from all over the brain and controls CNS and hormonal activity. Having received the signal of a threat in the environment (as stressors), the hypothalamus thus signals the arousal of the sympathetic part of the autonomic nervous system, which then becomes more active than the parasympathetic part.

This activation signals the release of various hormones into the body, including stress hormones such as adrenaline, noradrenaline, and cortisol. The hypothalamus also sends messages to the pituitary gland, which produces another hormone (adrenocorticotropic hormone, or ACTH), which also signals the release of stress hormones. There are thus two paths through which the stress response is activated: the hypothalamus-sympathetic-adrenal route and the hypothalamus-pituitary-adrenal route.[4]

The stress response, in the form of this neurohormonal activity, creates a number of nonspecific changes in the body that adapt the organism for fight or flight:

1. Blood pressure is increased. Blood flows to the muscles and heart, and much is diverted from the peripheral (outer) parts of the body; this is why cold feet and hands are often a symptom of stress. Blood is also diverted away from functions, like digestion, not needed for fleeing or fighting.
2. Sugars and fats (including cholesterol) are released to give the body energy.
3. Immunity is temporarily depressed to allow the body to tolerate possible invasions, such as wounds.

These changes suggest how prolonged, uninterrupted stress might create physical problems. For example, does the continued release of fats and sugars into the blood help to explain the connection between stress and coronary heart disease? Can prolonged stress affect the mechanisms that regulate blood pressure? These are some of the issues investigated by stress research.

According to Selye (1975: 148), the GAS is "the manifestations of stress in the whole body as they develop over time." There are three stages in the body's adaption to a stressor. The first is an alarm reaction, which involves the neurohormonal changes described above. The second is a stage of resistance, during which the body adapts to a continuous threat. This adaptation, however, produces the risk of "diseases of adaptation," such as ulcers. If the body is not allowed to return to a state of rest, the adaptive response (or stress response) actually becomes maladaptive. The body is then depleted of resources and reaches a third stage, exhaustion.

[4]The stress response can never be measured directly. In a sense, a stress researcher is like an investigator who tries to deduce what is happening inside a factory on the basis of noises she hears while standing on the outside (Suter, 1986). Some measures of stress include the calculation of the amount of electrical activity in the nervous system and the biochemical analysis of blood and urine, but all of these methods have problems. For instance, while the quantity of cathecholamines in a person's urine reflects different levels of stress, it may also be a function of that person's unique way of metabolizing (processing) such substances, since some people will excrete such hormones more rapidly than others.

This brief sketch of the neurohormonal connection shows how stressful events in the social and physical world may be linked to changes within human bodies. A prolonged stress response can contribute to health problems. Researchers have linked chronic, unabated stress to lowered immunity, and increased blood sugar and levels of serum cholesterol (Suter, 1986). Events that are perceived as stressful may thus produce bodily wear and tear, particularly if the body cannot restore itself. The stress response gears the body up, increasing certain functions. Continued stress may wear out the body.

The stress response, in which the body is wound and sped up, has also been called an ergotrophic response. When this happens constantly, it may be hard to slow down. What is called the relaxation or tropotrophic response may become more difficult to evoke. To oversimplify somewhat, does the constant revving up make it difficult, after a while, for the body to unwind, to relax and slow down? Some investigators have developed techniques for eliciting the body's natural tropotrophic or relaxing response (Benson, 1979).

The events in modern life that elicit the stress response in humans are not usually physical but more typically social and symbolic in nature (e.g., the threat of being humiliated). Furthermore, modern conditions do not always make the adaptive response of fleeing or fighting a practical one. We may be provoked by a boss to fight or run, but we have learned that neither response would be appropriate. Thus the body may be continuously geared up for action but not allowed by the rules of "civilized" behavior to act.

Any demanding situation, such as climbing a dangerous trail for enjoyment or mining coal in a dangerous mineshaft for a living, can be stressful. Not all stressors are negative, however; some can energize and challenge. Stress itself is not inherently unhealthy. It is a part of life, and a totally stressless environment would be both impossible and boring.

Negative and positive stressors are not necessarily equal in their impact on us. Are there qualitative differences in how people respond to negative or positive stressors? Some research (Glass, 1977; Dohrenwend and Pearlin, 1982) suggests that it is not just change or environmental demands that are stressful. The uncontrollability of the stressor-event seems to increase its destructive consequences for the body. Stressors are likely to have a negative effect when the individual feels helpless in the face of them.

The Relationship Between Physical and Sociopsychological Stressors

There is evidence that physical and sociopsychological stressors interact with each other. By lowering immunity, stress can aggravate an individual's vulnerability to infectious microorganisms. Being physically run-down may also make it harder to cope with social stresses. Often different kinds of stressors interact with each other and may in fact *increase* one another's impact on the body. Such a mutually enhancing interaction is called a synergistic relationship. Each factor may "feed" into the other, amplifying effects that either one alone might have had.

The relationship between diet and stress exemplifies synergism. In our fragmented ways of looking at health and illness, we often focus on one factor (such as diet) as *the* determinant of health. Some think that eating properly will save them from heart disease and other woes, yet diet cannot be considered in isolation from other factors. A high cholesterol diet *combined* with high levels of social stress can increase the likelihood of atherosclerosis (hardening of the arteries), over and above the effect of diet by itself (Kaplan et al., 1983; Eyer, 1984).

House and his colleagues (1979) studied workers who were exposed to chemicals known to cause respiratory problems. They found that the workers suffered even higher levels of these disorders if, simultaneously to being exposed to the noxious chemicals, they were also exposed to "noxious" supervisory pressures. Social stress increased the effect of physical (chemical) stressors on the body. Supervisory pressure and noxious chemicals thus interacted in a synergistic fashion.

A Note on Measuring Stressors

How are we to measure stressors? Some are clearly more devastating than others. Being hit by a car is not the same as stubbing one's toe. Getting promoted (a positive event that produces stress) is not the same as getting a birthday card. Most of the instruments developed to measure stressors are usually paper-and-pencil questionnaires.

One widely used measure, developed by Holmes and Rahe (1967), is the social readjustment scale, or the schedule of recent experiences. A list of forty-three events was composed from the case histories of five thousand patients in Seattle. Other subjects then ranked these events in terms of the amount of readjustment they thought they required (i.e., the amount of stress they produced). Thus, the death of a spouse was assigned the highest value of 100, and taking a vacation was given a low value of 13 (see Table 4.1).

Subjects in a variety of societies (Japan, Mexico, Denmark, and Sweden) ranked the items very similarly (Lauer, 1973). One might argue that some events, such as divorce, are the *results* as well as the source of stress. According to this approach, the more high-impact events that a person had experienced recently, the more likely it would be that the person would become ill. High scores on the scale did in fact prove to be consistently related to the onset of illnesses such as respiratory and heart ailments (Liem, 1981: 65–66). These studies indicated that individuals faced with

TABLE 4.1   The Stress of Adjusting to Change

EVENT	SCALE OF IMPACT[a]
Death of spouse	100
Divorce	78
Marital separation	65
Jail term	63
Death of a close family member	63
Personal injury or illness	53
Marriage	50
Fired at work	47
Marital reconciliation	45
Retirement	45
Change in health of family member	44
Pregnancy	40
Sex difficulties	39
Gain of new family member	39
Business readjustment	39
Change in financial state	38
Death of close friend	37
Change to different line of work	36
Change in number of arguments with spouse	35
Mortgage over $10,000	31
Foreclosure of mortgage or loan	30
Change in responsibilities at work	29
Son or daughter leaving home	29
Trouble with in-laws	29
Outstanding personal achievement	28
Wife begins or stops work	26
Begin or end school	26
Change in living conditions	25
Revision of personal habits	24
Trouble with boss	23
Change in work hours or conditions	20
Change in residence	20
Change in schools	20
Change in recreation	19
Change in church activities	19
Change in social activities	18
Mortgage or loan less than $10,000	17
Change in sleeping habits	16
Change in number of family get-togethers	15
Change in eating habits	15
Vacation	13
Christmas	12
Minor violations of the law	11

[a]200 or more stress points cause physical illness

Source: Holmes, T. H. and Rahe, R. H. "The social readjustment rating scale" Journal of Psychosomatic Research 11, 1967: 213–218. Copyright © 1967 Pergamon Press, Inc. Reprinted with permission.

many and/or extreme changes in their lives may be at higher risk of illness in a subsequent six-month period (Rahe and Ransom, 1968).

While such research is valuable and demonstrates a relationship between life-event stressors and the onset of illness, it has several problems:

1. Such a measure is based on the subject's recall of events, but not all stressful events are remembered or noticed. For example, the scale does not measure the low-level chronic and diffuse stress that a person may experience daily. Many stressors tend to be taken for granted after a while, yet exact their toll.

2. Such a list preselects and precategorizes events in a way that a subject might not conceptualize them. A person using this scale thus passively chooses from among multiple-choice answers, which may discourage other possible responses.

3. The scale does not show how the same event may be experienced in a qualitatively different fashion by different subjects. Being fired may be a blessing if I have inherited money and hate the job, but a curse if it means I will suffer devastating unemployment and poverty.

4. The scale takes events out of the contexts of a person's life and does not show how various events and circumstances are interrelated.

5. Because the scale measures stress by the degree of readjustments events require, with "positive" events (e.g., getting a new job) equated with "negative" ones (e.g., getting fired), it is unable to distinguish between stressors that are manageable and those that are disempowering.

In short, such scales must be taken as very crude measures that make it difficult to assess, with any depth, how people experience and cope with these stressors.

A QUESTION OF SUSCEPTIBILITY

Why do two people react very differently to the same stressors? Some of us face stress with confidence; others with fear, despair, and a sense of hopelessness. While some people seem to weather life's crises without much damage, others break easily. Clearly it is not only the stressor itself that determines the reaction, but also how the individual experiences and deals with the stressor. Furthermore, some research suggests that even physiological reactions to stress vary from person to person. Some people's bodies react very strongly to a stressor; others' less so. What factors account for such variations in individual susceptibility?

Although there are important individual variations in reactions to stress, we should avoid individualistic interpretations that ignore the social circumstances contributing to these variations. Such approaches tend to blame the victim of stress rather than to examine the social situations that might account for variations in individual susceptibility. Three interrelated kinds of individual variations in stressor reaction exemplify this problem; the mere presence of a stressor does not account for a person's physical reaction to it. First, there are differences in the way people's bodies respond to stressors (**physiological reactivity**). Second, there are variations in how people perceive stressors and assess what is happening to them (**cognitive-emotional appraisal**). Third, there are differences in the way people manage stressors (**coping**).

Physiological Reactivity

While the basic pattern of the stress response remains essentially the same from person to person, researchers have found recurring *individual* patterns in the way people's bodies respond to stress. Some individualized physical responses are more fixed or rigid than others. Two people faced with the same stressor will show differences in the level to which their blood pressure rises. The pressure of persons who have hypertension tends to fluctuate more dramatically than that of those whose blood pressure at rest is "normal" (Suter, 1986; Buytendijk, 1974).

Individuals also differ in their patterns of neurological excitation. In some people the ergotrophic response, in which sympathetic arousal is high, is more easily elicited. Other people respond more quickly with a tropotrophic response, in which parasympathetic excitation predominates (Suter, 1986). Individuals may also differ in how readily their bodies shift between these two responses, physically changing from being in a state of fight or flight to being in a state of relaxation (Gellhorn, 1969).

Individuals have varying hormonal reactions (Bieliauskas, 1982: 5). In some laboratory studies, men produced more epinephrine in response to stressors than did women. Whether this difference is representative of naturally occurring responses is not clear (Polefrone and Manuck, 1987). It is possible, however, that men overreact to stress, thus producing an inefficient excess of stress hormones (Overfield, 1985). Some physiological variations may reflect differences in biological make-up. Perhaps men and women *do* differ biologically to some extent in hormonal reactions. Perhaps some individuals are genetically predisposed to hypertension or coronary heart disease. Such issues are by no means resolved, and the research results are mixed.

Variations in physiological reactivity, such as differences in catecholamine reactivity, may also be the result of social factors, at least to some extent. Men and women are socialized to deal with stress in different ways.

It may well be that these learned patterns also affect their way of responding physically (Birke, 1986; Lowe and Hubbard, 1983). The fight-or-flight response tends to elevate blood pressure. A long-term exposure to stressors and a learned typical way of responding to them might eventually lead to a regular pattern of reacting physically, as some animal studies suggest (McCarty et al., 1988).

Moss (1973) has argued that given a certain cognitive-emotional orientation to stressors, over time the nervous system might become "tuned" into a particular pattern of arousal. Thus the sympathetic nervous system's reaction to situations might become amplified and fixed in that amplified pattern. The parasympathetic nervous system would not, therefore, be as readily activated. The person could be easily excited and would find it hard to "unwind." Individual physiological patterns in responding to stress might be partly the result of learning and other social experiences (Suter, 1986: 84). The distinction between physiological factors (e.g., individual differences in hormonal output) and social factors (social situations which promote physical changes) in health is thus not always clear-cut.

Cognitive-Emotional Appraisal

Cognitive-emotional appraisal is the physiological impact of a person's interpretation and emotional reaction to a stressful event. In one study of this phenomenon, Lazarus (1966) and his associates showed male students different versions of a film that depicted ritual operations on the genitals: circumcision (cutting around the penis to remove the foreskin) and subincision (cutting the penis lengthwise). One version of the film had no sound and showed only the operations. Another version had a soundtrack that emphasized the harmlessness of the procedures and the fact that the participants in the rites saw them as an honor. A third version contained the narration of an anthropologist who, in an intellectual tone, constantly commented on events as the interesting and "exotic" customs of other societies. The researchers measured the level of physiological stress response of each member of the audiences. Those exposed to the second or the third version of this film showed lower physiological levels of stress. Lazarus concluded that one's physical reaction to a stressor is affected by how one interprets it. In this case, the soundtracks helped the audiences interpret the stressor as less threatening. Although watching a stressful event on a film is not the same as seeing it in person or having it done to oneself, such experiments illustrate that our interpretations of events have a significant effect on how we react to them.

Several theories emphasize the importance of an individual's cognitive-emotional appraisal of situations in linking stress to illness (see Moss, 1973; Totman, 1979). Antonovsky (1987: 13) proposes that people with a high "sense of coherence" are healthier, because they have a global orientation that expresses the extent to which one has a pervasive, enduring though dynamic feeling that 1) the stimuli deriving from one's internal and external environments in the course of living are structured, predictable and explicable; 2) the resources are available to one to meet the demands posed by these stimuli; and 3) these demands are challenges worthy of investment and employment.

Cultural factors and an individual's position in a social structure can affect this sense of coherence. Antonovsky does not, however, thoroughly examine the ways environments disempower people, nor does he systematically consider how conditions that attack a person's sense of coherence are built into the social organization of institutions such as the work place and the family. He also does not explore in sufficient depth the impact of social and economic systems such as capitalism on individuals' sense of coherence.

These theories emphasize the importance to health of feeling a sense of empowerment or control.[5] What they clearly do not distinguish is how a person feels or perceives the world, as opposed to conditions that lead a person to emotionally and mentally appraise the world a certain way. The emphasis on cognitive appraisal in the stress literature often implies that how one perceives an event is the result of a psychological attribute or quality inherent in the person, independent of the event itself. This approach treats *how* we perceive things as almost unrelated to *what* we are perceiving.

While individuals do vary in the way they appraise stressors at any given time, these differences are often the result of former social experiences with past stressors. Feeling helpless may come from some set of previous objective experiences. If, for instance, people were once overwhelmed and made to feel powerless by social class, economic, or familial events, later in life they may find it harder to believe that a stressor now confronting them is a manageable one (even if it is!).

Seligman (1975) observed that animals placed in laboratory conditions

[5]Antonovsky (1979: 127–128) claimed that it is important to differentiate a sense of control from one of coherence, because a sense of control implies that "I am in control," which reflects a cultural bias that equates a *sense* of control with *self*-control. However, people do not have to be in control to have a sense of coherence, but simply be participants in shaping their fate and believe that who or whatever is in control (e.g., their god or leader) is controlling events in the people's interest and is a legitimate authority. Indeed one can feel that the world is relatively safe and in control and yet not *be* in control.

But two issues must be raised: First, self-control *is* important in Western industrialized societies. Second, however much events can be "in the hands of the Lord," so to speak, individuals still must feel the world is manageable and not working against them. It is inconceivable that persons could tolerate feeling that they were puppets or that their actions were not their own. To be unable to connect one's actions with more or less predictable outcomes would be most disturbing. While control need not be totally in individuals' hands, they, as Antonovsky admitted, must feel themselves to be participants in their actions and that the world is being managed in their interest. It is in this way that we argue that theories such as Antonovsky's emphasize a *sense* of control, which we would agree is not synonymous with *self*-control.

of helplessness for a long enough period were unable to cope with subsequent stress or possible activity. He has linked such "learned helplessness" to depression, poor health, and a generally heightened susceptibility to stressors. The experience of powerlessness in everyday situations, such as work or home, may produce a similar learned helplessness in humans (Lennerlof, 1988). Other authors have introduced similar concepts, for example, the "giving-up complex" (Schmale, 1972) and the "paralysis of will" (Bakal, 1979). Likewise, the notion of "surplus powerlessness" (Lerner, 1979) suggests that if individuals were once made to feel powerless, the expectation that they will again be powerless builds up and keeps them from acting when confronted with stressors (even when they are able). People's present reactions to stressors are thus linked to their past experiences with empowering or disempowering situations. A lifetime of social exploitation or domination will certainly have an impact on whether a person feels empowered.

Coping

Coping refers to all of the ways of managing the tension a stressor produces (Mechanic, 1978: 51). As Syme and Berkman (1976: 6) observed:

> Generalized susceptibility to disease may be influenced not only by the impact of various forms of life change and life stress, but also by differences in the way people cope with such stress. Coping, in this sense, refers not to specific types of psychological responses but to the more generalized ways in which people deal with problems in their everyday life. It is evident that such coping styles are likely to be products of environmental situations and not independent of such factors.

One's cognitive-emotional appraisal of a situation is in itself a way of coping or managing stress. Some people "overact" emotionally; seeing the glass as half-empty, they give up. Others see a glass that is half-full and keep striving. Coping is not merely a matter of attitude, perception, or emotional response, however; it also involves action—that is, doing something about the stressor.

The focus of much stress literature on individual coping leads to two blind spots. First, these studies fail to consider how power affects people's ability to do something about stress. How does social class, ethnicity, gender, or work situation influence resources for effective coping? Second, much research tends to separate coping and stressor, thereby missing the fact that the conditions creating stress often also limit both the possibility of and options for coping. One's social position (such as one's status as a woman) often limits options for coping. In some areas of life, such as in friendships, certain personal styles of coping strategies are possible, but in much of everyday life people's options for managing stress are very limited. The world of work, for example, allows most people only limited coping strategies (Pearlin and Schooler, 1978).

The early literature on stress gives the impression that stress is a problem primarily for high-powered, white-collar workers. Yet research indicates that, while these groups do face a great deal of stress, they also have access to resources that allow them to cope with it more effectively than those who lack resources. Even among animals the "top dog" generally has more resources to handle stressors than the "bottom dog." One study of baboons found that, in response to stress, high-ranking males showed faster increases in cortisol, a stress hormone, than subordinate baboons; however, their basal level (i.e., the ordinary amount when not exposed to stress) of the hormone was lower than that of the subordinates. Furthermore, when the stressful event ended, the amounts of cortisol in high-ranking baboons returned more rapidly to the basal levels than did those of their subordinates. The more effective coping of these "top bananas" was attributed to such advantages as better choice of food, mates, and living conditions (Sapolsky, 1982). Another researcher found that rats that can control the source of stress or predict when stress will occur also cope more effectively and show fewer pathological effects of stress than do rats that cannot control or predict stressors (Weiss, 1972). Although animal studies cannot be used uncritically to generalize about human situations and behavior, executives and other "top bananas," whose job conditions allow for control and provide resources for coping (such as more control over the use of one's time), can probably cope with stress more effectively than those who do not experience such advantages.

One might argue that nonexecutive stress is a more serious health hazard than executive stress. A study of 5,100 Swedish and American men found the highest risk of coronary heart disease among workers with both heavy job demands (i.e., numerous stressors) and a "low ability to influence how their tasks are done" (Nelson, 1983; Karasek et al., 1981). Thus one's social position (such as on the job) may influence both the amount of stress one faces and the resources one has for coping. The most stressful occupations are those that combine high levels of stress with little control over those stressful conditions. Being a telephone operator or a waitress may therefore be more stressful than being a bank officer, sales manager, or physician. For example, a National Institute of Occupational Safety and Health study found that clerical women who had low control over their work with VDTs (video display terminals) showed higher levels of job stress than the highly pressured air traffic controllers, who also work with such terminals (Howard, 1985: 73). Thus the social circumstances in which people find themselves influence not only the demands to which they are exposed but also their ability to handle those demands.

In recent years, corporate health programs have proliferated in the United States. Sponsored mainly by larger corporations, they emphasize exercise, meditation, diet control, and smoke cessation (Pelletier, 1985; Conrad, 1988). While programs for blue-collar and lower-echelon white-collar workers exist, many are directed toward executives, who present potentially more expensive health-related losses for the corporation. These programs seem to have developed in an economic environment of escalating medical costs to corporations and governments (Alexander, 1988). However, there is no definitive evidence yet that, in the long run, they do prevent illness (Conrad, 1988).

While their overt function is to use prevention to reduce health care costs and loss of workdays, corporate health programs may also direct attention away from political and environmental issues in the work place. They do not generally encourage workers to examine critically the social conditions under which they work, such as work pace, vacations, breaks, or participation in decisions affecting their work. The implicit message to employees is that their health (and the costs they incur by being sick) are their individual responsibility (Glassner, 1989). Such programs may even be used to justify cutting back on medical benefits. The corporate image also benefits by such programs, and other parts of the business sector profit by selling the equipment and services for these programs (Alexander, 1988).

Stress and Power

Young (1980:133) observes that both scientific and lay discussions of stress tend to "subvert sociological reasoning" by removing people from their social contexts and from class and group conflicts. They tend to emphasize subjective factors and the way individuals *perceive* events, or in other words, psychological as opposed to sociological factors.[6] The way people see things gets confused with the way that things are (Young, 1980: 145). Instead of beginning analyses of stress and health by looking at coping responses, cognitive-emotional appraisal, or individual forms of coping, why not begin by examining social conditions of inequality or structural arrangements, such as those that force a person to work under pressure or do not allow time to relax?

Scheder's (1988) analysis of diabetes among Mexican-American migrant farm workers illustrates the relationship among psychosocial stress, limited options for managing stress, and social inequality. Much research on diabetes has focused on factors of nutrition, obesity, and health behavior. While these variables are important influences, exclusive emphasis on them obscures the role of such factors as social inequality. Diabetes is more common among low-status and low-income people (Scheder, 1988). The

---

[6]We therefore do not agree with Mechanic (1978:71), who after reviewing literature on helplessness and health, concluded that whether we in fact control our external environment is a "philosophical issue." What is significant, he said, is our subjective response to conditions, or our sense of helplessness.

exact role that psychosocial stress plays in the disease is not clear; however, some evidence suggests stress may influence its onset and course (Jacobson and Leibovich, 1984; Scheder, 1988). Stress can also affect health behavior, such as excessive eating and drinking. The neuroendocrinological arousal generated by high levels of chronic stress may also affect blood sugar metabolism (Jacobson and Leibovich, 1984). Scheder found that rates of adult-onset diabetes (Type II diabetes mellitus) were much higher among those who had spent a long time as migrant farm workers and had frequent experiences of stressful life events. Obesity did not distinguish those who got diabetes from those who did not. Scheder concluded that the high levels of stress experienced by these migrant workers as a result of their low social position, disrupted social networks, social marginality (i.e., being outsiders in American culture), discrimination, heavy workloads, job insecurity, poverty, and feelings of hopelessness and helplessness, contributed to catecholamine-produced impairments in glucose levels. This study suggests the kinds of questions we need to ask about the effects on health of power, psychosocial stress, and a personal sense of control.

SUMMARY

Material environments and our interactions with them affect our bodies. Symbolic and social factors, however, may also influence bodies through neurohormonal and other physical changes, which in turn may even mediate the interaction between our bodies and the physical environments they inhabit.

Stress is not merely in the eyes of the beholder, nor are the ways in which people handle stressors merely a matter of our individual resourcefulness. The economic organization of a society, the various social pressures to which its members are subjected, and their membership in sociological categories such as class, race, ethnicity, gender, and age are very important considerations. In the next chapter, we shall look at qualities of social environments that both empower and disempower to emphasize the effects of social-structural factors, such as stratification and social control, upon people's bodies and health.

RECOMMENDED READINGS

Articles

Howard Becker, "History, culture and subjective experience: An exploration of the social bases of drug-induced experience," *Journal of Health and Social Behavior* 8, 1967: 163–176.

George L. Engel, "Sudden and rapid death during psychological stress: Folklore or folk wisdom?" *Annals of Internal Medicine* 74, 1971: 771–782.

Robert Karasek, Dean Baker, Frank Marxer, Anders Ahlbom, and Tores Theorell, "Job decision latitude, job demands and cardiovascular disease: A prospective study of Swedish men," *American Journal of Public Health* 71, 1981: 694–705.

Lennart Lennerlof, "Learned helplessness at work," *International Journal of Health Services* 18(2), 1988: 207–222.

K. W. Pettingale, "Towards a psychobiological model of cancer: Biological considerations," *Social Science and Medicine* 20(8), 1985: 779–787.

Books

Aaron Antonovsky, *Unraveling the Mystery of Health: How People Manage Stress and Stay Well*. San Francisco: Jossey Bass, 1987. An elaboration and application of Antonovsky's "sense of coherence" perspective.

Rosalind Barnett, Lois Biener, and Grace K. Baruch, eds., *Gender and Stress*. New York: The Free Press, 1987. A good collection of articles dealing with gender differences in experiencing and responding to stress.

Martin Seligman, *Helplessness: On Depression, Development and Death*. San Francisco: W. H. Freeman, 1975. An introduction to the concept of learned helplessness that presents evidence for its various applications.

Steve Suter, *Health Psychophysiology: Mind-Body Interactions in Wellness and Illness*. Hillsdale, NJ: Laurence Erlbaum, 1986. An introduction to the psychophysiology of stress, basic relevant anatomy, and applications of the psychophysiological perspective to several illnesses.

Andrew Weil, *Health and Healing*. Boston: Houghton Mifflin, 1983. A very readable critique of biomedicine and presentation of a holistic perspective.

Chapter Five

Social Organization, Health, and Illness

In the previous chapter we described how a sense of manageability and control over our circumstances can affect our health. What kinds of conditions empower or disempower us? As we suggested in Chapter 4, the amount of stress a person experiences in the work place, for example, partly depends upon certain social conditions. Social status and the social organization and regulation of activities are crucial in structuring these social conditions.

ORGANIZATIONAL SETTINGS AND EMPOWERMENT: SOCIAL STATUS AND CONTROL

A number of factors can either contribute to our feeling of empowerment or erode our sense of coherence, and thus affect the stressfulness of life events and the effectiveness of our responses to those events. These factors include: (1) the ways activities are scheduled and the individual's attitudes toward time; (2) how social relationships and circumstances either affirm or assault a person's sense of self; (3) whether social environments provide sufficient information important to individual well-being and security; and (4) the quality of social support systems.

Social stratification and control are closely linked with both empowering and disempowering situations in the social production of health and illness (Freund, 1982). They shape whether we experience time as stressful; how we feel about ourselves, our abilities, our competence, and our ability to predict the outcomes of our behavior; and the quality of social relationships that support us.

Our examples of social stratification and control are generally drawn from Western capitalist societies, with an emphasis on the illness-producing organizational properties of capitalism as a socioeconomic system. These properties are, however, by no means confined to such societies. The USSR, for instance, has experienced a significant deterioration in life expectancy and infant mortality since the mid-1960s (Feshbach, 1984; but see also Cooper, 1987). Lifestyle factors, such as a high rate of alcohol consumption and smoking, and a poorly functioning health care system contribute to these problems (Feshbach, 1984). Some observers have speculated, however, that Soviet health problems are caused by social organizational properties similar to those found in capitalist societies. Large social status differences, for example, affect health and access to health care (Cooper and Schatzkin, 1982). As in monopolistic capitalist societies, the thrust toward "the efficient accumulation of capital" (Eyer, 1977: 38), productivity, and control over workers takes precedence over workers' health. Soviet industry has eagerly appropriated capitalist techniques of increasing labor productivity, such as the assembly line (Braverman, 1974). Social inequality and oppressive forms of control are thus not exclusive to capitalism.

KILLING TIME AND BRIDLING MOTION

Control over time—our own or other people's—is a form of power. Powerful persons have the ability to regulate other people's time and labor. The ability to manage our own schedules is limited by our position in society. Wealthy persons have more resources for managing the stress of demanding schedules. A teacher can keep a student waiting, but students should not be late for their appointments with a teacher, since a teacher's time is assumed to be more valuable. *Time is socially organized, and the ability to schedule time and to manage it is socially distributed.* Those with more power have more control over time.

From the moment we enter the world as babies, we are subject to a social calendar that is not of our own making, and we are taught to respect the constraints of time. The fragmentation and structuring of time and space in adult terms begins early. In some societies, however, adults and children do not experience such sharp time distinctions between work and play (Cherfas and Lewin, 1980).

In our society, the emphasis is on productivity. The social organization of our economic life is the basis of much of our social scheduling of time. This organization demands intense productivity and encourages us to internalize certain attitudes toward time. **Internalization** is the process by which people take on and make their own the attitudes, beliefs, and ways of looking at and acting on the world held by others. The work ethic, one such internalized complex of attitudes toward time, affects us not only at work but even at leisure.

The social organization of time and learned attitudes toward time can have a profound effect on our health. The rhythms of time and motion demanded of people and the way people respond to these demands are very important sources of stress; they also shape our ability to cope with these stressors. Personal ways of responding to environmental demands are socially learned. The family, for instance, can teach its members to become obsessed with time. Controls over time can be both externally and internally imposed. The time clock at the factory, the doctor's appointment, the classroom bell, and the income tax deadline exemplify externally imposed controls over time. The so-called Type A way of responding to time is an example of a self-imposed, or internalized, form of control over time. Type A behavior is the result of socialization during which some individuals learn to respond to time in a socially approved way.

How members of a society collectively use time and the different degrees of control over their own or other people's time are central sociopsychological factors in health. They determine the frequency and intensity of stressors as well as the effectiveness of means of dealing with those stressors. For example, work time can be stressful for many people; factors such as social or occupational status influence how well they can cope with work time.

Time and Work

In the beginning of the twentieth century, the intense control by employers over work time, which had characterized the growing capitalist society of the nineteenth century, was further extended. Workers became more and more paced by the rhythms of the machine. With the emergence of the assembly line and "scientific management" of work activity, new, more systematic, "scientific" or rationalized forms of control predominated in the work place. For instance, standards for workers were increasingly set by time-and-motion studies.

The work of Frederick Taylor epitomizes the attempt to impose rationalized, scientific controls over time and motion. In *The Principles of Scientific Management* ([1911] 1947), Taylor argued for a sharp division between those who *plan* work and those who *do* it. The planning was to be carried out exclusively by managers trained in scientific management. Jobs were to be divided and subdivided into the smallest, easiest-to-learn unit of activity. Time-and-motion studies would determine the most efficient way to move and the optimum unit of time each subdivided task should take. These studies would then set standards for precisely how and how fast all the workers would move. Taylor argued that such a system of management should take precedence over the idiosyncratic rhythms and needs of individual workers. While his system is no longer widely applied in most work places, the attitudes and assumptions of Taylorism still prevail among many managers.

Work in industrial manufacturing in particular was highly regulated by machines and specific, limiting instructions. Tasks were broken down into short, simple, repetitive units of activity (Braverman, 1974). The result of this form of control, used in the pursuit of productivity, was to place workers increasingly into environments that moved too fast, were deadeningly boring, and controlled the motions of the body in an unnatural and uncomfortable way.

The quest for increased productivity has been most intense in industrial manufacturing. This drive has put greater pressure on industrial workers in the form of ever-increasing demands on pace and the effective use of working time, and decreasing options for variety, relaxation, and social interaction at work. Various studies show that poor mental health, psychosomatic disorders, and sick leaves are most common in low-status industrial manufacturing jobs (Frankenhaeuser and Gardell, 1976).

The pace and motion of factory work has been extended to white-collar office work. The movements of some typists, key punch operators, and other office machine operators have taken on "automaton-like characteristics" (Stellman, 1977: 55). The growth of computer technologies since the 1950s has opened up new work possibilities, but it has also led to more highly repetitious, boring, machine-paced work in the office. Computer technology provides for increased control over individual workers. A terminal on a supervisor's desk can monitor the number of strokes made by each individual key-punch operator (Garson, 1988).

Bell Telephone computers print fifteen-minute summaries of how many operators were on duty, how many calls each operator handled, the average speed of an operator's answer, and how long they spent talking to each customer (Howard, 1985: 63). Citicorp Bank uses Management Information System (MIS) software, which provides management with data about work places hundreds of miles away. Each clerk's printout shows the amount of time spent processing records, talking on the phone, and the like. The records are then evaluated according to standards set by Citicorp's time-and-motion specialist (Howard, 1985: 30–31). A National Association of Working Women's survey found that 35 percent of its members, in jobs as diverse as bank teller, data entry clerk, waitress, and truck driver, were monitored by computer (Howard, 1985: 62). Even middle-level managers and executives are subject to closely monitored time controls; some must submit accounts of work done every half-hour (Garson, 1988). Thus the tendency in office and professional work, as in factory work, is toward greater standardization of work and control over time (Garson, 1988). There is a growing de-emphasis on skill and on individual control over the work process (Glenn and Feldberg, 1977).

Load Balance.   Some environments demand too much, too fast, while others demand some degree of involvement but make too few demands and are boring. The different rhythms of working (and of living in general) may be conceived of in terms of load balance: Do they demand too much or too little? How much pressure (or how much of a load) is imposed on a person? A load imbalance may involve either overload or underload, or both, as temporal rhythms. A chronic load imbalance may adversely affect one's health. While our examples of time rhythms are drawn from the work place, the problem of load balancing may apply equally to the lives of the unemployed, the elderly, homemakers, and persons with disabilities (Frankenhaeuser, 1981).

Underload and **overload** are products of the degree of control one has over the rhythm of one's work. Temporal demands are not as stressful when self-generated. However, they are stressful when they are imposed and combined with little control over how one's work is done (Karasek et al., 1981). Such jobs are likely to be held by low-status workers. Overload may involve piecework, such as being paid by the number of letters typed each hour. Overload usually results from a work environment that moves too fast for comfort. Underload often involves machine-paced work, such as an assembly line. Workers' movements are standardized but also demand their attention. Underload tends to be boring and tiring work. Clearly some boring work need not be stressful. A night watchman can read, walk, and chat; this work may thus not be as stressful as boring work that requires sustained alertness and attention, such as watching a machine.

Work often involves both underload and overload (Frankenhaeuser and Gardell, 1976). A woman who is a felter (a person who makes felt linings) in a luggage factory provides a dramatic example:

> In forty seconds you have to take the wet felt out of the felter, put the blanket on—a rubber sheeting—to draw out the excess moisture, wait two, three seconds, take the blanket off, pick the wet felt up, balance it on your shoulder—there is no other way of holding it without tearing it all to pieces, it is wet and will collapse—reach over, get the hose, spray the inside of this copper screen to keep it from plugging, turn around and walk to the hot dry die behind you, take the hot piece of felt with your opposite hand—set it on the floor, this wet thing is still balanced on my shoulder—put the wet piece on the dry die, push this button that lets the dry piece down, inspect the piece we just took off, the hot piece, stack it, count it—when you get a stack of ten, push it over and start another stack of ten—then go back and put your blanket on the wet piece coming up from the tank . . . and start all over. Forty seconds (Terkel, 1974: 384–385).

One can imagine the multiplicity of stressors that characterize this job, which entails the danger of burns and the discomfort or even ill health (e.g., arthritic joints) from the wet felt the worker must balance on her shoulder. There is also the psychosocial stress produced by the pressure of time and the boredom coupled with the demand for constant alertness. Many jobs involve such a combination of extremes of hectic and boring work, together with strict control over time and movements that is physically and psychologically uncomfortable.

Overload and underload have been linked to increased excretions of catecholamine, a stress hormone (Spillane, 1984; Frankenhaeuser, 1981; Kahn, 1981). A study of sawmill workers found that those whose jobs were characterized by a lack of control over their situation (as a consequence of overload and underload) were most likely to have increased catecholamine excretions in their urine. These workers also reported feeling tired, tense, anxious, and ill more frequently than other workers (Frankenhaeuser and Gardell, 1976).

At times the pace and lack of control over motion may even produce a "stress epidemic" that is manifested through mass symptoms of dizziness, nausea, headaches, and hallucinationlike phenomena (Chase, 1980). This is most common where the work is routine, repetitious, and boring (Alexander and Fedoruk, 1986). Similar group outbreaks have also occurred in schools (Small and Borus, 1983). Some observers have noted that women are more susceptible to stress epidemics. However, this is not really due to gender but to the fact that women are more likely to end up with the lowest-status industrial manufacturing jobs (Chase, 1980).

The machine-paced nature of much work means that, in a sense, the human body must function like a machine. Since machines can tolerate what humans cannot, the gearing of the body to the rhythm and movements of a machine may have destructive physical effects. A sociologist who worked in a Hungarian tractor factory described how the time pressure of machine-paced work affected the way workers paid attention to physical signs that they are tired or uncomfortable:

> The best way I can put it is like this: *I* cease to exist. When the huge side doors of the workshop are opened and the transporters rattle in loaded with material, I *know*—without having a thought as such, I simply *know*—that I am in a freezing draught, but I do not *feel* that I am cold. My back aches, there is a cramp in my fingers, the piece rate is ridiculous: I don't feel or think any of this (Haraszti, 1978: 112).

One's working conditions can thus put one out of touch with one's own body.

Social class may be related to the individual's degree of sensitivity to illness (Koos, 1954). The fact that lower-class persons show decreased sensitivity to such symptoms as backaches, headaches, chronic tiredness, and coughing may be due to social conditions that deaden awareness of the body's messages. Tight and complex schedules, long hours, and shift work are the results of attempts to control workers' time in the interests of productivity. They often do so at the expense of workers' control over the quality of their lives.

To argue that our contemporary work hours are long may seem absurd in comparison to the nineteenth-century workweek of around seventy hours (Friedmann, 1961: 105). That period, however, was not typical. Industrial capitalism was then becoming a dominant force in Western society, and productivity was being enhanced mainly by lengthening the workday. By contrast, in agricultural societies the workweek was shorter (around thirty hours a week) and more in gear with seasonal rhythms, and workers frequently labored only about fifteen weeks a year (Johnson, 1978; Eyer and Sterling, 1977).

Shift Work.   Working on shifts is another kind of temporal rhythm that is utterly unknown in many societies. As capitalism became the predominant form of economic and social organization in Western society, shift work became more common. By 1980, 11 percent of full-time U.S. workers were on late shifts (U.S. Department of Labor, 1981). Roughly 20 to 25 percent of U.S. workers are on some form of shift work (Blyton, 1985). In Europe the proportion of workers on shifts has increased overall since World War II, with the greatest increases among women and nonmanual (white-collar) workers (Blyton, 1985). Shift work became more common as the investment in machinery became greater and as it became profitable to sustain production around the clock. Some shift work is needed for technical reasons, such as a specific manufacturing process that cannot be interrupted. Certain service jobs (like those in hospitals) also require round-the-clock coverage. Most shift work, however, is instituted because it increases profits by maximizing the use of the equipment and space in which capital has been invested.

There are many different systems for arranging shifts. The most common is to have an early morning, late afternoon, and night shift (e.g., 5 A.M. to 1 P.M., 1 P.M. to 9 P.M., and 9 P.M. to 5 A.M.). The number of days worked on the same shift is called the rotation period. The most common rotation period is one week (Baker, 1981: 109).

Shift work often goes against the rhythms governing many bodily functions. Heart rate, body temperature, the production of various hormones, and metabolic rates all vary with the time of day, and seem to follow a twenty-five–hour cycle called a circadian rhythm (Baker, 1981: 116). One researcher suggests that shift work often violates workers' physiological rhythms by not giving them enough time to adjust from one cycle to another (Levi, 1981, 1978; see also Luce, 1971). One study exposed one hundred volunteers to rotation periods that shifted between three days and three nights of continuous work. It was found that the circadian rhythms, geared to being awake during the day, persisted. The author concluded that although the endocrine system will eventually adapt to the shift, *long* rotation periods are necessary to adapt (Levi, 1978). However, most shift arrangements do not allow for this.[1] Other studies show higher rates of sleep, mood, and digestive disorders among shift workers (Baker, 1981).

The time of the day a person must work affects sensory-motor performance (e.g., quickness of reflexes). It also has an impact on the metabolism (i.e., the body processing) of various chemicals and toxins to which individuals are exposed in the course of their work. How quickly the body absorbs a medication depends on what time of day it is taken. Similarly, how chemi-

---

[1]Some individuals adjust better than others; some prefer certain time cycles, and there are sometimes ways of arranging shifts so that workers have an opportunity to adjust. However, most workers, as opposed to owners or managers, do not have sufficient control over these matters and cannot set up temporal structures compatible with their individual needs.

cals and other physical stressors affect the body may depend on the time of day of exposure, an issue that has not received much attention in research on time, work, and health (Baker, 1981: 117). Social factors often interact with physical stressors in complex ways.

Shift work, like overtime, may be formally voluntary in the terms of a union contract, but often financial pressures or fear of denying a superior's request may make what is formally voluntary in practice almost compulsory (Pfeffer, 1979: 87–88). Working overtime or on different shifts, furthermore, has social consequences for workers and their families. Shift work often intrudes into the worker's personal life, affecting leisure and social networks such as family and friendships. These changes in turn influence eating habits and sleep patterns, and may produce such adverse health consequences as digestive disorders. For these reasons, some countries, such as Sweden and Belgium, have laws that strongly limit the prevalence of shift work.

Some experiments allowing employees to have some control over their own time (e.g., "flextime"), by choosing to work longer days and shorter weeks or other alternatives to nine-to-five daytime hours, have been tried in the United States and Europe. In West Germany and Switzerland about 40 to 45 percent of the work force is on flextime; it is mainly a white-collar prerogative, but more blue-collar workers are on flextime in those countries than in the United States. About 8 percent of the U.S. work force has flextime, and those workers are concentrated in the service sector and among nonmanual workers in large-scale business enterprises (Blyton, 1985). Unfortunately, flextime experiments are often limited by overriding fears of declining productivity and managerial control.

Internalized Time Pressure

In addition to the workers' *externally* imposed time pressures, which are related to health problems, individuals also *internally* impose such pressures on themselves. Certain social structures, especially the hierarchical division of labor in modern societies, encourage and reinforce individual motivation to overwork. These hierarchical and manipulated job settings reflect larger societal stratification and cultural values (Garfield, 1980). Self-motivated workers, however, have internalized these values, becoming their own "slave drivers." The "workaholic," sometimes described as having a "Type A" personality, displays a behavior pattern produced by cultural values and social pressures experienced in the contexts of school, family, work, and other settings (Ivancevich and Matteson, 1988).

One of the dimensions of Type A behavior is a "time sickness"—an obsession with time and a constant time urgency. The physicians Friedman and Rosenman (1974) first became aware of this distinct pattern of behavior when they noticed that, in the waiting room for their heart patients, the front of the seats were all worn down: Their patients were literally sitting on the edge of their seats. Other dimensions of Type A include a competitive attitude, hostility, repressed anger, and a compulsion to be perfect.

Some studies have linked Type A behavior with health problems, especially coronary heart disease (Rosenman et al., 1975; Haynes et al., 1980; Suls and Sanders, 1988). Other research found that, in response to high demands and loss of control, Type A persons show more elevated heart rate, stress hormones, and blood pressure than Type B persons (Ivancevich and Matteson, 1988). Although research on the connection between Type A behavior and health problems has produced conflicting results (see MacDougall et al., 1985; Shekelle et al., 1985; Suls and Sanders, 1988), the concept is suggestive of some ways that cultural values and social pressures encourage the internalization of "sickening" attitudes.

People's socialization to these attitudes leads them to become their own source of time pressure. Type A is a personal style that motivates people to overload themselves constantly. Such personality patterns are encouraged by the norms and patterns of socialization characteristic of the future orientation, restlessness, and driven quality of modern capitalist-industrial societies. In our society, with its work ethic and emphasis on constantly producing, getting ahead, and being competitive, many people incorporate such traits into their personality and practice them in extremes (Drummond, 1980).

Type A behavior is not simply a personality trait belonging to certain types of *individuals;* rather, it is produced in certain *social situations.* Many researchers see it as "in the nature of Type A people to produce Type A behavior" (Young, 1980: 139); however, this approach treats the style as an attribute, existing independently of the person's social situation. Nobody's behavior is totally independent of the situation that they are facing at a given moment. Even a Type B person will be more anxious if supervisory pressure is high. Some studies suggest that coronary-prone behavior patterns can be elicited by work settings (McQueen and Siegrist, 1982), especially those that are time pressured and competitive, and threaten personal control (Ivancevich and Matteson, 1988). Type A behavior may not be a *significant* risk factor in coronary heart disease unless combined with such stressful situations. The distinction that is often made between personality and social forces is a misleading one, however, since much of our personality is shaped in the course of our social experience.

Work Time, "Free" Time

A "time urgency" characterizes behavior not only in work time but also in *free* time. In fact, the character of leisure time is affected by work time. The two-week vacations that are common in the United States (compared to the average of four to six weeks in many other industrial countries) are directly affected by the other fifty weeks of work. Temporal rhythms of underload and overload affect life experiences other than work (Antonovsky, 1979: 187). A college professor who worked in a factory on his year of academic leave observed:

> Except for shopping at supermarkets that are open all kinds of hours, I could hardly run errands, go see a doctor, or do anything in the community. . . . I found myself torn between spending those few precious hours of waking leisure with my son, with my wife or by myself. I found myself, in short and with some important differences no doubt, trying to live with drastically curtailed and compressed free time as millions of American workers have learned to live, snatching moments of personal satisfaction largely from time not sold to others (Pfeffer, 1974: 41).

People who work in dull and restricting jobs tend to be less likely than those with interesting jobs to engage in "leisure activities requiring planning, participation and effort" (Frankenhaeuser, 1981: 492). Workers do not typically compensate for dull jobs with exciting, challenging leisure-time activities.

Not only may the rhythms of work time seep into the lunch hour, weekends, and holidays, but the *physiological* responses to work stress may also continue long after the workday is done. One study indicated that even after a stressor had been removed, monkeys continued to show physiological stress responses at the same time of day that the animals had originally been exposed to the stressor (Luce, 1971: 106).

Some researchers suggest that the nervous system may retain a "memory" of stressors (Luce, 1971: 150). The physiological effects of work overload may thus spread to leisure hours, thus delaying their full impact (Frankenhaeuser, 1981: 499). Many of us have experienced a form of work time carrying over into our free time when we are unable to adjust our sleep patterns during vacations and continue to wake up to an inner "alarm clock" geared to the memories of work time. The inability to unwind is accompanied by the hormonal system's inability to slow down, even in the absence of environmental demands. Thus workers who have been working overtime show elevations of catecholamines not only at work but through the next evening as well. The process of unwinding may be accompanied by an increase in psychosomatic problems (Levi, 1981: 53).

The inability to relax during free time is also the consequence of media and peer pressures to consume frenetically. While some people may shop as a way of relaxing or even as a means of affirming themselves ("I shop, therefore I am," is one mock motto), often free time ends up as rigidly scheduled as work time. The activity of consuming requires that commodities be bought, kept, and maintained. More time must be scheduled and compartmentalized to allow for shopping, getting to sales on time, and having goods repaired, waxed, shampooed, trimmed, and polished. Because time spent consuming must to some extent be scheduled, leisure time is therefore, regimented. Sports and amusements may also mirror the rhythm and movement of the work world. One observer commented:

> Even days ostensibly outside daily routine, holidays, are occupied with "organized" sports and amusements which, far from being liberating forms of leisure facilitating participation in subjective atemporality, are ritualistic reaffirmations of the daily grind, veritable sermons or morality plays on the value of efficient use of "on" time and the rewards of synchronized cooperation. Indeed, unprogrammed, "idle," or "non-productive," time, eagerly sought and jealously safeguarded in more subjective cultures, is experienced as malaise in machine culture (Dye, 1981: 58–59).

A disciplined worker and a disciplined consumer go together hand-in-hand in our society.

So-called leisure time is often consumed by unpaid labor in the form of housework and the care of dependent children and elderly. In our society, this burden falls disproportionately on women. Parenting and housework are work, even though they are not socially recognized as paid, "productive" labor. These forms of work are characterized by recurring, boring, repetitious tasks; long hours; social isolation in the home; and many features, such as underload and overload, that characterize factory work (Stellman, 1977; Chavkin, 1984). Working mothers thus carry a double burden from both paid work and housework.

The standardization of work time (such as the practice of working for eight hours from nine to five) also means that many people are excluded from paid work, including mothers who cannot afford child care, elderly people who must rest more often, and disabled people who may not function as effectively on a nine-to-five schedule. Since the industrial "revolution," there has been a trend to separate spheres of activity. Paid work is increasingly done *outside* the home, while in earlier days it was often done *at* home. This segregation of activities of work and home, together with the standardized workday, makes it difficult or impossible for mothers and others who cannot function on "normal" time to participate in the paid labor force.

It would be simplistic to assume that the unemployed poor merely have "time on their hands," without examining the quality of this time. The poor, both unemployed and employed, are unable to enjoy the privileges of time use that go with higher social class levels. For example, they spend a great deal of time waiting for various services in places such as emergency rooms, clinics, welfare offices, and courts. Such waiting can cost precious wages, especially since many services are not available after working hours. Middle-class people can take time off, and upper-status people can have the service brought to them (Henley, 1977). One's social position also influences the degree of access to other people's time and control over one's own use of time (Henley, 1977; Schwartz, 1973).

Elderly or disabled persons sometimes find themselves in surroundings that overwhelm them, because they are unable to function at the speed demanded. In the right context, however, they might still be able to function well. Older people's disorientation and inability to function are sometimes interpreted as signs of senility; others' inability to function at "full speed" may be seen as a sign of mental or social disturbance. Thus, instead of seeing these problems as responses to environments that move uncomfortably fast or slow, we tend to treat them as personal, *internal* states of mind. When the environment of college students was experimentally sped up so that they could not maintain the pace, they also began to show irritability and the inability to function (Kastenbaum, 1971). Retirement and institutionalization lead people to experience "standard" time as irrelevant, thus atrophying time-related coping skills and contributing to behavior that may be incorrectly interpreted as evidence of senility.

There is an important relationship between time and health. The standard ways of socially scheduling activity often conflict with one's personal pace or biorhythms. A sharp discrepancy between the two will have an impact on one's health. Such a split between social time and our ability to keep up is prevalent in time-pressured, production-oriented Western societies. In a society as productive as ours, a shorter work week with longer breaks, more flexible hours, and less time-pressured work should not be impossible. Despite two-day weekends and labor-saving devices, we seem to live in a world that is more time pressured than past societies and many present ones.

HEALTH AND SELF: BEING HELPLESS, FEELING WORTHLESS AND HOPELESS

What is the relationship between our sense of self and our health? Our sense of self is our experience of ourselves as unique and distinct persons. Our self-concept refers to our thoughts and feelings, both positive and negative, about ourselves as individuals. Much of our sense of self is developed during our socialization in response to other people's attitudes and treatment of us. How we feel about ourselves depends very much on both the extent to which various social interactions validate or affirm our sense of self and our social position (e.g., class, gender, and age). How competent and capable we feel to manage various stressors also contributes to our sense of self and health (Ben-Sira, 1985). Similarly, our self-image is related to ways we display ourself to others, or our presentation of self (Goffman, 1959). Some social settings force us to present ourselves in ways that are incompatible with our fundamental sense of who we are and what we are feeling; they may affect our sense of self and health. For example, a salesperson who must smile in the face of insults and tirades from rude customers may experience this as an assault on her feelings about herself and possibly also her health.

Our health is affected by our sense of self or self-presentation. An empowered self, one experiencing a sense of coherence (Antonovsky, 1979, 1987), can produce health. By contrast, "giving up" on life can be a significant catalyst for disease (Schmale, 1972; see also Engel, 1976; Seligman, 1975). A "dispirited" self (Jourard, 1964), characterized by a poor sense of self, a lack of a sense of control, and a feeling of being overwhelmed by events, has been linked to depression and anxiety (Johnson and Sarason, 1978). People with a poor conception of themselves take longer to recover from mononucleosis (Anderson, 1978). A study of West Point cadets found those who were unable to live up to their expectations of themselves were at higher risk for infectious mononucleosis (Kasl et al., 1985). Other studies found a sense of failure and self-devaluation to be characteristic in heart patients, patients with respiratory problems, and those suffering from ulcerative colitis (Totman, 1979). These and related studies suggest that intense and prolonged social invalidation, particularly when it is incorporated into a person's self-concept, may contribute to weakened bodily defenses, make it harder to cope with stressors, or heighten the sensation of such symptoms as pain (Feuerstein and Skjei, 1979).

Structural Sources of Self-Invalidation

Attacks on one's identity can be stressful (Cockerham, 1978), because the self is regarded as a sacred object in modern Western cultures. While being degraded or treated as incompetent has always been painful, the importance attached to the self has varied historically. Only in recent times has the self been conceived as an object, much less as a sacred object. How we feel about ourselves and who we are has become significant only in the last few centuries; the idea of a self-concept in psychology emerged in the twentieth century (Burns, 1979). The significance that people attach to the self, how they think about it, the importance they attach to various aspects of the self (such as self-control), and above all the social standards by which they judge themselves all depend on social and historical circumstances. As psychologist Fromm (1965: 311) observed,

> Thus modern man, instead of having to be forced to work as hard as he does, is driven by the inner compulsion to work which we have attempted to analyze in its psychological significance. Or instead of obeying overt authorities, he has built up an inner authority—conscience and duty—which operate more effectively in controlling him than any external authority would ever do.

The inability to live up to the demands of this "inner authority" leads to a sense of personal failure, even when the causes of failure are beyond an individual's control. This is particularly true given our society's emphasis on each individual's responsibility for one's fate. While modern Western society puts a value on the self and self-expression, it also systematically produces assaults on the self and limits self-expression. To some extent, the invalidation of people is built into the characteristic structure of economic and social inequality.

The effects of social inequality are aggravated in America by the myth that everyone can succeed and that if they fail, it is their own fault. In the nineteenth century, when this myth had somewhat greater basis in reality, American economic structure was more fluid and open, but now success may be harder to attain. Only a few achieve any measure of success in this system, while many are left behind. Sennett and Cobb (1972: 58) observe that "the creation of badges of ability requires the mass to be invisible men." The success ladder is endless, without a top rung, and plastic images of greater and greater success are flashed before people as constant reminders of their inadequacies. The media create superstars and celebrities of the moment. Even those who do achieve moderate success pay psychic costs in terms of their own guilt and the resentment of others. Sennett and Cobb argue that such guilt and resentment are built into the competitive social relationships that characterize our society. Because society pressures people to keep striving to escape a damaged sense of self, and because defeated people are more likely to blame themselves rather than the existing social arrangements, "American society benefits when it makes people feel anxious, defeated and self-reproachful for an imperfect ability to command the respect of others" (Sennett and Cobb, 1972: 153). These assaults on the self are attributed to personal deficiencies rather than to the *condition* of individual powerlessness. Many situations in our society make people feel powerless. One of the major sources of identity is work, yet significant assaults on people's sense of self take place in the work place.

Work, Self, and Health.   A sociopsychological approach to work is based on the assumption "that challenge and pride in work are fundamental ego needs and that any serious threat to these needs will endanger the individual's total well being" (Frankenhaeuser and Gardell, 1976: 39). Much work undermines workers' sense of self-esteem and job satisfaction. The absence of these two interrelated psychological factors, however, is a more important predictor of the risk of coronary heart disease than the presence of other relevant factors, such as poor diet, a lack of exercise, and smoking (House, 1974).

Pride and challenge in work are increasingly absent in many work places. Some surveys indicate that in the 1970s and early 1980s, workers have been more dissatisfied and discontented with their work than in previous decades (Pelletier, 1985). The reasons for increased dissatisfaction are not clear, but may include changes in the kind of people in the work force, lowered motivation, or greater willingness to voice criticism. Some of the increased dissatisfaction, however, may be due to changes in the work place itself.

Worker autonomy is being destroyed under bureaucratic and scientific management. Since World War II, more jobs have been "deskilled" (i.e., they require fewer skills, and are less complex, less challenging, and more boring). The rhythms and motions of the assembly line have come to characterize even white-collar work and help to erode self-esteem and job satisfaction (Braverman, 1974; Glenn and Feldberg, 1977; Howard, 1985).

Workers may perceive the stressfulness of machine-paced work conditions but see their inability to cope as a sign of their own lack of competence. Insofar as they take the situation as natural and accept company production norms as demands that *should* be manageable, their inability to manage stressors erodes their sense of self. The impersonal nature of controls in places like the computerized work place, described earlier, makes it harder to locate the actual agent responsible for imposing stress. The problem is "in the system," and since it is hard to get angry at a system, workers often fault themselves (Howard, 1985: 89–90). One author observed that "to the degree that workers internalize the values of corporate culture, they tend to blame themselves for its contradictions" (Howard, 1985: 137).

Supervisors may constantly remind many workers of their childlike status. They address workers in terms appropriate for children, such as calling women "girls." Some workers have to ask their supervisor for permission to go to the bathroom and are reprimanded for overly lengthy bowel evacuations (Garson, 1977; Terkel, 1974; Pfeffer, 1979; Howard, 1985). *Reader's Digest* gave its employees report cards, perpetuating a childlike treatment typical of school settings (Garson, 1977). One phone company manager, referring to women working in his department, stated: "These girls are just an interface between the customer and computer" (quoted in Howard, 1985: 56). Thus workers may be treated not only as children ("these girls"), but even worse, as a *thing* ("an interface").

Unemployment and Health.   If work can be a health hazard, so too can unemployment. In our society work is an important source of many people's sense of self. The loss of one's job involves more than a loss of financial resources; it may also result in loss of part of one's work-related social network. The stress of unemployment can place a strain on one's relationships with family and friends (Atkinson et al., 1986). Nonemployment, as well as loss of employment, may adversely affect health. Some studies show that women who are employed outside the homes (even if they also do housework) tend to have better health than those who are not employed (Cleary, 1987). Underemployment may also affect self-esteem, because people who need to work settle for jobs that do not utilize their abilities or pay adequate wages and fringe benefits. People with disabilities and women with children are especially likely to be underemployed, since the work place seldom accommodates their special needs (see Serrin, 1989).

Massive unemployment, such as a factory closing, can rip apart the social fabric of a community, affecting not only those who are laid off but also neighborhoods where workers owned homes and local businesses patronized by workers. Unemployment statistics do not adequately capture the concrete psychophysiological effects of unemployment on health. As one author observed,

> Unemployment, with its associated alienation and loss of self-esteem, takes a heavy toll on the lives of Western psychotics. The negative symptoms of schizophrenia—apathy, withdrawal, restricted emotions and lack of interest in the world around—may be to a degree the common psychological effects of long-term unemployment. Every time the economy goes into a decline, mental-hospital admissions for psychosis in working-age people increase. Economic stress and unemployment, by triggering the onset of new cases or worsening already apparent illness, may well account for this phenomenon (Warner, 1986: 51–52).

Brenner (1976) has estimated that between 1970 and 1975, a 1.4 percent increase in unemployment was related to an additional 1,500 suicides, 26,000 deaths from cardiovascular and kidney diseases, 870 deaths from cirrhosis of the liver, and 5,500 mental hospital admissions. A relatively small increase in unemployment thus produced extensive human mental and physical costs. Because he found that there is a consistent relationship, over a number of decades, between an increase in unemployment and higher mental hospital admissions and stress-related diseases, Brenner (1979) argued that economic instability and insecurity increase the likelihood of unhealthy habits and that the stress of unemployment disrupts social networks. In addition to having a direct physiological impact on people's bodies, the stress of unemployment may increase the tendency to adopt destructive coping habits (e.g., smoking and drinking) and may strain social relationships. Brenner's research has been questioned, however, because it is not clear whether the factors he implicated were actually the cause or the result. Perhaps poor health itself tends to produce unemployment, rather than the reverse. Although his findings need to be supplemented by more small-scale and detailed qualitative studies, on the whole, such studies seem to confirm the general relationship between unemployment and illness (Buss and Redburn, 1983; Liem, 1981).

Case studies of particular communities have documented the link between unemployment and some mental problems such as suicide, schizophrenia, and depression (Buss and Redburn, 1983; Jahoda et al., 1971).

Detailed analyses of small samples also confirm the connection between unemployment and health. Cobb and Kasl (1977) applied sophisticated psychological and physiological measures to study a small group of people before and after a plant closing. They found that job loss increased the likelihood of suicide. The workers' levels of cholesterol, norepinephrine, and epinephrine (i.e., stress hormones) were also higher after the layoffs, which suggests that unemployment may increase the likelihood of such physiological problems as coronary heart disease and hypertension.

Another study found that the economic recession in the early 1980s had significant health-damaging effects (Kessler et al., 1987). One advantage of this study was that the researchers controlled for the possibility that during periods of layoffs, workers' psychological and physical health might affect how quickly they would be laid off, a selection bias that would obscure the relationship between unemployment and health. Unemployment itself should not be treated as a stressor utterly independent of a host of other factors affecting the stressfulness of the unemployment experience. High levels of social support may buffer a person against the stressful effects of being out of a job, although unemployment may also put a strain on social support resources.

Some researchers have suggested that health is adversely affected not only by unemployment and downward swings in the business cycle but also by periods of relative prosperity when unemployment is *low*. Eyer (1977) argued that in these "boom" times, mobility and the attendant social dislocation, as well as job stress and pressures to succeed, are especially high; all of these factors increase health risks. Eyer noted that death rates are lower during periods of high unemployment and higher in times of rapidly expanding employment (Eyer, 1977; Eyer and Sterling, 1977). Is this difference due to greater exposure to job-related physical risks or increased psychosocial stress? Relationships between the fluctuation of business cycles and changes in health status are difficult to assess, in part because there are often time lags between the experience of a stressor and its health consequences. Such studies, while raising intriguing questions, are done on such a broad and general scale that they can yield only crude results that must be interpreted cautiously. Numerous studies, however, confirm at least some connection between unemployment and illness.

Other Contexts of Self-Invalidation.   Social conditions encountered later in life can reinforce a lack of self-esteem that often builds upon an already injured sense of self that developed as a part of the individual's early family experience. Pearlin (1983: 6) concluded that

> the family does have a dimension to its place in the stress process that sets it apart from occupations, however. It is, of course, a major reservoir of prob-

lems and tribulations. Multiple facets of marital relations, parent-child encounters, and the transitional points along the family life cycle have been
viewed as fertile ground out of which stress can grow. It is likely, too, to be an
arena in which problems generated elsewhere are transplanted. But the family domain, unlike occupation, is also the place where the wounds that people
incur outside are most likely to be healed. The family is truly many things to
its members: it is commonly an active and rich source of pain, and it it just as
commonly where people turn to find relief from pain. In the stress process, it
stands in a uniquely pivotal position.

Several studies suggest that those whose families make them feel powerless,
force them to surrender their autonomy, or inhibit their displays of anger in
response to arbitrary authority will experience subsequent health problems.
Severe asthma in children, for example, has been linked to low self-esteem,
difficulties in expressing aggression, and complaint behavior (Panides and
Ziller, 1981). The skin disease eczema often involves a struggle for independence from overcontrolling parents (Pratt, 1976: 127). These studies are
exploratory, but point to the role that feelings of helplessness, low self-
esteem, and a poor self-concept that are generated in some families may play
in precipitating various childhood and adult diseases (Chesler, 1972;
Doherty and Campbell, 1988; Laing and Esterson, 1965; Pratt, 1976; Sagan,
1987; Schmale, 1972; Schneider, 1975; Seligman, 1975).

Those who display physical or mental "brokenness" are particularly
likely to experience attacks on their sense of self. Our society, with its strong
values on the ability to work, has little use for those who are not productive
by these standards. Thus it devalues physically or mentally handicapped,
aged, and disabled persons. One of the primary goals of self-help movements, such as the Gray Panthers, an activist organization for the young
and old, and the Center for Independent Living in Berkeley, California,
has been to escape the trap of being treated as invisible, socially dead, and
nonexistent.

Some invalidating consequences of the social structure are amplified
by total institutions (such as hospitals) and social service organizations. An
ethnographic study of a nursing home provides an excellent example of
such structurally produced invalidation (Gubrium, 1975). In this institution, as in others, top staff, floor staff, and patient-residents inhabited very
different social worlds; the communication that passed between them was
distorted by hierarchical arrangements. In making room assignments and
other decisions, the top staff worked from simplified, one-dimensional pictures of patient-residents that were constructed with input from the floor
staff, but very little input from the patients themselves. Some evidence
suggests that individuals' freedom of choice in entering a nursing home is
an important predictor of their longevity (Seligman, 1975). A sense of

control over one's life affairs—a sense of being empowered—may be crucial in dealing with institutional stressors, such as those found in hospitals (Volicer, 1978, 1977).

In the course of people's experiences in the family, work situations, and other institutional settings, they may be "persuaded" that they are incompetent or worthless as they simultaneously learn to value competence and control, and to regard the self as a sort of sacred object. Invalidation of our selves can be stressful, even when it is not internalized and made part of our self-conception.

Dramaturgical Stress

One author suggested that "stress could be induced when an individual perceives his chosen face or performance in a given situation to be inconsistent with the concept of self he tries to maintain for himself and others in that situation" (Cockerham, 1978: 49). **Dramaturgical stress** is generated by being forced to keep up social appearances that are inconsistent with one's real feelings and concept of self. Some research suggests that there are physiological consequences to situations of great discrepancy between the way one must present oneself to others and the emotional-psychological reaction to others that the situation elicits. In one experiment, some subjects responded to provocative situations by expressing overt hostility ("anger out"). Persons displaying "anger in" responses were more likely to blame themselves and not express overt hostility. "Anger in" respondents exhibited more extended physical stress reactions than the "anger out" group (Funkenstein et al., 1957).

In a laboratory experiment, anger was induced experimentally by having a colleague arbitrarily harass and insult subjects while they were trying to solve a problem. The subjects' anger resulted in increases in their blood pressure. Those who could express their hostility toward the experimenter's colleague by giving him what they believed was a mild electric shock (actually a fake one) had their blood pressure return to normal more rapidly. Those who were not allowed to display anger in this fashion continued to show signs of elevated blood pressure long after the harassment had stopped (Hokanson and Burgess, 1962). Similarly, when a person's overt physical movements (such as jumping up) in response to a stressor (such as hearing a gunshot) are repressed, it takes longer for that person's physical functions to return to a prestress response state (Gellhorn, 1969). Such laboratory experiments only suggest how everyday life situations that continuously require certain people, such as powerless social minorities, to repress their anger in the face of the arbitrary exercise of power, might lead to permanently elevated blood pressure.

Minority Status.   Fanon, the Algerian psychiatrist, has dealt with the connections between racial and colonial domination and psychological and physical well-being. In the following passage, he linked muscular tension and illness in Algerians to their powerlessness in the face of French colonial authority:

> This particular form of pathology (a generalized muscular contraction) had already called forth attention before the revolution began. But the doctors described it by portraying it as a congenital stigma of the native, an "original" part of his nervous system where it was stated, it was possible to find the proof of a predominance of the extra-pyramidal system in the native. The contracture is in fact simply the postural accompaniment to the native's reticence and the expression in muscular form of his rigidity and his refusal with regard to colonial authority (Fanon, 1963: 293).

Since it was not possible for the colonized Algerians to express anger openly toward colonial authority, it was held in but manifested itself in in the form of muscular tension. Note also that the effects of a social problem (colonial rule) were viewed by the colonial doctors as an inherited, individual problem.

Encounters with authority, particularly when it is experienced as arbitrary or oppressive, can be stressful, even when the invalidation stemming from such situations is not internalized. Some researchers suggest that the high rates of hypertension among black males cannot be explained by diet, genetic, and other factors alone. They speculate that since black males may be exposed to more anger-provoking encounters with arbitrary authority (e.g., in regard to housing, employment, and the law) than other groups but cannot express their anger, the invalidation of their emotional responses might well contribute to their greater incidence of hypertension (Harburg et al., 1973). Socialization to suppress hostility may be especially high among the "respectable poor" of the upwardly mobile, upper-lower class, who emphasize the importance of politeness, or those who respect and emulate upper-status people (Harburg et al., 1973). The demand that one always be polite and civil—no matter how rude someone else may be—represents a form of social control. The strict control over anger is a norm in our society (Elias, 1978, 1982; Stearns and Stearns, 1986).

Other relatively powerless minorities also experience much dramaturgical stress. Those who must cope with a social stigma by concealing their identity under a cloak of "normal" appearances face special stresses. For example, in our society the widespread fear of homosexuality (homophobia) pressures homosexuals to hide their true selves in order to survive psychological and social expectations, yet trying to "pass" as heterosexuals may place them under considerable dramaturgical stress. In addition to the self-hatred that comes from internalizing antigay values and the repressed anger that results from discrimination, they may suffer from the constant fear of disclosure:

> Visible lesbians are treated as outcasts or queers. They are ignored, fantasized about, and played with. Lesbians are subject to verbal and physical harassment. Closeted lesbians live in fear of being found out. A lesbian's family may be a source of stress for her as coming out to one's family can often mean risking anger, pain or exile. Drifting apart from one's family may be the result of not coming out (O'Donnel, 1978: 14).

"Closets" are the refuge of the powerless, but the use of this refuge has its price. "Closets are a health hazard" was the slogan used by the physicians marching in the 1981 Gay Freedom Day Parade in San Francisco.

Dramaturgical Stress and Work

As more and more people work in corporate and bureaucratic settings, a great deal of control over the presentation of self becomes an important part of their work skills. To get along, manners and politeness become tools for the efficient and effective accomplishment of work (Mumford, 1963: 139). Many skills of self-presentation require what Hochschild (1983) calls "**emotion work**," or the activity through which we control how we show our feelings. Emotion work involves both repressing "undesirable" emotions, such as displays of anger, and forcing oneself to appear happy and enthusiastic, even when one does not feel that way.

The proportion of jobs providing services has increased in our economy. Those that involve some form of selling (e.g., salesclerk or stockbroker) or provide emotional services such as friendliness or reassurance (e.g., social worker or flight attendant) have especially increased (Hochschild, 1983). These service jobs demand elaborate skills in self-presentation and in managing one's emotions (both of which entail emotion work). As Fromm (1965: 268) observed,

> If you do not smile you are judged lacking in a "pleasing personality" and you need to have a pleasing personality if you want to sell your services whether as a waitress, a salesman or a physician. Only those at the bottom of the social pyramid, who sell nothing but their physical labor, and those at the very top do not need to be particularly pleasant.

In his description of the white-collar stratum that has replaced more entrepreneurally oriented middle class, Mills (1956: xvii) noted that the management of one's personality has increasingly become an essential work skill "of commercial relevance and required for the more efficient and profitable distribution of goods and services." This demand for "pleasing personalities," particularly in the face of job conditions that are anything but pleasing, can be highly stressful and often require workers to deny their emotional responses to those stressors.

A study of bank employees found that, when the emotional and physical appearances demanded of workers conflicted with their own sense of self, they began to experience self-artificiality. Bureaucratized structures, particularly those with commercial goals, are most likely to produce this tension between the public face and private self (Jackall, 1977). The rude customer who "is always right," the demand for geniality in the face of social isolation within the office, the interpersonal competitiveness, and the hierarchical pressures all produce dramaturgical stress in the work place (Freund, 1982).

Emotion work entails more than merely assuming a smiling mask, because that would come across as insincere. Rather one must convince oneself, to some extent, that one's angry reaction is not valid. Hochschild (1983) describes how flight attendants are taught to see the nasty customer as a victim and one's own angry response as unnecessary. In other words, they are expected to convince themselves that they feel something other than what they are feeling. Such invalidation of one's emotions may have long-term health consequences, especially as the split between what one feels and what one shows may become automatic, not merely a temporary mask that one assumes voluntarily.

Furthermore, one may lose touch with one's visceral ("gut") reactions because of the constant work requirement to "sell" a certain kind of personality and feelings.[2] Emotion work may short-circuit the experience of signals about people and places that feelings provide (Hochschild, 1983), and put people out of touch with their own bodily reactions.

INFORMATIONAL TROUBLES AND INSTITUTIONAL CONTEXTS

Appropriate and adequate information about our environment can significantly help us manage our lives and their stressors and strains by providing a sense of security as well as feelings of efficacy and competence. **Informational troubles** occur when people do not get enough feedback about their actions or about potential threats in their environment, and can seriously affect our health. Workers, patients, students, inmates, and other relatively powerless groups often may not understand the rationale behind actions

[2]Those prone to high blood pressure may respond to stress neuroendocrinologically in a more dramatic fashion. They are "high reactors" who in their demeanor show a "cool" exterior, are more controlled emotionally, and do not experience sudden and large fluctuations in their blood pressure; for instance, they usually do not blush (Lynch, 1985). It would be worth investigating how these psychosomatic splits are encouraged by such work conditions as the ones just described.

such as firings, hirings, reprimands, parole denials, and tenure denials. Chronic discrepancies between an institution's logic and individuals' understanding of reality is a source of informational troubles.

The following story of institutional life illustrates the impact of short-circuited information on a resident's sense of personal efficacy and health:

> A female patient who had remained in a mute state for nearly 10 years was shifted to a different floor of her building along with her floor mates, while her unit was being redecorated. The third floor of this psychiatric unit where the patient in question had been living was known among the patients as the chronic, hopeless floor. In contrast, the first floor was most commonly occupied by patients who held privileges, including the freedom to come and go on the hospital grounds and to the surrounding streets. In short, the first floor was an exit ward from which patients could anticipate discharge fairly rapidly. All patients were given medical examinations prior to the move, and the patient in question was judged to be in excellent medical health though still mute and withdrawn.
>
> Shortly after moving to the first floor, this chronic psychiatric patient surprised the ward staff by becoming socially responsive such that within a two week period she ceased being mute and was actually becoming gregarious. As fate would have it, the redecoration of the third-floor unit was soon completed and all previous residents were returned to it. Within a week after she had been returned to the "hopeless" unit, this patient, who like the legendary Snow White had been aroused from a living torpor, collapsed and died. The subsequent autopsy revealed no pathology of note, and it was whimsically suggested at the time that the patient had died of despair (Lefcourt, 1973: 422).

This woman may have given up on life because of the way she *perceived* her return to the chronic ward. Her previously learned helplessness may have aggravated her despair. Another important element, however, is how the social structure of the hospital contributed to her death. The institution was unaware of her perceptions, the implications of her changed behavior, and the consequences of returning her to a "helpless" chronic ward. Her inability to make her needs known to the staff and the staff's inability to perceive her needs were linked to two factors that were to some extent built into the hospital: her social status as a resident and her powerlessness in the face of how the institution regulated behavior and made decisions about her life. Her "giving up," while an extreme reaction, was thus not simply a feature of her personality or state of mind but also her response to institutional conditions that were neither created nor readily changeable by her.

Informational Troubles and Illness

Uncertainty about information important to one's security has physiological consequences that in the long run may adversely effect one's health. Studies suggest that social environments may be damaging when they leave a person uncertain in the face of a threat (Kiritz and Moos, 1974). Similarly, situations in which individuals receive inadequate or inaccurate feedback from their environment are especially stressful, because people literally cannot know what to expect and hence how to act (Levin and Idler, 1981). Ambiguities about one's appropriate role and one's effectiveness in that role may also be unhealthful (Garfield, 1980). Unsatisfactory connections between expectations and actual experience have been linked to stress and eventually to lowered immunity (Moss, 1973). While some informational troubles are due to disturbances in the individual's own perceptions, many organizational settings generate or amplify informational uncertainty. Similarly, structural factors (such as social class and age) contribute to informational troubles by creating chronic discrepancies between expectations[3] and experience, and between actions and their consequences:

> An individual's appraisal of his own performance, his self-esteem and sense of identity are partly dependent on his value system and the information feedback he received from his social milieu. When the promulgated values are discrepant and conflicting, the individual will have greater difficulty in choice and decision-making as well as in attaining a sense of competence, which enhances self-esteem and satisfaction (Lipowski, 1973: 523).

In short, the lack of information and adequate feedback from one's environment has an impact on one's self-esteem and sense of competence.

In some cases the cliché that "what you don't know can't hurt you" might be true, but in other cases, as Selye wrote (1956: 229) "knowing what hurts you has an inherent curative value." Having adequate information, for example, affects recovery after an operation; patients who were given clear information as to what to expect after surgery required less postoperative medication for pain (Feuerstein and Skjei, 1979). Yet doctors are often reluctant to give much information because they fear that giving the patient too specific a prognosis would commit them to a course of action that they may not later wish to follow. As discussed further in Chapter 10, in the doctor-patient relationship, the "physician's ability to preserve his own power over the patient . . . depends largely on his ability to control the patient's uncertainty" (Waitzkin and Stoeckle, 1972: 187). Such asymmetrical, unbalanced situations between those who are "in the know" and those who remain "in the dark," which are characterized by the use of information to control others, have come to characterize many contemporary institutional settings, including the work place.

---

[3]Although Moss (1973), Antonovsky (1979, 1987), and Totman (1979) have suggested that informational troubles can affect health, they do not adequately demonstrate how the degree of power that accompanies one's social status and the way behavior is regulated in various social settings create informational troubles. Further research needs to establish more clearly the connections among social structure, controls specific to that structure, various kinds of informational troubles, and the stress they produce.

Informational Troubles in the Work Place

Informational troubles are generated by features inherent in various bureaucratic and corporate structures of everyday modern life. In work settings, much production is characterized by a marked organizational split between those who manage work and those who execute various tasks. On an informational level, the split is between knowledge about the planning and control of production and about its execution.

One of the "social functions of ignorance" is the maintenance of control over clients or workers (Moore and Tumin, 1949). As a college teacher who worked in a factory during his sabbatical observed:

> As indicated, the factory worker's subordinate and related vulnerability is affected in part by the company's keeping from the workers sufficient advance information about the factors of production and intentions of the company so likely to affect their lives. . . . Keeping workers ignorant also helps management control them. Ignorance particularly in the face of economic instability, makes workers insecure, hanging on for information in company handouts that consistently come too late for a meaningful response. Management treats information as a part of its private property and uses information to protect its own authoritarian rule (Pfeffer, 1979: 103–104).

Workers, for example, are seldom told the rationale for establishing production goals (Haraszti, 1978: 61), even though they structure and affect the quality of working life.

Management also controls information about dangers in the work environment. Many companies do not tell their workers, or the workers' doctors, the generic names of the chemicals to which workers are exposed. Because these substances as well as dangerous production processes are often protected as "trade" secrets, only the trade name, a code number, or a general description of its use is provided (Howard, 1985).

Workers who experience symptoms such as nausea, rashes, or headaches may suspect that the cause is the substances they work with, but they cannot get definitive information from management (Scott, 1974; Berman, 1978; Nelkin and Brown, 1984; Howard, 1985). Their only knowledge about the effects of these chemicals may come from rumors or indirect indicators, such as the fact that those working in high-risk areas are asked to "spit in the can" (i.e., give specimens for sputum cytologies) or give urine samples (Kingsport Study Group, 1978: 61). A local doctor in a Tennessee Eastman (a part of Eastman Kodak) "company town" reports seeing tell-tale symptoms of work-related health problems in many of his worker-patients or hearing accounts of illness their co-workers are experiencing. He concluded, "But you never read about this in the paper. The only way you get it is through the grapevine. Some of the grapevine is probably inaccurate, but I have a feeling as a physician that I'm seeing the tip of the iceberg" (quoted in Kingsport

Study Group, 1978: 60). One worker in the microchip electronics industry (where the work often involves solvents and acids) remarked,

> People don't know what they are working with because they're never *told* what they're working with. I was never informed of the hazards. Oh, I was told that I was working with acid and that it could burn me, yes. But I was never told about the possible carcinogens or the effects of the solvent inhalation (quoted in Howard, 1985: 158).

Like the doctor-patient and professional-client relationships, the manager-worker relationship is characterized by unequal access to important information. Management's monopoly over knowledge is a resource that keeps management's options open, and protects against lawsuits, strikes, and other critical actions. Such managerial control over information, however, also affects client or worker security, autonomy, and often health.

Imagine feeling some symptoms, having an uneasiness about the substances you work with, or hearing rumors, and yet being uncertain of how those substances might affect you.[4] Such uncertainty aggravates an individual's sense of powerlessness and insecurity. These informational troubles often result in an inability to predict and plan or know the sources of one's distress. To remedy some of this uncertainty, Norway has legislation requiring that workers be informed about systems used in planning and controlling of production, that they be given training to understand such systems, and that they be able to influence their design. In Sweden, the law requires that workers on all levels be given comprehensive information about working conditions and their hazards (Levi, 1981: 119–120).

SOCIAL SUPPORT

As discussed in Chapter 4, humans' biological make-up makes them open to influences from the social environment, including relationships with other people. The loss of a spouse or intimate friend can be a stressor of such magnitude that it precipitates something like voodoo death (Engel, 1971). Bereavement can increase the risk of coronary problems (Pilisuk and Parks, 1986: 33) and lower immunity (Bartrop et al., 1977). Mourning and separation from loved ones can affect levels of stress hormones (Pilisuk and Parks, 1986: 45). Yet although the withdrawal of social support or a diminished quality of social relationships can have a sickening impact on us, social bonds also have the potential to heal us.

[4]Recall the study by House et al. (1979) cited in Chapter 4 (page 84). How might informational stress interact with the respiratory effects of the chemical (i.e., the chemical stressor)?

Social support is one source of the individual's sense of empowerment. It may seem strange and perhaps a bit clinical to think of our relationships with lovers, family, friends, and fellow workers or students in terms of power, yet social ties can serve as nets that hold us up or keep us from falling when we are threatened. They function as sources of information and financial or other kinds of aid, and as mirrors that help to reflect back to us messages of self-affirmation. Just as a fetus needs a womb to receive nourishment, shelter, warmth, and life support, human beings cannot function effectively as isolated individuals.

Social support is a general term for the many different resources that aid persons in times of crisis and help them cope with life. Social relationships empower individuals by making them feel that they are part of a larger social order. They are also a source of self-validation and a sense of personal security (Pilisuk and Parks, 1986). As symbols of those relationships, physical contact and intimacy can be empowering. Other people can remind us that we are alive and have someone to lean on and depend on when necessary, and generally enhance our sense of security and self-confidence. Emotional support is one of the most important ways social support empowers individuals (House, 1981).

This support may involve touch. Since many measures of social support use paper-and-pencil methods such as questionnaires, human touch has not been adequately investigated as a medium of emotional support. Giving social support may involve subtle cues like body language and tone of voice, which often go unnoticed by the researcher-observer (Pilisuk and Parks, 1986: 39). While the effects of social contact may not be mentally perceived, they still may have an impact on our bodies. Lynch (1979) cited some clinical observations that a nurse's touch can affect the blood pressure of even a comatose patient. Under the stress of electric shocks, dogs who were petted responded to these stressors with fewer pathological consequences than animals who were not touched. Another study found that rabbits on a high fat diet that were not touched were more likely to develop heart disease than those that were cuddled and petted (Thoits, 1983). While animal experiments should be used cautiously when generalizing to humans, these studies suggest that nonverbal aspects of social relationships may have health consequences.

Pearlin (1983) emphasizes that social support reduces strain by preventing the loss of self-esteem and aiding a sense of mastery that overwhelming stressors can erode. Social support empowers by giving individuals a sense that they are valued, esteemed, cared for, and belong to a network of mutual obligation. These are primarily *emotional* functions of social support, which also serves an *instrumental* purpose. Social support can provide useful information and material resources (such as financial aid) as well as other help (Levin and Idler, 1981). Support can also encourage recovery from a an illness, for example, by encouraging a family member to do therapeutic exercises. Other social networks also promote such health habits as regular exercise, good eating habits, and adequate sleep.

Social Support and Health

In the classic study *Suicide,* Durkheim ([1897] 1951) found a relationship between rates of suicide and the degree to which individuals were integrated into their group, which he measured with indicators such as divorce rates. Thus a group with high rates of divorce should show a high rate of suicide. Conversely, a more integrated group should have a lower rate.[5] Durkheim was the first social scientist to demonstrate that suicide was not simply an *individual* psychological issue but also to some extent a social and cultural phenomenon influenced by such factors as the strength of social bonds. Much of the literature on social support and health follows in this tradition by making similar associations between social isolation and poor health (Thoits, 1983).

Social isolation itself can be stressful. Some research indicates that low integration into social networks contributes to poor health, even when significant stressors are absent (Gore, 1978: 158). A comprehensive study showing the link between social factors and health was conducted by Berkman and Syme (1979) on a large population in Alameda County, California. They used measures of four types of social contact: (1) marriage partners, (2) close friends and relatives, (3) members of a church, and (4) informal or formal associations. Those who had contacts with any of these groups evidenced lower mortality rates than those who did not. The authors of this study recognized the problem of *causal direction.* Does illness cause a person to withdraw and others to withdraw from that person, or does social isolation generate sickness? Therefore, they analyzed groups with every kind of health status and found that even among those who were sick, persons with higher levels of social contact had lower mortality rates. Persons with extensive social connections were likely to smoke and drink less, and to eat and sleep more regularly than those with few social connections. This finding suggests that social relationships also protect health by encouraging good health habits (Wallston et al., 1983).

Another study, analyzing pregnancy complications, found that neither high stress nor the lack of support, in and of themselves, increased such problems. When major stressors were combined with a low degree of social support, however, there were significantly higher numbers of complications. Women who had high stress and high levels of social support experienced fewer difficulties than those who had a lot of stressful events but not much support. When the levels of stress were low, the absence of social

---

[5]Durkheim also recognized that groups fostering *too much* integration could encourage what he called "altruistic suicide," such as the deaths of Japanese Kamikaze pilots who crashed their planes into Allied warships during World War II.

support did not have a notable impact on complications (Nuckolls et al., 1972). This evidence suggests that social support helped to buffer women against the effects of high stress. Most research finds social support to be either a primary *causal* factor (i.e., a *main* effect) in determining health or a *mediating* factor, which may protect the person from the full impact of the stressor.

Lynch (1979) argues that social isolation can both contribute to coronary heart disease and adversely affect a person's recovery from a heart attack. Although much of his evidence is indirect and the quality of his data uneven, as a whole it provides compelling evidence that social isolation can influence us physiologically and hence affect our health. Lynch emphasized that social contact (or what he calls "dialogue") is of chief importance for health. Two people may bicker and fight, yet need this conflictual relationship to keep them going. Interaction, a sense of purpose, and connectedness to something (or someone) outside of oneself—but not necessarily "love"—are the important factors for health.

Mortality rates are considerably lower among those who are married than among those who are single or formerly married. Some studies also show differences between those who are married and those who are not in death rates from cirrhosis of the liver, tuberculosis, and pneumonia (Levin and Idler, 1981; Lynch, 1979). While such evidence is in line with our cultural assumptions about the importance of family life, it must be interpreted cautiously. Marital status tells us nothing about the quality of social contact. Many people are formally married but psychologically live alone and feel isolated from each other, whereas divorced and other single people may participate in rich social lives.

Social support is also a potential mediator of negative effects of unemployment on health by offering a sense of empowerment. A longitudinal study of men who were laid off from work found that those with higher degrees of social support reported fewer symptoms of illness and showed lower levels of cholesterol. Conversely, those with lower levels of support had higher levels of cholesterol and reported more illness symptoms (Gore, 1978).

Social support is also important in the work place, where it buffers work-related stress (House, 1981; see also LaRocco and House, 1980). A study of NASA workers found that good work relationships protected them from the effects of such stress (Caplan, 1972). Further investigation is needed on how particular organizational forms encourage or discourage social support. For example, how do cultural factors, such as an emphasis upon competitiveness and individualism, affect the possibility for supportive relationships in the work place? As two authors observed, "social currents of careerism, autonomy, mobility, privacy and achievement that disrupt our traditional roots and ties also make difficult the continuity of new bonds" (Pilisuk and Parks, 1986: 59). Do stressors in the work place, such as high noise levels, also inhibit social interaction? While social support may be empowering, it is also important to examine how control over work conditions makes social support possible.

Limitations of Social Support Research

Much of the social support literature makes two assumptions that are problematic. First, social support should not be treated as a stable, constant factor; levels of social support do not necessarily remain the same over time. Second, stressful events (stressors) and social support are not independent factors, but rather interact with each other (Atkinson et al., 1986). Just as social support may protect a person against a stressor (such as unemployment), so too may a stressor (such as unemployment) affect levels of social support. For example, a spouse's unemployment may put a strain on the entire family relationship and in turn reduce the support given by family members. Some evidence further suggests that economic stressors *and* the amount of support available are socially distributed by class: "It's as simple as that. If you are poor, you have more stress and less supportive resources" (Pilisuk and Parks, 1986: 58).

The research tends to focus only on the *beneficial* aspects of social support. Although it is popularly believed that it is always good to have family and friends around in times of trouble, social support is not necessarily helpful and at times can be counterproductive. For example, persons experiencing a health crisis can be overprotected, which slows recovery. Family members may also try to communicate supportive messages ("You can do it!") that may be interpreted by the ill person as a form of pressure to get well (Horton, 1985a). Social support may undermine sick people's sense of personal competence by making them feel that they cannot do anything on their own or that they cannot possibly reciprocate the help they have been given (Pilisuk and Parks, 1986: 39). One study indicates that *perceived* support may be more important than *received* support in coping with stressful events.[6] It concluded that it is possible that "the perception of one's network being ready to act can be as important—if not more important—than actual supportive behavior" (Wethington and Kessler, 1986: 84).

Perhaps the most significant blind spot in this area of research is the failure to consider the larger contexts of the power in which social support takes place. For example, people in economic need may have difficulties with their social networks. Their social and economic powerlessness in turn places a strain on their social networks, and may also limit their access to supportive social relationships. Working-class people on the whole have less developed social networks and group affiliations than middle-class people

---

[6]A problem in this study is that measures of both perceived and received support were based on the recall of subjects; they are therefore subjective and may have been perceptually modified by the respondents.

(Fischer, 1983). One study showed how poverty limits social involvement because of a lack of funds for transportation, recreation, or association dues (Pilisuk and Parks, 1986: 60).

The notion of social support is very much in fashion in stress research (McQueen and Siegrist, 1982), partly because of its appeal to common sense: We would all agree that "we get by with a little help from our friends." The thrust of many studies is that people who have—or perceive themselves to have—access to emotional, material, and other kinds of support are healthier and are at an advantage when dealing with life's crises, including sickness. One group of researchers reported, "We found that individuals showed a greater level of depressive symptoms if they experienced a most important and undesirable event. This effect was reduced if help came from strong rather than weak ties" (Lin et al., 1985: 259). This interpretation seems to represent a scientific way of saying something that we all know, yet the evidence does not always support this conclusion (McQueen and Siegrist, 1982: 359). One researcher observed that "it appears that lack of support in combination with deficiencies in self-esteem or mastery may account for differential vulnerability to life difficulties" (Thoits, 1983: 90). Thus an important factor in determining individuals' ability to cope with stress is how empowered they feel themselves to be.

The current emphasis on social support seems to be in tune with some of the other ideological biases we have discussed. Social support puts the emphasis on the individual and institutions such as the family in which individuals have some power. One consequence of the focus on the importance of social support may be to force people to fall back on their own *private* resources (Fischer, 1983), for it is in the private sphere of family life and friendship in which people have some control (Pearlin, 1983). In such public settings as the work place or school, social support may not be available, and individual coping mechanisms may not be effective. Thus coping difficulties and limits to social support derived from societal structures outside the private sphere are seldom addressed.

Studies on the availability of social support make little mention of class and power. For example, how does capitalism, as a social system, help to generate competitiveness, individualism, and social mobility that make social support difficult? How do controls in the work place affect social support as well as self-esteem and self-mastery? How does the distribution of power in existing social networks such as families affect social support? Social support can be a means of empowering the individual, but it is also a part of the social and cultural environments that determine its quality and availability. The research emphasis on social support should not blind us to the many other ways in which these social environments empower or disempower individuals, making it more difficult for them to control their own bodies.

SUMMARY

In this chapter we have examined social-organizational conditions of disempowerment, and how these conditions create psychosocial stress and affect the individual's responses to stress. Social stresses that attack one's sense of self and self-concept are particularly problematic in modern society, given the extreme importance attached to both concepts. Social class and work situations affect our self-concept. Dramaturgical stress also affects health, especially because contemporary society puts a great deal of emphasis on the importance of self-presentation as part of social and work skills. When people must "grin and bear it" under the most uncivil conditions, health problems may ensue.

Appropriate and adequate information is a significant source of security and help in coping with environmental demands. Institutional settings (such as the work place or a hospital) can generate informational troubles, which are related to illness and the inability to cope adequately. Social support is a means of being and feeling empowered. The absence of such support can itself give rise to stress and deprive individuals of a resource for coping with stress. The sociopsychological conditions of modern life reviewed here are related to chronic degenerative diseases—the "diseases of civilization."

RECOMMENDED READINGS

Articles

Joseph Eyer and Peter Sterling, "Stress-related mortality and social organization," *Review of Radical Political Economics* 9(1), 1977: 1–44.

Marianne Frankenhaeuser, "Coping with stress at work," *International Journal of Health Services* 11(4), 1981: 491–510.

James S. House, "Occupational stress and coronary heart diseases: A review and theoretical integration," *Journal of Health and Social Behavior* 15, 1974: 17–27.

Peter L. Schnall and Rochelle Kern, "Hypertension in American society: An introduction to historical materialist epidemiology," pp. 73–89, in P. Conrad and R. Kern, eds., *The Sociology of Health and Illness*, second edition. New York: St. Martin's Press, 1981.

Books

Peter E. S. Freund, *The Civilized Body: Social Domination, Control and Health.* Philadelphia: Temple University Press, 1982. An elaboration of the perspective of this chapter.

Arlie Hochschild, *The Managed Heart: Commercialization of Human Feeling.* Berkeley: University of California Press, 1983. Introducing the concepts of emotion work and emotional labor, this study of flight attendants discusses the increase of emotion work in the service sector.

Robert Howard, *Brave New Workplace*. New York: Penguin, 1985. An examination of social control, alienation, and health hazards in computerized work places and in the computer industry.

James Lynch, *The Broken Heart*. New York: Basic, 1979. A highly readable discussion of the relationship between social isolation and coronary heart disease.

Richard M. Pfeffer, *Working for Capitalism*. New York: Columbia University Press, 1979. The account of a college professor's experiences working in a factory.

Chapter Six

The Social Meanings of Sickness

What does it mean to be sick? In some ways a tree's disease is similar to a human's disease: Trees can recover or they can die of disease; branches become lifeless, leaves wither, and roots and trunks function poorly. Unlike trees, however, humans must also grapple with the experiential aspects of sickness. Humans are capable of reflecting upon themselves, their bodily conditions, and their self-perceptions. This reflexiveness means that humans typically suffer not merely from disease but also from their experience of illness and the meanings that they and others attach to it.

Sickness is upsetting to the social group too. Because it is a breech of the ideals or norms of the society, it is disruptive. Illness represents a threat to the order and meanings by which people make sense of their lives and organize the routines of their everyday existence. Sickness also raises moral questions, such as, "Who (or what) is responsible for this misfortune?"

ILLNESS AS DEVIANCE

The very notion of health is a social ideal that varies widely from culture to culture or from one historical period to another. For example, in the nineteenth century the ideal upper-class woman was pale, frail, and delicate. A woman with robust health was considered to be lacking refinement (Ehrenreich and English, 1978). In other periods, cultures, or subcultures, however, the ideal of health might be identified with traits such as strength, fertility, spirituality, righteousness, the absence of pain, the presence of certain pain, fatness, thinness, or youthfulness. The ideal of health thus embodies a particular culture's notions of well-being and desired human qualities. Standards of health in any culture reflect that culture's core values. Through ritual action and symbols (especially language), the social group continually reproduces these central, shared meanings (Durkheim, [1915] 1965).

Durkheim ([1895] 1938: 68–69) observed that deviance serves to remind the entire social group of the importance of certain collective values. Like crime, sickness is a form of **deviance**, or departure from group-established norms. Society typically imputes different kinds of responsibility for crime than for sickness. Durkheim asserted that the very existence of social norms—however defined—means that there will be deviance in all societies. The way a society reacts to sickness and crime reaffirms its core values. Furthermore, the practices for sanctioning deviance (such as punishing the criminal or treating the sick person) reaffirm and revitalize the collective sentiments and maintain social solidarity. Durkheim ([1893] 1964: 108) argued that societal reaction against deviance "is above all designed to act upon upright [nondeviant] people. . . ." This function suggests that the treatment of the sick in all healing systems serves to reaffirm cultural norms and ideals for the sick and the well alike.

Thus deviance is more a description of the social group that defines it than a quality of the individual considered deviant. In fact labeling of an attribute or behavior as deviant is a social product (Becker, 1963; Waxler, 1980). Cultures vary widely as to whether they consider deviant such bodily conditions as facial scars, obesity, shortness, and paleness. One cultural standard, for example, considers a certain amount of hair on a man's chest to be desirable, representing fortitude, robustness, and manliness. Much less hair on the chest is treated as too effeminate; much more is considered coarse and animallike. Other cultures (and subcultures), however, have different definitions of desirable body hair and different connotations of deviance from those norms.

As Chapter 9 illustrates, defining deviance is a social process involving factors such as power and stratification. Power in a society includes having significant influence in setting social norms and labeling deviance. It also involves having control over the social mechanisms by which these norms are taught and enforced. Indeed, one function of social control is to perpetuate the dominance of those in power in establishing the norms. Socially established norms are *imposed* on people, regardless of their own beliefs. Power is a factor in both the creation of a deviance label and its application to some individual persons.

The Sick Role

Society must deal with individuals who differ significantly from its norms. As indicated in Chapter 1, the concept of social control refers to all mechanisms a society uses to try to contain its members' behavior within various norms, including deterrents, incentives, rewards, and punishments. How society responds to an instance of perceived deviance depends largely upon its determination of the individual's responsibility for the deviant behavior.

Like all social roles, the **sick role** is primarily a description of social expectations (including those of the sick person). While these expectations strongly influence behavior, the sick role does not describe how sick persons actually behave (cf. Twaddle, 1981: 56–58).

According to Parsons (1951: 428–447), the sick role entails certain responsibilities as well as certain privileges:

1. The individual's incapacity is a form of deviance from social norms, but since it is not deliberate, the individual is not held responsible;
2. The sickness is legitimate grounds for being exempted from normal obligations, such as work or school attendance;
3. The legitimacy of this exemption is, however, predicated upon the sick person's intent to get well;
4. The attempt to get well implies also seeking and cooperating with competent help to treat the illness.

The sick role of someone with pneumonia exemplifies Parson's use of this concept. A person with serious pneumonia would not be expected to report to work, to do housework, or to keep an appointment. Failure to perform such basic social obligations is a form of deviance that is typically sanctioned, for example, by firing an employee. Having pneumonia, however, is usually considered an acceptable, but temporary, excuse for not meeting these obligations. The employer does not hold the sick person immediately responsible. This part of the sick role concept is thus connected with Parson's larger concern with how societies maintain their equilibrium in the face of deviance and disruptions such as sickness.

Although having pneumonia is a legitimate excuse for not reporting to work, the sick person is expected to "act sick" and try to get well. The employer would be less than happy to see the "sick" employee at a baseball game later that day, for example. According to Parsons, part of trying to get well involves seeking competent health care from a trained physician. The social expectations for a person with pneumonia thus include going to a doctor, obtaining and taking the doctor's prescription, and otherwise conforming to whatever regimen the doctor ordered. Thus he tied the sick role inevitably with the role of medical professionals. (Parsons was especially interested in the development of professionalism as a feature of modern society.) In his usage, the sick role directly implies the patient role; by contrast, we explore the patient role as a separate role, which sick persons may or may not enter, depending upon whether their sickness is brought to the attention of medical professionals (see Chapter 10).

Parson's concept of the sick role is valuable in that it highlights the social control functions of how society treats sickness. It also emphasizes the extent to which social definitions of sickness reflect larger cultural values of modern Western societies (Parsons, 1972: 124). Some of the cultural narrowness of Parsons's sick role concept is due to his explicit focus on American values, such as the emphasis upon individual achievement and responsibility. His conception of the sick role was thus primarily a description of American modes of dealing with the problems of deviance and motivation in the face of the potential disruptions when individual members feel unable to meet normal obligations. The sick role, however, is not as clear-cut as Parsons's model suggests. Four problems with his approach are discussed below.

The Sick Role Is Not Necessarily Temporary.   Parsons' conception of the sick role is based upon only one, relatively narrow class of health problems. The obligations and exemptions described in his model appear to fit serious, acute illnesses reasonably well. **Acute illnesses** characteristically occur suddenly, peak rapidly, and run their course (i.e., result in death or recovery) in relatively short time. Examples include influenza, measles, and scarlet fever.

Chronic illnesses, by contrast, are of long duration—typically as long as the sufferer lives. They often result in the steady deterioration of bodily functioning. Examples include emphysema, diabetes, multiple sclerosis, epilepsy, and heart disease. Furthermore, some acute illnesses are considered chronic when they become a continuing pattern in an individual's life; examples include chronic bronchitis, asthma, and ulcers. Additionally, a number of chronic, disabling conditions (e.g., paraplegia from a car accident) do not involve any ongoing disease, but may result in an ambiguous, lifelong sick role.

While many acute conditions can be cured (or are self-limiting), most chronic conditions are permanent. Treatment of chronic illness is aimed at best at controlling the deterioration caused by the disease and at *managing* the illness. Many of the most dangerous acute (usually infectious) diseases of earlier generations have been brought under control in developed countries through improved sanitation, nutrition, housing, and the like. Inoculations, antibiotics, and other medical treatments have also had some effect in curing infectious diseases (although, as Chapter 2 shows, their role has been somewhat overstated). By contrast, the proportion of persons suffering chronic illnesses has greatly increased, and modern medical intervention does not appear so potent in the face of such conditions.

The nature of chronic illness does not fit Parsons's sick role pattern. Obviously, his assumption of the necessity of an "intent to get well" is irrelevant if the illness is, by definition, permanent. His sick role conception presumed that the benefits were conditional, but chronic illnesses make most of the conditions meaningless (Alexander, 1982). Unlike infectious disease, chronic ailments are more likely to be considered partly the fault or the responsibility of the sufferer. Whereas few people consider a case of chicken pox, for example, to be the sick person's fault, lay and medical conceptions of many chronic conditions, such as lung cancer, high blood pressure, and cirrhosis of the liver, are believed to be brought on—at least partially—by the sufferer's own lifestyle.

Feelings about whether a chronic illness is sufficient grounds for exemption from normal responsibilities are also ambiguous. Since the condition is not temporary, the exemptions are all the more problematic for both the sufferer and those who would grant the exemptions. Just how disabling is the condition? Is a partial exemption feasible? Often persons suffering chronic illnesses do not want total exemption from normal responsibilities, but the illness prevents them from fulfilling some usual duties. For example, a person with emphysema may be able to work but at a much slower pace, and a person with chronic back pain may need more frequent breaks. Societal values enforced by the sick role suggest why persons with chronic illness have considerable difficulty negotiating such concessions.

As a means for maintaining stability and social control, the sick role allows temporary exemptions from normal role requirements without changing those requirements. Routine deviance from the requirements is, however, far more disruptive if judged by criteria of maximizing productive efficiency. If, for example, an employer expects all clerk-typists to put in eight-hour days, it would be highly disruptive to adjust work expectations to accommodate several workers' various chronic illnesses (e.g., by allowing one worker to work only six hours with frequent breaks, another to type at a very slow pace, and yet another to work only those days when the chronic condition was not flaring up). Thus the legitimate exemptions of the sick role are not readily granted to many chronically sick persons.

Similarly, many other "deviant" health conditions do not fit the sick role model of acute diseases and thereby lead to ambiguities about expectations. Should a person born with a physical handicap be treated as sick? What about accident victims or the mentally ill? In a process known as the medicalization of deviance, more and more problems that do not fit the sick role model are being defined as sicknesses (cf. McKinlay, 1972). Medicalization produces a proliferation of sicknesses, few of which can be medically cured. Like chronic illness, these conditions are typically only medically controlled or managed. The individual may be identified as sick, but the benefits and responsibilities of the sick role simply do not apply. Thus there is considerable ambiguity over the role expectations of those deemed to be "sick" with such conditions as pregnancy, menopause, hyperkinesia, alcoholism, pyromania, and PMS (premenstrual syndrome).

The Sick Role Is Not Always Voluntary.   Parsons's model holds that the sick person, in exchange for the advantages of the sick role, is motivated to assume that role and voluntarily cooperate with the agents of social control in the appropriate therapy for the deviant condition. In the above case of the worker with pneumonia, for example, the person's discomfort and fear of complications would presumably motivate the individual to see a doctor, have blood tests and x-rays, get bed rest at home or in a hospital, and take medications. Parsons thus assumed that, in contrast to the criminal deviant, the sick person voluntarily enters the socially prescribed role.

Not all persons, however, want to enter the sick role, even when they feel ill. Many people resist the expected childlike dependency the role often entails; many others have strong aversion to medical treatments, especially in the hospital. A Scottish study of lower-class women found considerable negative moral evaluation of persons who give in, or "lie down," to illness (Blaxter and Paterson, 1982). Some people, furthermore, simply cannot afford to withdraw from normal obligations; the sick role is a threat to their subsistence (Kasl and Cobb, 1966).

Some sicknesses carry a negative connotation or stigma. While the sick person would obtain some benefits (such as exemption from work or other duties) from the sick role, these negative attitudes toward that illness could be worse than the condition itself. For example, a person suffering epilepsy may actively avoid being socially identified as having the disease because of the repulsion and often outright discrimination associated with the illness (Schneider and Conrad, 1980).

Many persons are placed into the sick role by others, regardless of their own wishes. Children and the dependent aged are generally not considered competent to decide for themselves whether to assume the role; instead their caretakers make the decision for them. Likewise, some conditions force an involuntary entrance into the sick roles. The most straightforward example is a loss of consciousness. Other ambiguous situations arise when someone's family (or unrelated caretakers, such as doctors, social workers, or police) decide that an individual is too "sick" to have good judgment and then place the person into the sick role. Because many people thus do not enter the sick role voluntarily, their cooperation with the medical regimen cannot be assumed. In many such cases, the social control functions of the sick role are more coercive and less benign than portrayed by the model.

By contrast, some persons seek to enter the sick role and are denied access. A process of subtle social negotiation occurs when an individual claims the sick role. This claim must then be accepted as legitimate by others, especially authoritative others. Often medical personnel such as the school nurse and the company doctor are the critical gatekeepers who have the power to determine who will be admitted to the sick role in their institutional setting. Informal negotiation also typically takes place as the person claiming the sick role attempts to convince family and others of the legitimacy of the claim, and the others judge—and sometimes test—that legitimacy. Entry into the sick role is thus essentially a social and political process.

Variability in Sick Role Legitimacy.   Parsons's conception of the sick role also presumes that a single, stable value system is operative for all persons in a society. Historically, however, the legitimate exemption of sick persons from various obligations is highly variable. The criteria for such an exemption may also differ according to gender, social class, and subcultural expectations.

Legitimate exemptions from work obligations, for example, vary enormously, typically according to social class. Unskilled workers, for example, may not have any paid sick days, whereas white-collar workers may have a given allowance of such days proportionate to their rank or seniority. Indeed, the idea that absence due to sickness should not be a basis for dismissal is relatively recent; even today sickness is not a legitimate exemption for many workers, and they have no legal protection of their jobs.

The meaning of the sick role itself varies considerably according to social class. The same sickness has different connotations according to the class or gender of the sufferer. For example, in the nineteenth century consumption (tuberculosis) was a romanticized illness among the middle and upper classes. This sick role implied a "consuming" passion as expressed in artistic sensitivity and creativity. Some of the physical effects of tuberculosis were considered beautiful: slenderness, fever-bright eyes, pallor, and a transparent complexion accompanied by pink cheeks. One young woman with consumption wrote in her diary:

> Since yesterday I am white and fresh and amazingly pretty. My eyes are spirited and shining, and even the contours of my face seem prettier and more delicate. It's too bad that this is happening at a time when I am not seeing anyone. It's foolish to tell, but I spent a half-hour looking at myself in the mirror with pleasure; this had not happened to me for some time (Marie Bashkirtseff's Journal of 1883, quoted in Herzlich and Pierret, 1987: 81).

The well-to-do sufferer was " 'apart,' threatened but all the more precious for it" (Herzlich and Pierret, 1987: 25). While the disease was more prevalent and devastating among the lower classes, no such privileged or positive sick role was available to them.

The sick role was considered especially appropriate for women of that era, because it was thought to reflect ladies' refinement and delicacy. It was expected and even stylish for well-to-do women to faint frequently and to retire to bed for "nerves," "sick headaches," "female troubles," and "neurasthenia." Lower-class women, by contrast, were considered to be more robust, as evidence of their coarseness and less civilized nature (Ehrenreich and English, 1978).

Upper-class Victorians could obtain exemption from normal obligations by claiming the sick roles of neurasthenia or hysteria, illnesses of the "nerves" believed to afflict particularly intellectual or sensitive persons. The label of neurasthenia appears to have been especially useful for men, whose normal role expectations of fortitude and active participation in the world outside of the home made it difficult for them to exhibit dependency or weakness. The vague symptoms identified as neurasthenia, however, were a legitimate basis for men to assume the sick role (Sicherman, 1978; see also Drinka, 1984).

Cultural expectations of the sick role also vary, perhaps widely. There is some evidence that cultures differ in the degree of legitimacy they accord various illnesses and their resulting claims to exemption from responsibilities. For example, neurasthenia is a legitimate basis of the sick role among contemporary Taiwanese, whereas in the United States it is a far less common diagnosis or culturally recognized reason for assuming the sick role (cf. Kleinman, 1980). Similarly, persons of Hispanic background would be more likely than those of Anglo-Saxon heritage to consider a certain "fright" (*susto*), such as being startled by an animal or a possible assailant, to be a legitimate basis for the sick role (Rubel et al., 1984). Since cultures vary in how they understand various illnesses, they also have different expectations for the behavior of persons occupying the sick role, such as the amount of pain and disability they may experience (cf. Angel and Thoits, 1987). These examples illustrate that the expectations identified as a sick role change; problems that were identified in the past as a legitimate basis for claiming the role are no longer appropriate, while other problems—formerly unrecognized or discounted—are now accepted as legitimate.

Responsibility for Sickness.   Parsons's model of the sick role held that, unlike crime, sickness was not the responsibility of the deviant person. Furthermore, he considered the professional diagnosis and treatment of medical deviance to be purely technical, neutral, and unbiased. As Chapter 9 illustrates, however, the very definition of illness is socially constructed, and social groups often impute responsibility for illness to the sick person.

Freidson (1970) observed that certain conditions are typically viewed as the responsibility of the sick individual and thus are treated relatively punitively, like crimes. Examples include various sexually transmitted diseases as well as substance abuse and conditions derived from such abuse. Freidson noted that the attitudes of both the society and the medical profession, while greatly expanding the range of conditions considered to be properly "medical" problems, do not necessarily abolish the negative moral connotations attached to these conditions. He also described another category of sicknesses that, while not technically considered the fault of the sick person, are nonetheless stigmatized (Freidson 1970: 234–237). *Stigma* is a powerful discrediting and tainting social label that radically changes the way an individual is viewed as a person (Goffman, 1963: 2–5). For example, being an illegitimate child was (historically more than currently) an enormous barrier to presenting oneself as a "normal," upright citizen.

Many sicknesses carry a stigma. Leprosy, epilepsy, and AIDS, for example, all carry connotations of disreputability and even evil. The sick role for someone with a stigmatized illness is clearly different than that for a person with a "neutral" sickness. Stigmas can result in various forms of discrimination: Persons with epilepsy, for instance, have experienced job discrimination, difficulty in obtaining a driver's license, prohibitions against marrying, and difficulties in obtaining insurance (Schneider and Conrad, 1980). Even after someone has been treated and pronounced "cured" of such a condition, the stigma often remains on that person. Furthermore, the stigma frequently spreads to the family and close friends of the sick person in what Goffman (1963: 30–31) calls a "courtesy stigma." For example, families and friends of persons with epilepsy, cancer, or AIDS sometimes find themselves being shunned or harassed (Conrad, 1986).

The source of stigma is not the disease itself but rather the social imputation of a negative connotation. Leprosy is highly stigmatized in India, but far less so in neighboring Sri Lanka. Lepers in India are treated as outcasts, whereas many lepers in Nigeria remain in the village and carry on normal social lives (Waxler, 1981). Because cultures vary in the stigma imputed to different sicknesses, the sick role for those illnesses vary accordingly.

The degree of stigma and responsibility attached to a sickness may also change over time, often as notions about an illness change. In the nineteenth century, when tuberculosis was considered to be a somewhat romantic sickness resulting from an inherent disposition of passion and creativity, the illness had relatively little stigma. Later, however, when tuberculosis was considered infectious, those with the disease were seen as carriers to be avoided, isolated, and feared (Herzlich and Pierret, 1987).

Specific social and historical conditions lead to the stigmatizing of a sickness. Before the middle of the nineteenth century, leprosy in Hawaii was of minor importance and not stigmatized. As international trade and colonialism began to change the islands' social and economic situation, however, many outsiders came to the islands. Large numbers of Chinese immigrants arrived to work on the plantations, and the Hawaiians believed that they had brought leprosy. Although the Chinese immigrants were hard working and frugal, they were viewed as an inferior ethnic-racial group that threatened the jobs of other working-class persons. In 1880 Hawaii enacted laws to exclude the Chinese, partly on the basis of a belief that they carried disease. Health data suggest that the Chinese were not, however, an important source of leprosy, which more likely came to the islands through the ethnically mixed crews of ships from countries where the disease was prevalent. The Chinese were stigmatized in part because they were thought to be the source of leprosy, which at the same time became stigmatized because it was identified with the Chinese. Thus a relatively unknown and unimportant disease was transformed into a morally threatening sickness (Waxler, 1981).

The stigma attached to AIDS in recent years is a parallel situation. AIDS can and does affect all kinds of people, including many newborns. However, since most people identify the disease with homosexuals and drug users, it carries a considerable stigma. The widespread imputation of responsibility and stigma to sick persons suggests that Parsons's sick role model understates the moral judgment and social control aspects of sickness.

The Medicalization of Deviance

Religious, legal, and medical institutions have all contributed to the definition of deviance in society. For example, "Thou shalt not steal" is a religious norm: Stealing is a sin. Legal systems define similar norms of behavior, and violation of the norms is a crime. In a process called the **medicalization of deviance**, medical systems increasingly also define what is normal or desirable behavior: Badness becomes sickness.

The relative influence of religious, legal, and medical institutions in defining deviance has shifted in Western societies. As the Middle Ages waned and these three institutions became increasingly differentiated from each other, the religious organizations still had the greatest weight in defining deviance. This preeminence continued into the eighteenth century, but in America and France (and later in other European countries), the legal mode of defining deviance gained ascendancy (see Freidson, 1970: 247–252). In America, the increasing preeminence of the legal definitions was promoted by religious pluralism and by the increasingly rational organization of the nation-state (cf. Hammond, 1974).

The significance of legal definitions of deviance has diminished somewhat in the twentieth century, and medical definitions have gained in importance. This shifting balance is clearly reflected in the 1954 precedent-setting case *Durham* v. *United States* (214 F.2d 863), in which the court ruled that "an accused is not criminally responsible if his unlawful act was the product of a mental disease or mental defect." The shift in balance favoring medical definitions of deviance corresponds chronologically with a period of the rapid professionalization of medicine, when medical discoveries and technology proceeded quickly, and public faith in science and medicine was increasing.

Part of the reason for the declining importance of religious definitions is that they appear too nonrational and, in a religiously pluralistic country, lack societywide acceptance. Legal definitions, while more rational, seem to hinge too greatly upon human decisions, such as the judgment of twelve ordinary citizens on a jury. Medical definitions, by contrast, appear to be more rational and scientific, and based upon technical expertise rather than human judgment.

The concept of sickness, however, far from being a neutral scientific concept, is ultimately a *moral* one, establishing an evaluation of normality or desirability (Freidson, 1970: 208). The medical profession (especially its psychiatric branch) has defined a wide range of disapproved behavior as "sick": alcoholism, homosexuality, promiscuity, drug addiction, arson, suicide, child abuse, and civil disobedience (Conrad and Schneider, 1980). Social stigma adheres to many sicknesses, such as leprosy, AIDS, pelvic inflammatory disease, and cirrhosis of the liver. Moral judgment is also applied in the evaluation of "good" patient behavior, defined as acknowledging the necessity of medical care and following "doctors' orders" for various conditions, which may include receiving prenatal care, accepting blood transfusions, obtaining inoculations for one's children, and following prescribed drug and dietary regimens. Issues of moral judgment and responsibility are at stake.

When sicknesses thus labeled are defined as "bad," the doctors who join or organize efforts to eradicate or control them function as "**moral entrepreneurs**" (Becker, 1963: 147–163), or those who make an enterprise out of moral concerns.

The "discovery" of an illness category called hyperkinesis (or minimal brain dysfunction) involved such entrepreneurial action in a recent example of the medicalization of deviance. Virtually all of the persons labeled with this syndrome have been children; most are boys. The characteristic behaviors identified with hyperkinesis include excess of motor activity, short attention span, restlessness, impulsivity, and inability to sit still in school and comply with rules. These behaviors, however, have been frequently observed among schoolchildren, probably since the invention of the institution of the school. While no organic basis for "minimal brain dysfunction" has been identified, the "discovery" of hyperkinesis is explained in part by social factors such as the development and vigorous promotion of psychoactive drugs (specifically, Ritalin [methylphenidate]) for controlling hyperkinetic behavior, and the crusading efforts of moral entrepreneurs, including doctors, educators, and parents. Although hyperkinesis has been a medical category for only a brief time, it rapidly became an attractive diagnosis, and the drug Ritalin accounted for significant proportions of the pharmaceutical industry's profits (Conrad and Schneider, 1980: 155–161; see also Conrad, 1975).

Moral entrepreneurs engage in considerable political efforts to get their definitions of sickness accepted and implemented. Professional colleagues must be convinced; related professionals who could make referrals must be informed; and relevant regulatory agencies must be persuaded. The recent attempt to medicalize participation in religious cults (Robbins and Anthony, 1982) illustrates how the illness label is a product of such political efforts. The 1980 edition of the American Psychiatric Association's *Diagnostic and Statistical Manual of Mental Disorders* (DSM-III) contained several changes from the previous edition in order to characterize participation in new religious movements as a disorder. For example, in the definition of paranoid personality disorder, the revised manual stated that "individuals with this disorder are over-represented among leaders of mystical or esoteric religions and/or pseudoscientific and quasipolitical groups" (American Psychiatric Association, 1980: 308). Thus an evaluation of someone's mental health includes a judgment as to whether the individual's religious, scientific, or political persuasion is deviant. Interestingly, the efforts to define participation in new religious movements as "sick" were primarily those of a relatively small number of therapists who made their living "deprogramming" former members or testifying as expert witnesses in court cases involving such religious or other social movements. These moral entrepreneurs were establishing a specialized professional territory for themselves by creating illness labels (Richardson, 1987; Maloney, 1987).

While the boundaries of what is called mental illness are generally more malleable than those of physical illnesses, similar political processes are often involved in the classification of physical ailments. Ideas about the etiology of an illness (and, by extension, responsibility for it) are often politically debated. For example, a syndrome called miners' nystagmus has been the subject of continual political negotiation as a medical category. In the nineteenth century, this syndrome, characterized by oscillation of the eyes and spasms of eyelids, frequently accompanied by other complaints such as tremors of muscles of the neck, dizziness, headaches, sensitivity to light, and troubled sleep, was a recognized diagnostic category. Later, however, it had become an expensive item of compensation, so the British mining industry engaged in continual medical-legal debates as to whether it was a legitimate illness. The incidence of nystagmus complaints was often related directly to changes in conditions of work (e.g., production schedules) in the mines. As the result of complex social interactions involving doctors, management, labor, and government agencies, this illness was eventually psychologized, and thereby both recognized as a problem yet invalidated as a compensable illness (Figlio, 1982).

Zola (1983: 261) argued that "if anything can be shown in some way to affect the workings of the body and to a lesser extent the mind, then it can be labelled an 'illness' itself or jurisdictionally 'a medical problem.'" Thus even normal processes, such as menstruation, pregnancy and childbirth, child growth, and aging, have been brought under medicine's jurisdiction. The recent medicalization of menopause and premenstrual syndrome are examples of this tendency.

The Medicalization of Moral Authority

The same historical processes that brought about the preeminence of medical definitions of deviance also led to a much stronger role for medical authority in moral issues, such as what is right or wrong?, what is good or bad?, and whose good should prevail? Sometimes court events involve a clash of several sources of authority.[1]

In one representative court case, claims were made from legal, medical, parental, and religious bases of authority. A young person had been comatose for months, and was "as good as dead" in the common-sense view. Her body was being kept alive by technological intervention, and eventually her parents sought legal permission to terminate these "extraordinary" measures. Because no single authority held uncontested legitimacy, the case was complicated. Medical experts gave their opinions on the medical definitions of death. Legal experts raised issues of the legal rights and guardianship of comatose patients. Theological experts offered briefs on the borderlines of life and death, and the girl's father made a thoughtful personal statement about his request. The relevant issue is not merely the uncertainty of the outcome but also that it was the court in which medical, legal,

[1]This section is adapted with permission of the publisher from *Religion: The Social Context*, Second Edition, by Meredith B. McGuire, © 1987, 1981 by Wadsworth, Inc.

religious, and parental figures vied to have their statements taken seriously (Fenn, 1982; Willen, 1983).

The situation of difficult childbirth illustrates the growing role of physicians as arbiters in several such moral issues. For example, sometimes the infant's head is too large for the pelvic opening, making vaginal delivery difficult or impossible, and jeopardizing the lives of both the mother and the infant. In the late nineteenth and early twentieth century, several medical technologies were developed to deal with this crisis: high forceps (instruments to reach and reposition or pull the fetus), symphysiotomy (surgical severing of cartilage to separate the pubic bones), pubiotomy (cutting of the pubic bones), Caesarian section (surgical opening of the abdominal wall), and craniotomy (surgery on the fetal head to enable it to fit through the pelvic opening). Because none of these procedures was without risk to the woman or the fetus or both, each operation involved some moral concern for whose good was paramount.

Particular moral problems developed, however, in dire cases in which an emergency craniotomy was the last resort to save the mother's life. Initially, these moral decisions involved the doctor, the woman and her family, and sometimes the family's religious advisers as well. Gradually, however, the medical experts successfully asserted their autonomy and authority by their exclusive control of the relevant technical knowledge and by removing childbirth from home to hospital (and therefore out of the arenas of influence of family or clergy). Physicians tried to justify their own authority in this moral decision on the grounds of technical expertise and presumed rationality, but analysis of their rhetoric shows that their decisions were often based on social attitudes about women's childbearing role as much as were the previous decisions of other moral authorities (Leavitt, 1987).

The growing legitimacy of medical authority, relative to other sources of judgment, is further illustrated by contemporary court decisions upholding medical judgments to perform Caesarian sections. Caesarian sections are increasingly common, now accounting for about one in four births in the United States. They involve major abdominal surgery, with its concomitant risks and complications. An investigation of court cases between 1979 and 1986 showed that courts often accept physicians' decisions to operate over the objections of patients, their families, or religious persuasion, even though subsequent medical developments suggest that many of these operations were not necessary (Irwin and Jordan, 1987).

Medical dominance has effectively reduced the legitimacy of actions of other "encroaching" institutional areas such as religion and the family. Several courts have overruled religious or moral objections to various medical procedures. Jehovah's Witnesses, for example, believe that blood transfusions are forbidden by scripture, but the courts have generally upheld the medical authorization of such treatments, even for unwilling recipients

(*United States* v. *George*, 239 F. Supp. 752, 1964). Medical authority was also ruled to supersede parental authority in decisions presumed to determine life or death (precedent cases in 1952, 1962, and 1964 are cited in Burkholder, 1974: 41). Even in instances in which the medical ability to prevent death is doubtful, greater legitimacy is given to medical rather than parental authority. In 1977, for example, a Massachusetts court ordered that parents of a child dying of leukemia submit the child to medically prescribed chemotherapy, rather than to a less unpleasant (but also less respectable) nonmedical alternative therapy.

Social Control and Power

The labeling of deviance is an issue of legitimacy on another level as well, for the power to define sickness and to label someone as sick is also the power to discredit that person (Zola, 1983: 276–278). If a person's mental health is called into question, the rest of society does not have to take that person seriously. The individual then becomes the locus of the "problem." During the Vietnam War, a physician refused to train medical personnel for the army, claiming that his religious conscience compelled him to refuse this service. The army insisted that his compulsions were psychological rather than religious (Fenn, 1978: 57). By thus raising doubt about his psychological health, the army was able to evade his religious dissent as well as his legal claim to protection under the First Amendment of the Constitution.

Medical control in defining deviance also produces medical power in certifying deviance, which is another aspect of social control. The societal acceptance of medical definitions of deviance gives the medical profession unique power to certify individuals as sick or well. If a back disorder is a legitimate basis for taking the sick role (and thus to be excused from work or to claim insurance), a physician is considered to be the appropriate agency for certifying a valid claim. One study found that sick persons typically use "feeling" terms to describe internal states that they experience as illness; they say, for example, "I don't feel good" or "I feel too dizzy to stand." Thus, especially when the bodily condition of sickness is not obvious to their audiences, they need doctors' substantiation to legitimate their claims to being sick (Telles and Pollack, 1981). One of the functions of physicians, then, becomes the role of gatekeeper (Stone, 1979a, 1979b). Similarly, from 1952 to 1979, when homosexuality was a legitimate basis for denying a person U.S. citizenship, psychiatrists were given the power to certify that a homosexual should be thus denied (see Szasz, 1970).

When a person is certified as deviant, the agency of social control must then deal with this offender. Religious responses to deviance include counseling, moral indignation, confession, repentance, penance, and forgiveness. Legal responses include parallel actions, such as legal allegations, confession, punishments, rehabilitation, and release with or without the stigma of a record. In the medical model, the responses entail other parallels: diagnosis and therapy.

The process of reintegrating the deviant individual into the social group is therapy, which for even relatively minor deviance involves a form of social control (such as getting a young mother "back on her feet" so she can resume her family responsibilities). The social control functions of therapy are clearly evident in their grossest forms, such as the kidnapping and forcible "deprogramming" of persons with deviant religious or political views (Robbins and Anthony, 1982), and the mental hospitalization of political dissidents in Russia (Medvedev and Medvedev, 1971); similar use of medical definitions for political purposes in the United States is exemplified by the treatment of Ezra Pound and General James Walker (Freidson, 1970: 246; see also Turner, 1977).

The use of psychoactive drugs for social control is one area of particular concern. The above example of drug prescription for difficult-to-manage children shows how matters of social control are medically managed. Similarly, several United States and Canadian studies have documented the very large proportion of the elderly receiving drugs that affect the central nervous system, such as tranquilizers, analgesics, antidepressants, sedatives, hypnotics, and anticonvulsants. One function, deliberate or not, of the use of these drugs is the management of elderly persons. For example, older persons need shorter but more frequent periods of sleep than younger adults, but sedatives are often prescribed in many institutions to try to keep the elderly in an eight-hour sleeping pattern, so the staff can better supervise them at night (Harding, 1981; see also Harding, 1986).

Social control is also involved in the use of drugs to make it possible for persons to accommodate themselves to an unsatisfactory social role. When workers experience severe stress in the work place, treating their stress-related health conditions with drugs keeps them performing their roles without challenging the work conditions or the appropriateness of those roles.

In 1987, a pharmaceutical company was investigated by the U.S. Food and Drug Administration for sending doctors an advertising brochure depicting on the cover a very tense air traffic controller at the computer monitor in a hectic control tower. The caption reads, "He needs anxiolytic [tranquilizer] therapy . . . but alertness is part of his job." Inside the folder, the worker is portrayed as cheery and smiling, and the text reads, in part, "BuSpar. . . . For a different kind of calm." While the ad was criticized as misleading in its downplaying of negative side effects of the drug, the more serious sociological issue is the notion that a tranquilizer is the solution to work-place stress brought on by specific policy decisions. According to a U.S. Government Accounting Office study, air controllers suffer very low morale, extreme overwork, and other pressures due to chronic and serious understaffing—a major problem since President Reagan fired 11,000 striking air traffic controllers in 1981 (Hinds, 1987; *Health Letter,* 1987).

Research in the United States, Canada, Germany, and Italy showed that women were the overwhelming majority of recipients of prescriptions for tranquilizers and sedatives (Harding, 1986). Pharmaceutical company advertising to doctors specifically recommended such psychoactive drugs to deal with women's dissatisfaction with their social roles. An advertisement for Valium (diazepam) showed a troubled young woman sitting at a table in a school gymnasium; the photo was labeled,

> Symbols in a life of psychic tension: M.A. (Fine Arts), PTA (President-elect), GYN repeated examinations normal (persistent complaints). . . .
> Rx: Valium . . . M.A. (Fine Arts) . . . PTA (President-elect) . . . representations of a life currently centered around home and children, with too little time to pursue a vocation for which she has spent many years in training . . . a situation that may bespeak continuous frustration and stress: a perfect framework for her to translate the functional symptoms of psychic tension into major problems. For this kind of patient—with no demonstrable pathology yet with repeated complaints—consider the distinctive properties of Valium (diazepam). Valium possesses a pronounced calming action that usually relieves psychic tension promptly, helping to attenuate the related somatic signs and symptoms.

Like the air traffic controller, this young woman is identified as suffering from the stress and frustration of her social role. The solution of prescribing tranquilizers serves the social control function of keeping people in their roles without questioning the role demands themselves.

Social control may seem more pleasant or humane when the deviance is treated as sickness rather than as crime or sin, but the potency of the control agencies is just as great. Certain medically defined deviance can permanently spoil the individual's identity (cf. Goffman, 1963). Even when the condition is considered medically "cured" or under control, stigma still adheres to such "illnesses" as alcoholism, drug abuse, mental disorders, syphilis, and cancer. This problem of stigma is especially evident in the case of epilepsy and other conditions involving deviance from one very important cultural norm: self-control. Chapter 7 further examines the problems of stigma and control in chronic illness and handicaps.

Sickness and Social Dissent

The social control functions of the sick role and of some medical interventions demonstrate that society's constraints on individual behavior are real, even when individuals do not agree with the norms for behavior. Although social control measures may be objectively powerful in a society, their effect is never total. Society's members are never fully socialized and compliant. Thus deviance such as sickness can also be a form of social dissent—usually unorganized, but sometimes organized—against existing social arrangements.

Sickness is, as the sick role concept shows, an act of refusal that is potentially threatening to the established order. In effect, the sick person is saying, "I will not any longer." By claiming the sick role, the individual may refuse to go to school or work, to be responsible for dependents, to serve in the armed forces, and to participate in everyday social obligations. Indeed, in its extreme form sickness is a refusal to cope, to struggle, and to endure. As such, claiming the sick role resembles the activist strategy of passive resistance (Lock, 1986; see also Herzlich and Pierret, 1987: 183–184). Taking the sick role is thus often a way of expressing dissent from other social roles. Many social historians consider the epidemic of hysteria among Victorian women to be an expression of their dissent against the constraints of their social roles (Ehrenreich and English, 1978; Sicherman, 1978). Similarly, workers' job dissatisfaction is often expressed by high rates of absenteeism for sickness.

Sickness is, however, not necessarily an effective form of dissent. Waitzkin (1971) suggested that the sick role has latent (i.e., not recognized or intended) functions that maintain the status quo in society and reduce conflict and change. For example, if disgruntled workers take sick leave to relieve the tensions of their job satisfaction, the sick role reduces the likelihood that those tensions would be addressed politically, such as in a confrontation with management. The sick role instead provides a temporary safety valve to reduce pressure in various institutional settings, such as the family, prisons, and the military.

While the sickness may not be able to change social arrangements, such as social class or gender hierarchies, it may be effective in obtaining actual advantages or relief for the sick person. Some secondary gains of sickness, such as receiving extra attention in the family, may be such a result. For example, in many African societies there are special healing cults for women, such as the *zar* cult of the predominantly Moslem peoples in Ethiopia, Egypt, Sudan, and Somalia. Some anthropologists have interpreted the *zar* affliction, in which the sick person is believed to be possessed by spirits, as women's assertion of dissatisfaction with their lack of social and economic power. While these periodic afflictions and their accompanying healing rituals do not substantially alter women's subordination in the society or household, they do achieve for the sick person extra attention from fellow cult members and the family, a respite from normal household duties, and frequently a party, new clothes, or other economic benefits at the expense of the male head of household (Lewis, 1971). Taking the sick role is thus a relatively successful (albeit manipulative) assertion of power of the subordinate members of the society. It poignantly expresses women's dissent, but does not fundamentally alter the social arrangements.

Similarly, sickness is sometimes the attempt to cope (although not always constructively) with an intolerable social situation, as discussed in Chapter 4. Sickness expresses frustration, dissatisfaction, and anger turned against oneself. Alcoholism and other substance abuse, depression, and suicide exemplify this potentially self-defeating attempt. To interpret, for example, the alcoholism of a middle-aged, unemployed, impoverished Native American on a reservation as a purely individual sickness is thus to miss the likelihood that it is the expression of his frustration and hostility in the face of his utterly marginalized social condition (Lock, 1986). Lock argued that modern medicine has so thoroughly individualized its image of sickness that it has lost sight of the extent to which sickness may be the expression of social dissent about frustrated and unmet human needs. She stated:

> In summary, we wish to stress that while illness symptoms are biological entities they are frequently also coded metaphors that speak to the contradictory aspects of social life, expressing sentiments, feelings, and ideas that must otherwise be kept hidden (Lock, 1986: 26).

These metaphorical aspects of the body and sicknesses are described in more detail below.

PROBLEMS OF MEANING AND ORDER

Illness is upsetting because it is experienced as a threat to the order and meanings by which people make sense of their lives. Suffering and death create problems of meaning not simply because they are unpleasant, but also because they threaten the fundamental assumptions of order underlying society itself (cf. Berger, 1967: 24). For the individual, illness and affliction can likewise be experienced as assaults on the identity, and on the ability to predict and control central aspects of one's own and one's loved ones' lives. Healing, in all cultures, represents an attempt to restore order and to reassert meaning.

Illness disrupts the order of everyday life. It threatens our ability to plan for the immediate or distant future, to control, and to organize. Even a relatively minor malady, such as a head cold, can disturb the order of daily life; how much more so can serious, potentially fatal, or debilitating illnesses, such as cancer or polio, throw our lives into disorder! A study of the impact of childhood leukemia found two characteristic experiences of sufferers and their families: uncertainty and the search for meaning (Comaroff and Maguire, 1981).

There are a number of ways by which medical systems in all cultures restore order in the face of illness. Diagnostic actions, whether accomplished by divination or CT (computed tomography) scan, divine revelation or physical examination, is a means of naming the problem and giving it a culturally recognizable form. Naming the illness imposes order on a previously chaotic set of experiences, thereby giving the sick person a set of expectations and some basis for acting. Etiologies likewise contribute to restoring a sense of order, because they reflect important values of the social group, especially by identifying a causal relationship between sickness and socially prescribed normal or ideal social relationships. In applying particular etiologies to a given illness episode, the medical process ritually reaffirms these values (Young, 1976).

In many cultures, the healing process addresses not only individual disruption but also disordered *social* relations. The healing role of the African Ndembu diviner is to identify (in symbolic guise) the agents of affliction. Sickness is understood as an eruption of social conflict and divisiveness in one symbolic place. For example, the Ndembu attribute menstrual disorders to *chisaku* (misfortune due to displeasure of ancestral shades or breach of taboo). The healing ritual propitiates the ancestors and exorcizes the evil influences of both living and dead. Significantly, it involves the woman's matrilineal kin, with whom there may be a problem for the woman and her husband. The larger aims of the healing ritual include restoration of problematic kinship ties, reconstruction of the woman's relationship with her husband, and enhanced procreation, thereby benefiting both the marriage and the lineage. Because the disordered body is the expression of disordered social relations, healing consists of reunifying and reordering the entire group, of which the sick person is only an individual expression (Turner, 1968, 1969).

Similarly, faith healing in many Christian groups restores order through healing the metaphorical body (McGuire, 1982). For example, troubled marriages are healed by bringing the "body" (wife and children) into proper relationship (i.e., submission) with the "head" (husband and father). The importance of the body as a natural symbol suggests that, even in Western cultures, illness and healing may be ways of symbolizing order and meaning on several levels.

The Body as a Symbol

The human body is a natural symbol. The meanings of the symbol are not intrinsic in it, but are socially constructed and attached to it. Douglas (1970: 93) stated that

> The social body constrains the way the physical body is perceived. The physical experience of the body, always modified by the social categories through which it is known, sustains a particular view of society. There is a continual exchange of meanings between the two kinds of bodily experience so that

each reinforces the categories of the other. As a result of this interaction the body itself is a highly restricted medium of expression.

Thus she argued that bodily control is social control and that attitudes toward the body reflect the social concerns of the group (Douglas, 1970: 11–18; see also Douglas, 1966).

Body symbolism works on several levels; often the body and its parts are used as metaphors. For example, when we say a man is upright, we are referring to both a moral evaluation and a physical posture. Similar body metaphors are applied when we evaluate people as spineless, under-handed, open-eyed, heartless, cold-blooded, brown-nosed, blue-blooded, sinister, thickskinned, or gutless. Social relations are likewise reflected in body metaphors, such as, "He is a pain in the ass," or "They are thicker than blood."

Consider all the symbolic meanings we give to various body parts and body products, including hands, heart, womb, hair, eyes, blood, spit, feces, and sweat. These meanings are not inherent in the physical properties but are applied by a social group. In socialization, we learn our society's mean-ings. A baby is not born with an aversion to the sight of blood. A young child must learn to be disgusted by the feel of feces (usually only after having played with them and receiving several reprimands).

Through the meanings attached to the body, social structure shapes individual bodily expression. At the same time, bodily expression reflects the social structure. There have been numerous studies of various cultures, including Western industrialized societies, showing how core values are revealed in body-related beliefs and practices, such as eating (Turner, 1982), beauty and adornment (Turner, 1980; Kunzle, 1981), birth and death (Comaroff, 1984), sex (Foucault, 1978; Turner, 1984), pollution and cleanliness (Douglas, 1966; Elias 1978), and health and healing (Comaroff, 1985; Crawford, 1984; McGuire and Kantor, 1988; Westley, 1983).

The Meaning of Affliction

Illness is also upsetting because it raises the questions of meaning: Why is this happening to me? Why now? Who's responsible? How could God allow this to happen? Why do the good suffer and the evil prosper? In many cultures, the medical system and the religious system are inextricably inter-woven. Religious meaning is thereby connected with illness explanations.

In his analysis of religious systems, Weber noted the importance of **theodicies**, or religious explanations of meaning-threatening experiences, for sickness, suffering, and death ([1922] 1963: 138–150). Theodicies tell the individual or group that the experience is not meaningless but is rather part of a larger system of order, a religious cosmology (see also Berger,

1967:24). Some successful theodicies are in fact nothing but assertions of order. A woman discussing her personal meaning crisis after her husband's premature death said, "I finally came to understand that it didn't matter whether *I* understood why he died when he did, but that God had a reason for it, and that was all that mattered." For this believer, knowing that an order exists behind events was more important than knowing what that order was. Theodicies do not necessarily make the believer happy or even promise future happiness; they simply answer the question, Why do I suffer?

At the same time that Western societies are experiencing the increasing medicalization of authority, Western medicine is having difficulty dealing with sufferers' problems of meaning. Anthropologists remind us that however well Western medicine deals with the symptoms the sick person suffers, it fails to address the problem of "who sent the louse" (Comaroff, 1978). Illness etiologies in Western medicine typically deal with proximate causes (e.g., germs, viruses, or genetic defects), but these notions are not adequate explanations for many people, since questions of meaning frequently beg for ultimate causes.

A foremost characteristic of the institution of medicine in modern Western societies is its differentiation from other institutions that provide meaning and belonging. **Institutional differentiation** is the process by which the various institutional spheres in society become separated from each other (see Parsons, 1966). For example, religious functions are focused in special religious institutions, which are separate from other institutions, such as the educational, political, and economic. The medical institution has limited itself to the cure of disease, as a biophysical entity, and to the physical tending of the diseased individual. The functions of healing that provide meaning and belonging are treated as relatively unimportant, and are relegated to the private-sphere institutions of family and religion. These private-sphere institutions are allowed, even encouraged, to handle the meaning problems of the sick, but only so long as their beliefs and actions do not interfere with the medical management of the disease (McGuire, 1985).

Just as the physical body is a potent symbol of one's selfhood, so too are experiences of suffering linked with one's identity, as discussed in Chapter 7. Practically, being unwell implies being disabled, in the sense of being made unable to do what one wants or needs to do; it implies reduced agency. It means losing some control (an especially important quality in this society), and it involves losing one's routines—the very patterns by which daily existence is ordered (Cassell, 1982; see also Comaroff, 1982).

Suffering is not connected with disease or pain in any precise causal or proportionate way. The pain of childbirth, for example, may be more severe than the pain of angina, but it generally causes less suffering because it is perceived as temporary and is associated with a desired outcome. A disease may be incurable yet cause little suffering if it does little damage to the person's sense of self and ability to engage in everyday life. For example, a chronic fungal infection of the big toe may cause less suffering than a temporary but disfiguring episode of Bell's palsy. Many people may seek help and healing less for disease itself than for suffering and affliction.

Cassell (1982: 639) has suggested that suffering poses difficulty for the biomedical system, because it is "experienced by persons, not merely by bodies, and has its sources in challenges that threaten the intactness of the person as a complex social and psychological entity." He observed that medical personnel can unknowingly cause suffering when they do not validate the patient's affliction, and when they fail to acknowledge or deal with the personal meanings the patient attaches to the illness. Cassell (1982: 642) noted that "people suffer from what they have lost of themselves in relation to the world of objects, events and relationships." One woman still suffered greatly from a hysterectomy she had undergone six years earlier. As she explained, "It meant losing a huge part of my future." Unmarried, childless, and only twenty-nine years old, she lost hopes and dreams for the future. She expressed enormous anger at the insensitivity of physicians and hospital staff who had treated her "like an ungrateful child, crying over spilt milk" (quoted in McGuire and Kantor, 1988). The medical personnel, even if thoroughly well intentioned, probably felt their sole duty was the correct treatment of her specific uterine problem; the woman's suffering was not their problem nor relevant to their tasks.

Whether brought on by a physical problem or not, affliction often results from a threat to the *coherence* of a person's world. As noted in Chapter 4, a sense of coherence itself is related to health and healing. People suffer from a loss of connectedness—links with loved ones, valued social roles, and groups that are important to them. As Chapter 7 shows, the illness experience often involves such losses. In the face of affliction, people seek meaning and order to address this essential coherence (Cassell, 1982; see also Antonovsky, 1984).

SUMMARY

Sickness is not merely the condition of an individual, but is also related to the larger social order. It is connected with moral issues and the imputation of responsibility for deviance from social norms. Society deals with such deviance through social control mechanisms, including the sick role. Sick role expectations, however, vary historically and cross-culturally. The discrepancies between the ideal image of the sick role, which is based upon certain forms of acute illness, and chronic and other nonacute conditions result in ambiguous expectations for those whom society defines as sick. The medicalization of deviance and the social stigma of illness highlight the social control functions of medicine, which are yet another connection between power and health. The medical profession has successfully asserted primacy in the defining deviance and the corollary function of certifying deviance, thereby becoming a primary moral authority in modern societies.

A related issue is the problem of meaning created by illness, suffering, and death. Because of the importance of the human body as a natural symbol, bodily control and healing practices reflect social relationships and concerns. The problems of meaning brought on by illness are particularly difficult in modern Western medical settings, due to the differentiation of medical institutions from meaning-providing institutions such as religion and family. The biomedical model, with its nearly exclusive focus on physical conditions, does not adequately deal with suffering and the subjective experience of affliction.

RECOMMENDED READINGS

Articles

Jean Comaroff, "Medicine: Symbol and ideology," pp. 49–68 in P. Wright and A. Treacher, eds., *The Problem of Medical Knowledge: Examining the Social Construction of Medicine*. Edinburgh: Edinburgh University Press, 1982.

Robert Crawford, "A cultural account of 'health': Control, release, and the social body," pp. 60–103 in J. B. McKinlay, ed., *Issues in the Political Economy of Health Care*. New York: Tavistock, 1984.

Ronald Frankenberg, "Sickness as cultural performance: Drama, trajectory, and pilgrimage—Root metaphors and the making social of disease," *International Journal of Health Services* 16 (4), 1986: 603–626.

Nancy Scheper-Hughes and Margaret M. Lock, "The mindful body: A prolegomenon to future work in medical anthropology," *Medical Anthropology Quarterly* 1, 1987: 6–41.

Nancy E. Waxler, "Learning to be a leper: A case study in the social construction of illness," pp. 169–194 in Elliot G. Mishler, Lorna R. AmaraSingham, Stuart T. Hauser, Ramsay Liem, Samuel D. Osherson, and Nancy E. Waxler, *Social Contexts of Health, Illness, and Patient Care*. Cambridge: Cambridge University Press, 1981.

Books

Peter Conrad and Joseph W. Schneider, *Deviance and Medicalization: From Badness to Sickness*. St. Louis: C. V. Mosby, 1980. This highly readable volume explains the medicalization process, illustrating it with detailed examinations of the medicalization of mental illness, alcoholism, opiate addiction, hyperkinesis, child abuse, homosexuality, and criminality.

Chapter Seven

The Illness Experience

Illness is a profoundly human experience that calls into question normal expectations about our bodies and capacities. When illness is not part of our life, we take the relationship between our bodies and our selves for granted. Indeed, we are not likely to think about our bodies or be particularly conscious of many bodily sensations. In health, we expect our bodies to be able to function and to sustain a presentation of our selves as normal, reliable participants in social interaction (Dingwall, 1976: 98). What we call illness is a disturbance in body processes or experience that has become problematic for the individual.

ILLNESS AND SELF

The experience of illness, even if only temporary, reminds us of our limitations, of our dependencies—present and potential, and of our ultimate mortality. When ill, our bodies inform us that they cannot always be counted on to be able for what we want them to do. Because our very sense of who we are and our important social relationships are intimately connected with our bodies and their routine functioning, being ill is disruptive and disordering. We identify our selves with our bodies, as evidenced by one physician's introspective account of his own accident and gradual recovery. He exclaimed, "What seemed, at first, to be no more than a local peripheral breakage and breakdown now showed itself in a different, and quite terrible, light—as a breakdown of memory, of thinking, of will—*not just a lesion in my muscle, but a lesion in me*" (Sacks, 1984: 67).

Thus the illness experience is much more than a biophysical event; it has far-reaching social, emotional, moral, and spiritual implications. Kleinman's (1978, 1988) distinction between disease and illness is useful. According to his definitions, **disease** refers to the biophysical condition—the problem as seen from the biomedical practitioner's perspective. The physician transforms the patient's and the family's expressions of illness into terms that fit the theoretical models of disease. By contrast, **illness** refers to "how the sick person and the members of the family or wider social network perceive, live with, and respond to symptoms and disability" (Kleinman, 1988: 3–6). Because doctors of Western medicine have been trained to focus almost exclusively on disease, they have difficulty in dealing with the illness experience (Kleinman, 1978).

This chapter focuses on the experiences of illness and pain, especially as shaped by social structure and culture. While even the most minor illness can be problematic for the sufferer, we shall emphasize those illnesses most likely to have a damaging effect on the person's identity and sense of self. Most everyday illnesses are not profoundly disruptive, although they too remind the sufferer of personal limits and dependencies. If I have a bout of the flu, I may be very miserable, fall far behind in my work, and be temporarily dependent on family and friends, unable to reciprocate their care; however, such illness does not significantly challenge my relationships and my identity. Likewise, many accidents wounding the body and many acute illnesses, while temporarily very discomforting or even seriously threatening, do not damage the ill person's sense of self. If I suffer acute pneumonia, the condition may be life-threatening and require dramatic medical intervention—hospitalization, antibiotics, and intense nursing care—but I emerge to retain my essential relationships and identity. Other illnesses, however, are deeply disruptive, threatening the ill person's important relationships and very sense of self.

Loss is one factor that can make an illness experience profoundly disruptive. People actively grieve, because the loss of body parts (e.g., amputation of an arm) or functions (e.g., partial blindness) represent loss of integrity—the wholeness of the person (Cassell, 1982). People suffer not only from the loss of present capacities and roles, but also from being robbed of their future: the teenager who is a paraplegic after a car accident, the childless young woman who has a hysterectomy, the middle-aged lawyer who loses her eyesight, the elderly musician whose arthritis makes playing a beloved instrument impossible.

Chronic illness and pain in particular force the sufferer to come to new terms with the experience of time. Sometimes a life-threatening acute illness or a serious accident has such impact, but an acute condition is—by definition—temporary. Chronic illness, by contrast, often leads to a radical reassessment, in light of changed and yet-changing capacities, of one's self in relationship to one's past and future. The experience of chronic illness thus involves both a sense of loss and a heightened self-consciousness (Charmaz, 1987).

Illness is especially damaging to the self when it is experienced as overwhelming, unpredictable, and uncontrollable, because it paralyzes the person's ability to manage life, to plan, and to act. Enormous attention must be given not merely to actual crisis periods in the illness but also to minute, mundane worries such as: Can I visit my friend's apartment without having an asthma attack? Can I make it to the bathroom quickly enough? If I attempt sexual intercourse, will my back pain flare up? Do I risk a heart attack if I take on this interesting project at work? Can I negotiate the path from my car to the store? (cf. Kleinman, 1988: 44). Unpredictability and uncontrollability result in a disjunction between the person and the body; the functioning that was once taken for granted is gone, and the person in effect feels, "I cannot count on my body. *It* fails *me*." The body becomes an "other"—at best an unpredictable ally.

Illness that results in ongoing social marginality is also particularly damaging to the self. Much of our web of social relationships is predicated upon the assumptions that members will be able to reciprocate, that one member will not be utterly dependent upon others, and that all give and receive. Some illnesses undermine the assumption of reciprocity and thus make social relationships precarious. Losing independence is threatening to one's sense of self not just because of pride in self-sufficiency (a related value in our culture), but more because it impairs one's ability to participate as an equal in important social relationships. Valued friendships and social roles become strained or lost altogether. Often the individual lives in a deliberately collapsed world, because the larger world becomes unmanageable or threatening. One woman commented:

> What is really so awful is that illness, I believe, really makes you very lonely. . . . One is really out of the world. *When there is illness one is, and one stays, alone.* It's very hard to get help. . . . It destroys what one would like to do, it isolates you. . . . If I got into very poor health, I could no longer take care of them as I do. . . . I would be cut off from my family, life would have to be organized without me, I would not play the role that I play now. I believe that one who is sick is outside of normal life (quoted in Herzlich and Pierret, 1987: 178).

Pain and treatment often become a focus for the chronically ill, forcing them to withdraw into themselves. Lack of access to everyday activities also fosters isolation. Others, unable to deal with chronic problems, socially withdraw, and thus a spiral of increasing isolation is set into motion: The less one can or wants to do, the less one socializes; but the less one socializes, the more others withdraw, and in turn the more the person with a chronic illness withdraws. One man with severe rheumatoid arthritis said:

> Now the only place I go now is down to the local club. Everybody knows me sort of thing. They might say it's a shame for him, but nobody bothers me, they accept me as I am. But if I go anywhere else . . . people are embarrassed. People say 'bloody hell, is that . . . ? Dear me, what's the matter with him?' And they try not to catch your eye, if you will. People tend to stay away from you. I don't know, they just don't want to be involved. You tend to do the same then (quoted in Bury, 1982: 176).

All the more marginalizing are illness experiences involving stigma, which by definition has the potential to discredit the self that the individual is trying to present to others. For example, one young woman had undergone a colostomy in which a large part of her colon was surgically removed, necessitating the perpetual wearing and cleaning of a device that collected and held the contents of her bowels. She exclaimed:

> I feel so embarrassed by this—this thing. It seems so unnatural, so dirty. I can't get used to the smell to it. I'm scared of soiling myself. Then I'd be so ashamed I couldn't look at anyone else. . . . Who would want a wife like this?

How can I go out and not feel unable to look people in the eyes and tell them the truth? Once I do, who would want to develop a friendship, I mean a close one? How can I even consider showing my body to someone else, having sex? (quoted in Kleinman, 1988: 163).

Since control is so strongly valued in our culture, loss of control is especially problematic. People experience an assault on their sense of self when their illnesses involve losses of control, such as incontinence, loss of bowel control, flatulence, seizures, stumbling and falling, tics and tremors, and drooling. We rely on relative control of our bodies to present ourselves in socially valued ways (Goffman, 1963; Schneider and Conrad, 1983), but chronic illness and disability disrupt that control. Furthermore, in a culture in which productivity, vigor, beauty, and youth are very important values, disability and aging are especially threatening (Murphy, 1987). Thus certain chronic illnesses and disabilities are especially likely to threaten the individual's sense of self and connectedness with others.

Illness is not experienced merely by the individual in whose body the symptoms are located; often the family and other close members of the sufferer's social network also feel the disruptiveness of illness. For example, a retired lawyer described the effects of his wife's ten years of decline with Alzheimer's disease:

Our children come and they cry. And I cry. We reminisce about old times. We try to recall what Anna was like before this happened. But I can see it wears them out just being here for a day or two. They've got their own troubles. I can't ask them to help out any more than they do already. Me? It's made a different person out of me. I expect you wouldn't have recognized me if you had met me ten years ago. I feel at least ten years older than I am. I'm afraid what will happen if I go first. I haven't had a half hour free of worry and hurt for ten years. This illness didn't just destroy Anna's mind, it has killed something in me, in the family, too. If anyone asks about Alzheimer's, tell them it is a disease of the whole family (quoted in Kleinman, 1988: 183).

The human response to illness is to give it meaning, to interpret it, to reorder the disordering experience. To make sense of what is happening to us, we draw upon socially available categories from a large cultural repertoire and from personal and family stories and meanings absorbed from our particular ethnic and religious backgrounds. In the case of minor illnesses, the interpretations might include our underlying definitions of health and illness, and our notions about why we got sick and how to get well. Seriously disruptive illnesses are likely to evoke further interpretations about the meaning of life, moral responsibility, suffering, relationships, and death.

LAY CONCEPTIONS OF HEALTH

How do you know you are sick? How do you know if your condition is potentially serious enough to warrant "doing something" about the illness? Long before any outside help (medical or otherwise) is sought, individuals interpret their own condition. Underlying all such evaluations is a set of ideas about health and illness. The concepts and logic of these ideas are not those of science or medicine, although they may be borrowed, accurately or inaccurately, from those formal systems of knowledge. Rather they are the concepts and logic of ordinary people whose experiences, socialization, cultural background, and immediate social network shape and continually develop their notions of health and illness.

Many people think of health as being simply the absence of illness. For example, a Scottish study of older persons found that key dimensions of health mentioned were an absence of illness, a reserve of strength, and a feeling of being generally fit or capable of accomplishing daily tasks (Williams, 1983). Corroborating evidence came from a study of middle-aged French subjects, who described health in terms of an absence of illness, an equilibrium in daily life, and a capacity to work (Herzlich, 1973; Herzlich and Pierret, 1987).

Other research found that while both working-class and middle-class persons shared the notion that health meant the absence of illness, working-class people tended to emphasize what was essential for their everyday lives: the ability to carry out their tasks, especially job and family duties (Blaxter and Paterson, 1982). Middle-class persons were more likely to mention broader, positive conceptions of health that included such factors as energy, positive attitudes, and the ability to cope well and to be in control of one's life (Calnan, 1987; Herzlich, 1973). These views are illustrated by the following comments of a middle-class woman:

> I think that [truly healthy persons] . . . are very spontaneous and flexible, and I think they have more options that they experience. . . . They are feeling connected to a larger purpose and connected with other people. . . . I would also say that being in power, feeling powerful in your life, feeling responsible for your life is a very important part of it (quoted in McGuire, 1988).

The sense of being in control may be particularly important to the middle class, for it meshes with their experiences of making decisions and having a degree of control in their work and daily life. By contrast, because working-class persons have control over far fewer areas of their lives, this value may be remote or inconceivable to them. Crawford (1984: 78) argued that middle-class values have expanded the notion of health to something that must be actively achieved and proven, since "to be healthy [in this culture, means] to demonstrate to self and others appropriate concern for the virtues of self-control, self-discipline, self-denial, and will power."

There are important differences in lay conceptions of health and illness within various subcultures as well. Persons raised in different ethnic subcultures—Chicano, Irish, Appalachian, or Polish, for example—typically learn their group's ideas about health and illness, including: What is health? What can cause illness? What does a given illness mean? How can I protect myself and loved ones from illness? How can I counteract illness when it occurs? What can I expect to experience with different illnesses? What resources can I turn to for help in the face of illness?

Religious subcultures likewise influence not only their members' responses to illness but also their very definitions of health and illness. One member of a Christian healing group stated, "Health, wholeness—all these words to me are Scripture and salvation. It all goes together. A healthy person to me would be one that was whole in spirit, soul, mind, and body" (quoted in McGuire, 1988: 39). A study of middle-class spiritual healing groups found that, as persons became more actively involved, they expanded their notions of what needed healing in their lives. Because health was an ideal encompassing all their religious ideals, healing was a continual part of the process of striving for those goals (McGuire and Kantor, 1987, 1988).

Although there are few studies about other kinds of subcultural groups, it is probable that they too influence members' conceptions of health, illness, and healing. For example, to what extent is an adolescent subculture (and not just chronological age) a factor in the health notions of teenagers? Are there health belief systems communicated by other subcultures, such as homosexuals or the military? We have only begun to explore the diversity of lay conceptions of health and illness. The sketches we have thus far, however, illustrate the importance of lay conceptions for understanding people's behavior in the face of illness.

LAY UNDERSTANDINGS OF ILLNESS

Just as laypersons' notions of health are shaped by their social and cultural background, so too are the ways people understand their illnesses. People seek to comprehend what is wrong with them: What is the nature of this illness? Where did it come from? Why me? Why now? What can be done about this illness? What can be done to protect myself from other illness? Individual belief systems about illness are typically drawn from, but not necessarily rigidly determined by, larger cultural belief systems, which give shape to the illness experience, help the individual to interpret what is happening, and offer a number of choices about how to respond.

Lay images of various diseases reveal why certain responses "make sense." A study of middle-class New Yorkers found that people regularly refer to disease and diseased body parts as "its"—as objects separate from the person. This image allows ill persons to distance themselves from their problems. The concept of disease as an "it" also meshed with notions that the problem had its source in some external agent that invaded the body (Cassell, 1976). Because lay images of illness reflect people's diverse experiences, they vary by such factors as social class, gender, ethnicity, and religion.

A study of Scottish women showed the predominance of the image of disease as a thing that one "has," "gets," or "catches." Accordingly, "it" attacks, strikes, or sets in. One respondent said, "My family wis never bothered wi' their chest . . . it wis always their throats. It always went for their throat, not their chest" (quoted in Blaxter, 1983: 61). The regional idiom of "taking" a disease distinguishes temporary (typically infectious) illnesses from chronic illnesses or a clear physical abnormality. One might "take" pneumonia, measles, bronchitis, or scarlet fever, but not a tumor, cyst, arthritis, or cancer (Blaxter, 1983).

People employ their lay conceptions to explain the nature and causes of specific maladies. In one English community, respondents tended to think of their illnesses in terms of hot or cold and wet or dry; for example, a chest cold fit the wet-cold image, whereas a fever was depicted as hot-dry. By extension, then, certain maladies were linked especially with damp, cold weather or house environment. People held explicit images of the germs and viruses to which they attributed some illnesses. They often depicted these agents as clouds of tiny particles or as minute, invisible insects. Medical professionals sometimes participated in the use of these images, for example by explaining a problem as "a tummy bug" (Helman, 1978).

The causal categories used by laypersons may not be correct in bioscientific terms but are generally rational and based upon the kinds of empirical evidence available to laypersons. One Scottish study showed the most commonly invoked lay causal categories were, in rank order: (1) infection; (2) heredity or familial tendencies; (3) agents in the environment, such as "poisons," working conditions, and climate; (4) secondary products of other diseases; and (5) stress, strain, and worry (Blaxter, 1983; similar categories were found by Locker, 1981: 67).

The interpretation of illness is an ongoing process. People reinterpret their situation at various stages of their illness. They look back at earlier experiences and actions, and reinterpret them to make sense of subsequent events and new beliefs. Interaction with important others is another source of new interpretations. One purpose for this ongoing reconstruction is to make sense of a whole sequence of events, rather than viewing each part as an episode that just "happened." Thus, for example, cardiac patients retrospectively noticed the symptoms which had built up to their heart attack. Their reconstruction of the meaning of the sequence of events made the heart attack seem less threatening and more understandable (Cowie, 1976).

Cross-cultural research suggests that several explanatory logics are used by laypersons, including those in "modern" Western cultural settings. One category of logic is that of invasion, in which an outside agent is believed to come into the body to cause the illness. Examples include notions of possession, germ theory, or object intrusions. Another logic involves degeneration, in which the illness is explained as due to the breakdown of the body or its parts from such causes as exhaustion or the accumulation of toxic substances. Mechanical models provide another logic, explaining illness as the result of misalignment of body structures, or blockages of digestive or nervous channels, for example. A fourth logic commonly used is the notion of equilibrium, which attributes illness to the failure to maintain harmony (individual or social), balance, and order (Chrisman, 1977). While these categories can be used to analyze the logics of other cultures, they are all used extensively by laypersons in modern Western societies.

Lay understandings of illness typically address the broader issues of meaning, such as those discussed in Chapter 6: Why must I suffer? Why me and not someone else? Why now? Have I done something bad to bring this upon myself? Indeed, in much lay thinking cause and meaning are not separate interpretive categories. Serious illnesses in particular evoke broader causal interpretations that are often used in combination with medical interpretations. For example, one young woman accepted the medical etiology of her vision problems, but simultaneously employed a broader causal meaning to her illness: " 'With my eye problem, there was something that I didn't want to see. I couldn't get well until I opened my eyes to that something' " (quoted in McGuire 1988).

NOTICING ILLNESS

How do people know they are ill? In addition to these underlying ideas about health and illness, a number of other social factors influence whether an individual will perceive a particular disturbance and come to define it as distressing enough to warrant further attention. People react to the meaning of a symptom, not merely the symptom itself. The significance of symptoms is not self-evident; the person must actively give attention and interpretation to them. Sometimes a bodily disturbance is sufficiently acute and obvious to merit certain treatment. A person with a gaping and painful wound that is bleeding profusely is not likely to ignore the bodily disturbance. Other disturbances, however, are more open to varying interpretations, including those that make the person less likely even to notice them. Mechanic (1976) suggested that the ordinary response to such disturbances involves testing hypotheses by observing the situation over time. Part of this process involves assuming a wait-and-see stance to test such hypotheses as: This is something minor, the body will heal itself, and further symptoms may develop to give a better idea of what this could be.

Typically, people try to normalize their symptoms. They interpret disturbances as within the range of "okay," or at least understandable. A man who was hospitalized for a heart attack stated:

> I just felt rotten and I had a pain in my chest and I thought it was indigestion. I'd been rushing in the lunch hour and lifted a heavy box and all this sort of thing, and it was, oh three quarters of an hour after the actual rush that I felt the pain (quoted in Cowie, 1976).

Normalizing a disturbance, however, does not necessarily make it unimportant or less real. For example, a person might normalize an excruciating abdominal pain by interpreting it as a bout of recurring gall bladder problems. For this reason, the response to acute illnesses is typically different from the response to chronic illnesses. One U.S. study found that for acute problems, people focus on the symptoms. The amount of effort the individual puts into some form of treatment often depends upon the severity of the symptoms themselves. For chronic problems, by contrast, people develop strategies of management over a long term. When problems flare up, the response is routinized and not necessarily directly related to the severity of symptoms of that single episode (Verbrugge and Ascione, 1987).

PAIN AND ITS PSYCHOSOCIAL DIMENSIONS

The sociocultural and psychological dimensions of pain demonstrate how profoundly greater the illness experience is compared to its mere biophysical aspect. Because the medical model does not adequately encompass these dimensions, it often fails to meet the needs of pain sufferers. Pain is a form of biofeedback essential to our survival. Occasionally someone is born without the capacity to feel pain. In one such case, the person was deformed by the age of twenty-five because he had severely burned his hand and suffered other injuries without feeling them. Further, the ulceration and wearing down of bodily extremities characteristic of leprosy were once thought to be symptoms of the disease, until it was discovered that they were produced by its deadening of the victim's ability to feel pain (Neal, 1978: 47–50). Although pain is an essential warning system for the body, it can also be a scourge and a terrible existential reality, a source of fear and anxiety that in some cases becomes all-consuming and overwhelming.

Pain is the symptom that people report most frequently when they see a doctor. Musculoskeletal problems (e.g., lower back pain, joint pain, or arthritis) are the leading causes of disability among people in their working years; back pain is second only to respiratory problems as a reason for missing work (Osterweis et al., 1987). Approximately 7 million Americans have serious back problems (Bogin, 1982). A nationwide sample of 1,254 adults revealed that about 75 percent of Americans suffer from occasional headaches and more than 50 percent from back and muscular pain. People who reported high levels of stress also reported high levels of all kinds of pain (Schmeck, 1985). Pain seems to be a very individual and personal matter. As a physical sensation, it does not seem to be subject to sociocultural influences, yet there are many ways in which the private world of pain interacts with the sociocultural world.

The clinical reality of pain is, however, complex, and involves three components: a person's actual sensation of pain; a person's tolerance *threshold* for pain; and a person's expression of pain. Pain is unique as a medical phenomenon, since its measurement relies on individuals' accounts of what they are feeling as well as the doctors' observations of pain-related behavior. The doctor can observe a person's gait or flex limbs to see if pain is inhibiting movement, but all indicators are based on what the patient says or does. In other words, pain measurement depends on patients' intended or unintended expressions of the pain they are feeling. Although of limited reliability, several laboratory techniques (e.g., thermography and positron emission tomography scans) attempt to measure organic signs of pain without relying on patients' reports, but these are only indirect measures of the manifestations of pain, such as the degree of sympathetic nervous system activity (Osterweis et al., 1987: 141–142). Thus clinicians must rely heavily upon the individual sufferers to describe or show what they feel.

Pain as a Biosocial Phenomenon

Pain is obviously a sensation; a cut finger produces a "simple" physical sensation. Pain generally involves more than simply a physical sensation, however, because it is imbued with meaning. For some ballet students or athletes, the pain that comes with a workout is "good pain," or a normal, acceptable consequence of well-done exercise, whereas a sharp, sudden new pain of unknown origin would signal that something fundamental has gone wrong. One doctor observed that the wounded soldiers he was treating during World War II complained of less pain and requested less pain medication than civilians who had suffered equally serious wounds. The soldiers, for whom the wounds meant leaving the battlefield and further danger of death, apparently experienced and tolerated pain differently (Beecher, 1956).

While pain obviously involves physical sensations, it is often more than just sensations. As something that accompanies disease or a serious injury, pain takes on meaning as a form of suffering. "People in pain report suffering from pain when they feel out of control—when the pain is overwhelming, when the source of pain is unknown, when the meaning of the pain is dire or when the pain is chronic" (Cassell, 1982: 641). In short, when pain threatens one's integrity as a person and one's physical existence, it becomes suffering (Cassell, 1982). These negative meanings of pain may in turn amplify the physical sensations the person experiences (Kleinman, 1988).

In Chapter 4, we argued that the mind and the body should be seen as an interrelated whole. Placebos, for example, do not merely relieve pain "in the mind" but can also generate physical changes by stimulating the release of pain relieving endorphins. The spinal-gate control theory of pain suggests another mind-body-society thoroughfare by proposing that activity in the nervous system affects the opening and closing of "gates" in the spinal cord that modulate the flow of pain messages. Most theories of pain hold that a specific pain stimulus produces an input in the form of a pain message that travels upward along the spinal cord to a pain center in the brain, where an "alarm" is set off. In contrast, the spinal-gate control theory argues that pain messages from the frontal cortex (a higher brain center), from the limbic system (a midbrain area that controls emotions), and from other parts of the body can affect the opening and closing of these spinal gates, and thus modify incoming pain messages (Melzack and Wall, 1983). The experience of pain is, however, more than an incoming sensation, since it is affected by emotional states and "higher" order cognitive mental functions (Osterweis et al., 1987). Indeed, pain does have important biopsychosocial and cultural dimensions (Bates, 1987; Freund, 1982).

There may be ethnic variations in the experience of pain as well (Bates, 1987). Some studies suggest that men and women may differ in pain tolerance, with the male threshold allegedly being higher. Racial differences have also been indicated; whites have the highest tolerance for pain, and blacks and orientals have less (Woodrow et al., 1972). Of course major individual variations within groups exist, and all of these measures of tolerance are based on pain expressions and the way they are interpreted. The research is by no means conclusive, but it strongly suggests that such variations exist. But are they biological, cultural, or biocultural (Bates, 1987; Overfield, 1985)?

Sociocultural Variations in Pain Expression

Pain expression refers to how a person shows and behaviorally responds to pain. Pain expression is clearly influenced by sociocultural factors. Cultures in which emotional control is valued encourage stoicism about pain. "Big boys don't cry!" reveals a cultural expectation that adult males should repress the expression of pain. The ability to control the social presentation of pain even under conditions that inflict a great deal of pain may be a sign of one's moral status (i.e., one's "manhood," moral uprightness, or reliability). An elder of the Kuranko society of Sierra Leone in Africa, for example, describes the circumcision of an adolescent going through a puberty rite:

Even when they are cutting the foreskin you must not flinch. You have to stand stone still. You must not make a sound from the mouth. Better to die than to wince or blink or cry out (quoted in Jackson, 1983).

In the Kuranko society, control over pain expression symbolizes the ability to assume an adult male role. Painful procedures such as tatooing and scarification are endured by adolescents partly because the expression of pain is negatively sanctioned, and perhaps because the meaning and honor of the procedure affects the experience of pain itself. Many athletes endure pain that most other people would not. On the whole, however, our culture teaches that pain can and should be avoided, and we tend to medicate it extensively (Kleinman, 1988; Bogin, 1982).

Under some situations, persons suffer excruciating pain, yet must quickly learn to manage their expression in order not to threaten a group's morale or its ability to function. Medical settings are an excellent example of this. Were one to scream hysterically in a dentist's chair, what influence would this have on waiting patients, especially small children? In hospitals the treatment for severe burns, which includes scrubbing the wounds, scraping away dead tissue, and applying new dressings and medication, inflicts a lot of pain in addition to the extreme pain of the burns themselves. However, burn victims are socialized into enduring the pain by the "coaching" of staff as well as of other patients who have been through similar experiences (Fagerhaugh and Strauss, 1977).

People from varying cultural backgrounds present their symptoms, including pain, in different ways (Good and Good, 1981). Zborowski's (1952, 1969) study of hospitalized male patients suffering from back pain and spinal lesions found that Jewish and Italian men were particularly vocal and disturbed about their pain. While Italians were concerned with immediate pain relief, however, the Jews worried about the pain's implications for their future. Anglo-American patients wanted the pain taken care of but were not as vocal in their pain expression. Irish patients were the most stoic and likely to deny pain. Zborowski's work has been criticized for its limited sample and the fact that subjects were studied only in a medical setting, but its main findings have been corroborated by subsequent research. Zola (1966, 1983), for example, also found ethnic differences in how people showed and talked about their symptoms. Italians, for instance, described their symptoms more expansively and emotionally.

Generalizations about different groups' responses to pain must be used cautiously and not become the basis of stereotyping. While we may have typical ways of expressing ourselves, social situational factors can affect how we will express ourselves. Expressing pain must not be confused with *feeling* pain; for instance, acting stoic does not mean that one feels no pain. Even if people from various social categories (e.g., social classes, gender, or cultures) do present their pain differently, social and cultural factors also influence how observers interpret their pain expressions.

Responses to other people's pain expressions are influenced by cultural assumptions about what those expressions mean. An African woman's response to stomach pain due to infection may seem exaggerated to a Western-trained male doctor, but the woman's response is reasonable given her fears about infertility, a source of shame in her culture. The same woman, however, may handle the pain of childbirth without complaints (Susser et al., 1985: 136). Zborowski (1952, 1969) and Zola (1966, 1983) found that because Italians expressed their pain so dramatically, non-Italian doctors tended to question the credibility of their Italian patients, interpreting their problems as "psychiatric." Such differences in the social and cultural backgrounds of doctor and patient can thus lead to very different interpretations of pain. One study found that

> the pain of women was treated later and less directly than the pain of men. Women suffered longer before being referred to the Pain Unit. They were less often treated with procedures specifically intended to cure the pain. The men in a shorter period since pain onset were operated upon twice as often as the women. Paradoxically, women reported twice as many surgical procedures unrelated to pain (Lack, 1982: 62).

Women were also given more minor tranquilizers, antidepressants, and analgesics, and fewer narcotics than men. This difference implies that the doctors took women's pain less seriously, interpreting it as of psychological origin; however, they accepted men's pain is "real" and prescribed pain-killers. Was this difference due to variation in how men and women showed pain, or because of how male doctors interpreted women's presentations of pain?

The visibility of the source of pain is another significant factor in determining how seriously people take another's pain symptoms. It is often hard to see the cause of pain. Patients with chronic back pain may, for example, learn to conceal signs of pain, such as masking a limp caused by sciatic nerve pain. Because they look healthy, their pain may not always be taken seriously (Fagerhaugh and Strauss, 1977). By contrast, a bloody gash—even on a part of the body with relatively little nerve sensitivity—is taken seriously as a source of pain.

Chronic Pain

By definition, chronic pain is recurring or ongoing. It is not simply continuous but is experienced qualitatively differently from acute pain episodes. Because it is ongoing, chronic pain often has profound implications for a sufferer's life and very identity. People with chronic pain face continuing problems in symptom management (Strauss, 1975). How does one deal with pain and live life as normally as possible? People in chronic pain may not be able to tolerate regular employment, to follow schedules, or even to meet the demands of home life. Chronic pain is not always constant, but is often intermittent and unpredictable, flaring up unexpectedly (Bogin, 1982). Each day sufferers must manage a host of problems associated with activities that are taken for granted by others: They must pace their activities in order to tolerate or not aggravate the pain, and they must balance the undesired side effects of medication against the benefits of pain reduction.

Chronic pain also poses basic problems for the sufferer's sense of self. One person explained:

> Our personalities have been shaken to the core, and what we most counted on—our close relationships, our marriages, our jobs—may well have fallen by the wayside. Our whole sense of life has radically changed since pain became a part of it, yet no one seems to understand our listlessness, our loss of hope, our lack of optimism. Other people can't *see* our pain, so how can they imagine what it's done to us? Only someone who has lived with chronic pain knows how insidious the process is (Bogin, 1982: 4).

Acute pain goes away and does not become an ongoing, major focus of everyday existence. Chronic pain, by contrast, is a "somatic reminder that things are not right and may never be right. This reminder, phenomenally situated in one's own body, is inescapable" (Hilbert, 1984: 370). The body as subjectively experienced is transformed into an object with pain. One "moment one is one's body, the next one has a body" (Bergsma, 1982: 111). Chronic pain demands constant attention and can become all-consuming.

People in chronic pain often face invalidating responses from others, particularly if their pain is not believable or if an organic basis of pain is not apparent. One sufferer stated that she had considered unneeded surgery so that she would have a scar to show (Hilbert, 1984: 373). Another believed his several surgical treatments had worsened the pain but at least gave him scars that symbolized, to himself and others, the physical reality of the pain (Kleinman, 1988: 68).

Invalidating responses often come from doctors (Hilbert, 1984: 368), particularly when they are frustrated by their inability to treat effectively or find an organic cause for the pain (Bogin, 1982; Kleinman, 1988). Chronic pain challenges doctors' sense of competence and control. Invalidation of the reality of the experience of pain is particularly disconcerting, because sufferers are being told that what their bodies are telling them is not real. Since our bodies and physical sensations are primary sources of our sense of reality, this invalidation is especially devastating (Hilbert, 1984; Kotarba, 1977). Chronic pain sufferers find themselves in a bind. On the one hand, concealing signs of their pain reduces the likelihood that their claims to being in pain will be taken seriously. On the other hand, persons who regularly display and dramatize their pain risk wearing down other people's sympathy, placing a strain on their social support networks.

Somatization

In all cultures, the body serves as a means of expressing and communicating cultural, as well as personal, messages. Pain is a legitimate reason to assume the sick role (described in Chapter 6), thereby perhaps avoiding some undesired activity. Pain is one way people communicate social distress or a sense of social powerlessness. Sometimes, being in pain may be a way of avoiding difficult decisions. For example, a young adult's parents may be stifling her autonomy, but to leave home means to alienate them and to face an uncertain, perhaps hostile, existence away from home. Pain may be both a way of delaying the difficult decision and a means of communicating something about the conflicts she is experiencing (Kleinman, 1988).

Somatization is "the communication of personal and interpersonal problems in a physical idiom of distress and a pattern of behavior that emphasizes seeking of medical help" (Kleinman, 1988: 57). Somatization does not mean that the pain is inauthentic, except in cases of outright malingering. Pain may be physical in origin but sustained and amplified by sociopsychological factors. Social distress may create the physiological changes that amplify existing pain or create an experience of pain (Kleinman, 1988). The particular idiom of distress used is drawn from a cultural repertoire. For example, in Iran "heart distress" is a meaningful expression linking an entire set of social concerns: infertility, attractiveness, sexual intercourse, pollution, and old age. Thus when an Iranian complains of a "pressed heart," that complaint must be understood in terms of its cultural meanings (Good, 1977; cf. Guarnaccia and Farias, 1988). Even when it has sociopsychological sources, however, pain is not simply "in the mind" but also is a bodily phenomenon.[1]

CHRONIC ILLNESS AND DISABILITY: THE POLITICS OF IMPAIRMENT

Because chronic illness and disability more seriously disturb the person's essential relationships and very sense of self, they result in a very different illness experience than acute illness. An **impairment** is the loss of some physiological or anatomical function, whereas a **disability** is the consequence of such an impairment, such as the inability to walk, climb stairs, or travel (Scheer and Croce, 1988: 23). Many people with disabilities object to the term *handicap* because of its negative connotations, especially when it

[1]While pain always involves sociopsychological aspects, this should not detract from the reality of the physical aspects. A doctor who cannot discern organic sources of pain should not assume that there are none; biomechanical causes, for example, that were not detectible by earlier technologies (e.g., x-rays or myelograms) may appear through newer technologies (e.g., CT scans and magnetic resonance imaging). Perspectives such as Kleinman's (1988), that stress the biopsychosocial aspects of pain recognize the relationship between social life and pain, including the subjective reality of somatized pain.

implies that the whole person is handicapped. We shall, therefore, speak of persons with disabilities.

Although some people with chronic illnesses are impaired and disabled, chronic illness does not inevitably lead to disability. For example, diabetes may interfere only minimally with some people's functioning. Some people with an impairment and a disability (for example, from an automobile accident) are not sick and may object to being defined as such. The sick role (described in Chapter 6) temporarily exempts people from normal activities; however, people with disabilities who are treated as though they were sick may find themselves prevented from participating in normal social activities and placed in a state of perpetual dependence. Nonetheless, many people with chronic illness have impairment and share problems with those who have experienced a loss of functioning at birth or due to a trauma (e.g., an accident).

Impairment is relatively verifiable in "objective" medical terms.[2] Disability, however, is not as easily defined separate from the social and cultural context of impairment. In a small Egyptian village, for example, trachoma (an infection that affects the eyelids) is widespread, but the "Western" standards of blindness do not apply to those who are afflicted. Instead, the social and cultural arrangements make it possible for many villagers with severely impaired vision to function without disability:

> Most visually impaired adults are illiterate, so they do not need signs to read. There are no street signs or house numbers to read in the hamlet. The structure of the village changes very slowly. If a new house is built every five years the visually impaired can learn to find their way around it. . . . Plowing, sowing seed and harvesting ripe produce do not require much vision. If there is some small task they are unable to do, their extended family does it for them. Thus, they do not perceive themselves as disabled (quoted in Cockburn, 1988: 13).

Thus whether an "objective" impairment becomes a disability depends on the environment, the expected daily activities, and the attitudes of others. A disability is not just the result of the limitations of a person's sensory, motor, cognitive, or other capabilities, but a "function of the interaction between the individual's condition and the environment, both physical and attitudinal—in which they live" (Gartner and Joe, 1987: 1). Impairment is universal, found among people in all societies; however, social and cultural responses and the "design" of social environments vary (Scheer and Croce, 1988). The sociological focus, therefore, is not on disabled people but on disabling attitudes and environments.

One definition used in the United States considers disability to be "an

---

[2]Even in this respect, there is still the question of what is a "normal" body.

inability to engage in gainful employment"; more broadly, it refers to a reduction of activity, a "restricted activity day" (Mausner and Bahn, 1985: 113). Such criteria are used in Section 504 of the Rehabilitation Act of 1973, the first comprehensive U.S. legislation banning discrimination against people with disabilities, and providing them with the legal right of access to those educational institutions and places of employment receiving federal funds (Osterweis et al., 1987: 34). The 1980 United States Census estimated that one in five adults has some type of disability. Most common is difficulty in walking and lifting (*New York Times*, 1986). Nonwhite disabled people outnumber white disabled people by a ratio of about two to one (National Institute on Disability, 1986). These figures suggest that disabilities are not as uncommon as many believe. Our perceptions are based partly on the fact that Western society, especially the United States, tends to deny and to segregate disability, old age, and death. Furthermore, the likelihood of having a disability is socially distributed, as are individual resources for coping with disability.

Categorizing people as disabled has implications for social policy, as Zola (1982: 242) pointed out:

> By trying to find strict measures of disability or focusing on "severe," "visible" handicaps we draw dividing lines and make distinctions where matters are very blurry and constantly changing. By agreeing that there are 20 million disabled or 36 million, or even that half the population are in some way affected by disability, we delude ourselves into thinking there is some finite, no matter how large, number of people. . . . Any person reading the words on this page is at best momentarily able-bodied. But nearly everyone reading them will, at some point, suffer from one or more chronic diseases and be disabled, temporarily or permanently, for a significant part of their lives.

Being disabled is a "normal" condition of humanity, and categorizing people can create misleading distinctions (Sutherland, 1981). Such definitions are social and political constructions, as illustrated by the fact that the boundaries are historically shifting and cross-culturally variable (Osterweis et al., 1987; Fine and Asch, 1988).

Chronic illness is, by definition, ongoing, recurrent, and often degenerative. Conrad (1987) suggested that there are different types of chronic illnesses, each with its own social implications: "lived-with" illness, such as asthma and diabetes; "mortal" illness, such as some cancers; and "at risk" illnesses, which include inherited, "environmental," or "personal" behavior risks. People with disabilities or chronic illnesses in our society face a number of common problems regarding the social organization of their environments, the attitudes of others, and their sense of self.

Disability, Chronic Illness, and the Social Organization of Space and Time

The organization of the spaces in which people move and the time arrangements of their activities are related to the quality of life and health. Building codes, government ordinances, financial considerations, and many other factors structure the qualities of the buildings in which we work, live, and play (Hahn, 1988). Social and political considerations influence the quality and accessibility of transportation. Zola (1982: 208) described the inhospitable nature of many environments for a person wearing a leg brace:

> Chairs without arms to push myself up from; unpadded seats which all too quickly produce sores; showers and toilets without handrails to maintain my balance; surfaces too slippery to walk on; staircases without bannisters to help me hoist myself; buildings without ramps, making ascent exhausting if not dangerous; every curbstone a precipice; car, plane, and theatre seats too cramped for my braced leg; and trousers too narrow for my leg brace to pass through. With such trivia is my life plagued. Even though I am relatively well off, mobility is a daily challenge.

Imagine trying to walk about in a physical space designed only for those in wheelchairs. The doors would be too low, the floors would be too slippery for walking, and no chairs would be provided for sitting. People with physical impairments simply have more specialized or individual physical needs than those without impairments. The failure of social environments to account for individual rhythms and patterns for comfortable movement contributes to problems in health and the quality of life. The same problems apply even more to people with impairments.

While technological advances have made it possible for many people with disabilities to survive and potentially to function, such advances have not generally been applied to the design of public, work, and living environments. We live increasingly in humanmade, artificial spaces that are not currently adapted to a wide spectrum of bodies but could be so modified. In recent years, however, there has been a slight shift toward creating more environments of "universal" or "transgenerational" design, geared to the needs of persons with some physical impairment. While no environment can accommodate everyone's needs, "universally" designed spaces are intended for use by the widest possible range of bodies. One example is a park recently built for access both by able-bodied and disabled people; its tennis, pool, and special swings are designed for use by people in wheelchairs (Brown, 1988).

Much research on chronic illness and impairment focuses on malingering and whether government financial benefits motivate people not to work; instead, however, research should examine how work conditions themselves discourage the chronically ill from maintaining their jobs. The nature of the job, such as the pace of work and the physical design of the work place, is an important determinant of work disability (Yelin, 1986; Osterweis et al., 1987). During World War II people with disabilities assumed many of the jobs vacated by those who went to war. For all workers during that time, there were lower rates of absenteeism, work-related accidents, and turnover, and higher rates of production. After the war, workers with disabilities were replaced by returning "able-bodied" veterans (Struck, 1981: 26).

People with chronic impairments do not usually challenge disabling time limitations and pressures. They do not generally question the arrangements of work and living spaces in which they must function; rather, they typically assume such arrangements to be natural and given (Charmaz, 1983). People come to believe that their inability to squeeze their bodies and rhythms of movement into inadequate social-spatial arrangements are signs of their *personal* inadequacy. Disabling environments and attitudes thus contribute to a loss of sense of self and to suffering among those who have chronic physical impairments (Charmaz, 1983).

Disabling Attitudes and Sense of Self

Our society often places people who violate somatic norms into institutions or segregates them behind the scenes of everyday life. One woman with multiple sclerosis commented:

> I once asked a local advertiser why he didn't include disabled people in his spots. His response seemed direct enough. "We don't want to give people the idea that our product is just for the handicapped," he said. . . . If you saw my blind niece ordering a Coke, would you switch to Pepsi lest you be struck sightless? No, I think the advertiser's excuse masked a deeper and more anxious rationale: to depict disabled people in the ordinary activities of daily life is to admit that there is something ordinary about disability itself, that it might enter anybody's life. If it is effaced completely or at least isolated as a separate "problem," so that it remains at a safe distance from other human issues, then the viewer won't feel threatened by her or his own physical vulnerability (Mairs, 1987: C2).

The suffering created by such discrediting attitudes is not just a matter of the personal attitudes themselves but also the social conditions that engender them (Charmaz, 1983).

The stigmatizing opinions of others have a strong impact on one's sense of self. A stigma is a deeply discrediting attribute that, when visible, can brand a person as less than human, as pitiable, horrible, and publicly discreditable. The degree to which an attribute is stigmatizing depends on its sociohistorical context and the status of the person who possesses such an attribute:

Conjure in your mind a military man with an eye patch. Is there not something romantic and heroic about the injury? Doesn't it suggest a dark and complex past, a will of uncommon strength, perhaps a capability for just enough brutality to add a trace of virile unpredictability to the man? Now replace the image of the mysterious man who wears an eye patch with the image of a 7-year-old girl who wears one. For most people, something strange happens. The romance and mystery disappear; what we see is a handicapped child. There is something sad and even pitiful about her; we fear for her future and worry about her present. We think: this poor kid is going to have a hard time growing up and making it in this world (Gliedman and Roth, 1980: 29).

In all societies, certain deviations from somatic norms are considered stigmatizing, but there are no inherently stigmatizing attributes. Rather, stigma is a social construction that depends on person and context.

In our society, those with "severe" impairments are sometimes viewed as

visually repulsive; helpless; pathetic; dependent; too independent; plucky, brave and courageous; bitter with chips on our shoulders; evil (the "twisted mind in a twisted body"); mentally retarded; endowed with mystical powers and much else (Sutherland, 1981: 58).

Some of these attitudes are changing. The mass media, however, perpetuate stereotypes that associate disability with evil and criminality (e.g., characters like Frankenstein's hunchbacked assistant), a loss of self-control, an attempt to compensate for their impairment, and a tendency to either be asexual or "perversely" preoccupied with sex (Longmore, 1987).

Media images project some heroic role models: the blind skier, the one-legged pitcher who made it to the major leagues, and Helen Keller and her many achievements.[3] These examples show people's ability to transcend the most limiting of conditions, and in that respect they are inspiring. They may, however, imply another message: "that if a Franklin Delano Roosevelt and a Wilma Rudolph could *overcome* their handicap, so could and should all the disabled. And if we fail, it is our problem, our personality, our weakness" (Zola, 1982: 204–205). Many media "success" stories similarly communicate a message in the tune with the American ethos of rugged individualism and responsibility for oneself. This imagery, however, deflects from an understanding of the mundane problems faced by those with impairments and the many barriers that most humans simply cannot overcome.

Sexual expression is an important source of pleasure, tension release, and sense of self. Until recently, however, the prevalent attitude, even among

---

[3]Very few people know that Helen Keller was displayed for a while as an exhibit, like the Elephant Man, in a vaudeville show!

many professionals working with people with disabilities, was to deny or avoid recognition of their sexuality. The deviation of persons with disabilities from somatic norms often arouses an aesthetic anxiety in others, particularly in Western societies, which put a high premium on "supernormal standards of bodily perfection" (Hahn, 1988: 42). Our sexual fantasies are saturated with images from advertising and the entertainment world. Media-driven standards of sexual attractiveness, particularly for women, result in even greater disadvantages for people whose bodies deviate from the ideal (Sutherland, 1987: 27). Zola (1982) described a Swedish experiment in which counselors acted as sex surrogates with their clients who had disabilities; the experiment was stopped, however, because the counselors began to enjoy their contacts. The fear that "deviant" bodies may be "deviant" only in the eyes of the beholder made this experiment a threat.

People with disabilities also face special problems in the management of such emotions as anger. First, the impairment itself may inhibit anger expression. Being physically weak or on crutches may make the direct, motoric, dramatic expression of emotions difficult. Furthermore, disabling attitudes and environments force people into a state of dependency beyond the biological consequences of their impairments.

People with disabilities are also socialized out of their anger. They are expected to be grateful for what help they receive and cannot "afford" the luxury of overt anger expression for fear of risking the alienation of the people on whom they depend (Zola, 1982). When people regularly and vocally respond to frustrating or disempowering conditions, they further risk having their anger treated as a by-product of their impairment rather than as an appropriate response to their social environment or living conditions. The docudrama "Captives of Care" depicted a resident of an institution who was angry with the staff for the arbitrary limits imposed by institutional life. In one encounter, he lashed out at a nurse for invading his privacy. The nurse did not understand his reaction, and a colleague explained to her that "that's the way he is because he is twisted." Because his physical impairment was thus seen as explaining his behavior, his protest over institutional conditions was invalidated.

The constant emotional work involved in managing anger often results in repressing the anger, and turning it inward and against oneself. Zola (1982: 222) argued that depression among those with disabilities is partly due to constraints against getting angry. This depression is often viewed as the individual's problem rather than a normal response to social pressures. Thus turning socially provoked anger inward is socially functional, but individually repressive.

One strategy for avoiding the potential stigma of some disabilities is *passing,* or concealing a discrediting social status or stigmatizing attributes. In some cases, disclosure or "selective telling" can act as a means of forestalling a negative reaction from another person. Schneider and Conrad (1983) described how people with epilepsy weigh the stigma potential of their condition against positive consequences (e.g., having someone to help in case of seizure) of revealing the fact. Concealing one's condition is sometimes a way of avoiding stigmatizing attitudes. Because people with impaired vision may consider a cane to be a stigma symbol or an overt sign of disability, they may prefer a less obtrusive folding cane, even though it may not be as effective an instrument. The refusal to use highly visible prosthetic devices, however, is not necessarily irrational, but may be based on well-founded fears of being viewed as a "cripple."

In Chapter 4, we suggested that assaults on one's sense of self may have physical consequences, including an impact on the immune system. Certain chronic illnesses, such as herpes, leprosy, epilepsy, and AIDS, carry a load of powerful negative meanings that define afflicted persons and our perception of them. In addition to the fear of death, disfiguring treatments, and the usual threats to one's self-concept that accompany any debilitating disease, sufferers of AIDS are also faced with highly stigmatizing responses from others. It has evoked irrational fears of contagion, not unlike leprosy did in the past. Because of its association with homosexuality, it has also evoked intense homophobic reactions. People with AIDS have been dismissed from their jobs, evicted from their homes, rejected, and isolated by friends and relatives. Even the family, friends, or colleagues of victims may become stigmatized by association, a pattern that Goffman calls "courtesy stigma" (Goffman, 1963). AIDS victims may also be ostracized by medical personnel whose fears override their knowledge about contagion. Studies indicate that the risk of spreading infection from AIDS patients to health care workers is minute (Heyward and Curran, 1988), yet one patient with AIDS commented,

> The nurses are scared of me; the doctors wear masks and sometimes gloves. Even the priest doesn't seem too anxious to shake my hand. What the hell is this? I'm not a leper. Do they want to lock me up and shoot me? I've got no family, no friends. Where do I go? What do I do? God, this is horrible! Is He punishing me? The only thing I got going for me is that I'm not dying—at least, not yet (quoted in Kleinman, 1988: 163).

Such attitudes contribute to distress and unneeded suffering; they may also have biophysical consequences. Further research is needed on the impact of the social stress produced by the stigma of AIDS in further assaulting a person's immune system (Kaplan et al., 1987).

Disability as a Minority Status

People with disabilities constitute a minority group because of their relative powerlessness and their identifiability, both of which promote discrimination and stigmatization. Unlike other minority groups, however, the disabled do not usually share a subculture, a geographical location, or history. Their cultural status is ambiguous: They are "betwixt and between," neither healthy nor sick. Murphy (1987) argues that because such ambiguity is threatening to normals, the isolation and discrimination faced by those with disabilities may come from their anomalous and ambiguous status in our system of cultural classification. Nevertheless, like other minority groups, such as women, blacks, Hispanics, and gays, they do experience similar problems of being powerless objects of stereotypes and discrimination. Specific words are used for the discriminatory attitudes and behavior toward other races (racism), women (sexism), and the elderly (ageism), but there is no term to describe such attitudes and behavior toward the disabled, although Zola (1982) has suggested the use of the term "healthism."

A Harris poll in 1984 showed that 74 percent of persons with disabilities do identify with one another, and that 45 percent consider themselves a minority in the same sense as blacks or Hispanics (Fine and Asch, 1988). Some studies suggest that physically "normal" people view those with impairments, such as blindness, as inferior to members of ethnic minority groups (Susser et al., 1985). One study found a hierarchy of attitudes toward persons with disabilities, with those who were blind ranked below those with cerebral palsy, total paralysis, or epilepsy. Other studies show that blacks as a group were ranked close to the blind in terms of social preference. Such biases develop as early as the age of six (Gliedman, 1979).

Perhaps the most important feature that people with disabilities share with racial and ethnic minorities is the tendency for others to attribute their perceived inferiority and "differentness" to biological factors alone, rather than to social conditions. Disabling attitudes and environments create a self-fulfilling prophecy that legitimates individualistic and biologistic assumptions about the disabled. Because such environments and attitudes exclude people with disabilities from the community and from work places, the nondisabled conclude that this exclusion is evidence that the disabled cannot function in such settings. "Like racists, able-bodied people often confuse the results of social oppression with the effects of biology" (Gliedman and Roth, 1980: 28).

Disability Civil Rights Movements: Recapturing Self and Access

Stimulated by the 1960s civil rights movement, people with disabilities became politically active, working from the assumption that they constituted a minority group deprived of their civil rights. Shifting their focus from individual problems to attacking unfair social structures, they began demanding equal access to housing, jobs, transportation, and health care. The activism of the 1960s had widened the definition of political issues to include the personal, everyday problems faced by various groups. Various forms of **identity politics** (Anspach, 1977) attempted to forge a new identity and sense of self (e.g., "Gay is proud," and "Black is beautiful"). Often these politics revolved around particular stigmatizing definitions. For example, women's groups resisted the medical definition of menopause as a disease (McCrea, 1983) (see Chapter 9). Similarly, disability rights activists realized that definitions of disability were sociopolitical (Scotch, 1988).

After World War II, environmental barriers kept people with disabilities from participating fully in society, despite technological developments that made such a life increasingly possible. Those who had *acquired* an impairment (e.g., from polio or war wounds) were not used to being dependent and had higher expectations than those who were *born* with an impairment. The struggle for civil rights represented an attempt by people with raised expectations to remove barriers by ending employment discrimination, increasing architectural access, opening admission to universities and other institutions, and pursuing other policy goals (Scotch, 1988). Groups like the Center for Independent Living in California and Disabled in Action on the east coast, which are staffed largely by people with disabilities, sought to define issues such as access not as charity or welfare but as basic civil rights. Many workers in human services, however, still view people with disabilities as clients with problems to be treated. By contrast, the disability rights movement emphasizes the involvement of citizens with disabilities in shaping their own fate (Gliedman, 1979: 63). One of the main contributions of the movement has been to heighten public awareness of discrimination and chronic illness as sociopolitical issues, not merely medical problems.

SUMMARY

Illness is the complex set of ways in which the sick person (and family and friends) perceive, manage, and respond to symptoms and disability. The experience of illness reminds us of our limitations, dependencies, and ultimate mortality. While ordinary, even minor illnesses disrupt one's life, certain illness experiences are likely to have a damaging effect on the sick person's identity and sense of self. Certain disabling conditions and chronic pain and illnesses are especially problematic, because they involve a sense of loss; they are overwhelming, unpredictable, and uncontrollable; and they produce social marginality for the sufferer. The chronic illness experience is not limited to the sick person but often involves family and friends as well. People interpret their illness, giving it meaning, form, and order. These meanings in turn shape their perception of their symptoms and pain.

Disability and pain are important features of the illness experience, especially chronic illness. Social and political factors are involved in both the definition and management of disability. Disabling social and physical environments and attitudes are responsible for many of the problems suffered by persons with chronic illness or impairments. Similarly, both the experience and expression of pain are linked with sociocultural factors. Suffering is often increased, however, when others invalidate the reality of the pain. Since the majority of serious illnesses today are chronic, in contrast to the acute illnesses predominant in the recent past, we need to appreciate their powerful impact upon the sufferer's daily life, social relationships, and very self.

RECOMMENDED READINGS

Articles

Linda Alexander, "Illness maintenance and the new American sick role," pp. 351–367 in N. J. Chrisman and T. W. Maretzki, eds., *Clinically Applied Anthropology*. Dordrecht, Netherlands: D. Reidel, 1982.

Kathy Charmaz, "Loss of self: A fundamental form of suffering of the chronically ill," *Sociology of Health and Illness* 4, 1983: 167–182.

Sharon R. Kaufman, "Toward a phenomenology of boundaries in medicine: Chronic illness experience in the case of stroke," *Medical Anthropology Quarterly* 2 (4), 1988: 338–354.

Jessica Scheer and Nora Croce, "Impairment as a human constant: Cross-cultural and historical perspectives on variation," *Journal of Social Issues* 44(1), 1988: 23–37.

Books

Shizuko Fagerhaugh and Anselm Strauss, *Politics of Pain Management: Staff-Patient Interaction*. Reading, MA: Addison-Wesley, 1977. A study of the social organizational contexts—especially power relations—for the perception of pain and pain management.

Arthur Kleinman, *The Illness Narratives: Suffering, Healing, and the Human Condition.* New York: Basic, 1988. A sensitive witness to narratives of illness experiences, especially those that are chronic and disabling or disfiguring.

Robert F. Murphy, *The Body Silent.* New York: Henry Holt, 1987. An anthropologist's account of his increasing paralysis due to a spinal tumor and his personal perspective on the sociocultural aspects of disability.

Joseph W. Schneider and Peter Conrad, *Having Epilepsy: The Experience and Control of Illness.* Philadelphia: Temple University Press, 1983. A sociological look at epilepsy, and the management of its symptoms and stigma.

Susan Sheehan, *Kate Quinton's Days.* New York: New American Library, 1984. The poignant illness experience of an elderly woman, showing the impact of the medicalization of growing old and dying.

Irving K. Zola, *Missing Pieces: A Chronicle of Living with a Disability.* Philadelphia: Temple University Press, 1982. An excellent combination of sociological insights and Zola's personal experiences with disability, as well as his participant-observations as a guest in a Dutch village adapted to the needs of people with disabilities.

Chapter Eight

Seeking Health and Help

How do people conclude that they are ill, and what actions do they choose to take in response? There are a number of implicit and often utterly incorrect assumptions about how people seek health and respond to health problems. Probably each one of us can think of instances in our own experiences when these assumptions did not hold:

People know for sure when they are ill.

As soon as they realize they are ill, they seek competent help, specifically a medical doctor (or dentist, psychiatrist, or other appropriate professional).

When they consult the professional, they give an explanation of the problem that is as medically correct as possible.

The doctor understands what they are saying about their problem.

The doctor's explanation of the problem makes sense to them.

When the doctor prescribes therapeutic action, they follow that advice carefully until it takes effect or until the doctor changes the instructions.

People know for sure when they are well, and are satisfied when this state of health is restored.

The fact that these assumptions are rarely accurate is a source of considerable tension and outright dissatisfaction on the part of both medical professionals and patients. One key reason for this tension is the enormous, and generally unrecognized, chasm between the medical models of illness and the conceptions used by lay-persons in understanding and making decisions about their own health and illnesses. This gap is built into the structure of professionalized medicine, where—by definition—the lay person does not share the specialized body of knowledge used by the professional (Freidson, 1970: 278–279).

Most modern societies tend to treat professional interpretations as vastly superior to lay understandings. Medical professionals tend to demean lay conceptions, often labeling them as superstition, ignorance, foolishness, or instances of persons being unwilling to take proper care of themselves. From this perspective, the doctor is viewed as the expert whose rational pronouncements are the result of legitimate authority, whereas the patient should be passive and obedient, deferring all judgment to the expert.

By contrast, West (1979: 162) argues that attention should be directed to "the person as a conscious, reflective actor engaged in the process of making sense of various kinds of body changes within the framework of his own 'lay' knowledge". Studies of decision making in health matters show that most laypersons *do* make conscious choices that are rational, within the framework of their understanding of the illness (Locker, 1981). We will examine the vast range of interpretations and decisions the ordinary person makes in seeking health.

Contrary to the common misconception, health seeking is largely *not* a process of getting professional medical care. Most health-enhancing or preventive measures are nonmedical, and only a very small portion of ailments are ever brought to a physician's attention. As Zola (1983: 111) commented,

> Virtually every day of our lives we are subject to a vast array of bodily discomforts. Only an infinitesimal amount of these get to a physician. Neither the mere presence nor the obviousness of symptoms seems to differentiate those episodes which do and do not get professional treatment.

This observation is corroborated by recent studies documenting the "iceberg of morbidity"—the vast majority of physical problems that are never brought to medical (or formal health statistics) attention (Verbrugge, 1986). The Health in Detroit Study found, on the basis of health diaries, that persons over eighteen experienced an average of twenty-three health problems in sixteen days within a six-week period (Verbrugge and Ascione, 1987). This means that people experienced discomfort sufficient to be considered a health problem more than one-third of the days of the study (which itself was scheduled to avoid the height of hay fever and winter colds seasons, so this figure is probably conservative). The *least* commonly mentioned action in response to these problems was medical care; on only 5 percent of days on which they experienced problematic symptoms did respondents have medical contact of any kind (office visit, appointment scheduling, medical advice by telephone, or hospital visit). The study found that people typically responded promptly to symptoms, but that "for most symptoms of daily life, people opt to do something on their own without medical help" (Verbrugge and Ascione, 1987: 549).

This society generally and medical professionals in particular hold an ambiguous norm: Responsible persons *should* get professional medical care for all serious, medically treatable ailments and, at the same time, *should not* bother doctors or use medical facilities for unimportant or nontreatable ailments. This norm furthermore assumes that people share the professional definition of which ailments are serious or treatable and are able to assess their own situations adequately to determine into which category they fit. While physicians strongly urge professional attention for health problems, they simultaneously dislike being bothered with trivial problems or problems that they do not know how to treat effectively (Klein et al., 1982).

A British study found that 25 percent of general practitioners surveyed complained that patients consulted doctors for unimportant reasons. At the same time, 56 percent complained that patients did not have enough humility in accepting the medical expert's judgments (Cartwright, 1967). The contradictory or ambiguous norm is that laypersons should be actively expert in judging correctly which ailments to refer to the professional, and then assume a humbly passive role when under the care of the professional.

SELF-TREATMENT AND THE DECISION TO GET HELP

The vast majority of actions people take to prevent illness or to treat everyday health problems are done without expert help, either medical or nonmedical. A British study found that women respondents most frequently listed the following ways of keeping healthy: good diet, exercise and fitness, no smoking, sufficient sleep and rest, and fresh air. Very few respondents (less than 10 percent) mentioned medical checkups or screening (Calnan, 1987: 101–130).

Likewise, the individual or family typically responds directly, without lay or professional help, to ordinary health problems. The Health in Detroit Study found that self-dosing with prescription or nonprescription drugs was the most common response, used during 58 percent of the days on which people experienced symptoms. Self-imposed restriction of activities (such as cutting down on errands and chores) was also common, used on nearly 24 percent of the days on which symptoms were noticed (Verbrugge and Ascione, 1987).

British researchers found that although 91 percent of adults studied reported symptoms during the two weeks prior to interview, only 16 percent had consulted a physician. Indeed, only 28 percent had consulted their doctor at all during the previous twelve-month period, even though, under the British National Health Service, the cost of consulting a doctor is not a deterrent, as it is for many in the United States. A far more frequent action in response to symptoms was taking medicine. In the twenty-four hours before the interview, 55 percent of adults had used some medicine; in the two weeks before the interview, they had taken an average of 2.2 different items of medication. Some were taken for preventive purposes, but most were taken in response to specific symptoms: a temperature, headaches, indigestion, and sore throats. Self-medication also includes the decision to take medicines prescribed and often kept for long periods, to be taken "as needed." Prescription drugs for the central nervous system (such as tranquilizers and sedatives) were frequently self-dosed. In a sample of households in England, Wales, and Scotland, 99 percent of homes kept one or more medicines; the average number was 7.3 nonprescribed and 3.0 prescribed. A fifth of the households kept sedatives, tranquilizers, or sleeping pills, and two-fifths kept some medication that the respondent could not identify (Dunnell and Cartwright, 1972).

Some responses to illness are not merely physical. If the person's belief system attributes illness to nonphysical causes, such as emotions or spiritual factors, then it is logical for a sick person to choose nonphysical approaches to treating the illness. If, for example, a person believes that she is especially vulnerable to infections when she is lonely or "blue," she might choose to treat an ailment by doing things that cheer her up or by visiting a close friend. Similarly, if someone believes that God will intervene to heal his illness, then prayer for healing constitutes a therapeutic action.

Such nonphysical responses are rarely done to the complete exclusion of physical treatments, and often they are meshed in interesting combinations. For example, when a person chooses to treat a bad case of the flu by consuming a bowl of steaming chicken soup or a concoction of milk toast, is the treatment merely the ingestion of a therapeutic substance or the soothing emotional connotations of the food, or both? Likewise, when a sick person says a blessing prayer over a bottle of prescription pills, is the treatment purely a physical response to illness?

The Health in Detroit Study found that about half the time people responded to their health problems by talking with family or friends (Verbrugge and Ascione, 1987). This response is both therapeutic in itself and also a way of consulting with other laypersons about what to do. Laypeople rely upon their own networks of contact for advice, including suggestions about where to seek further help. Family, friends, neighbors, and colleagues at work, school, a religious group, or a social club all constitute potential sources of advice. The sick individual, however, must decide whose advice is sought and whose advice is heeded. For example, your grandmother might be a valued source of home remedies, and her burn ointment may be more effective than any commercial salve you have tried, but you might not want her advice on what might be a sexually transmitted disease, since the advice is likely to come with a lecture on sin. Individuals are typically selective in their choices of lay advice.

There is some evidence that these lay advice networks rely especially upon women as knowledgeable sources of referrals and as the seekers of health advice both for themselves and for members of their families (Graham, 1985). The division of labor in many households allocates to women more than to men such duties as caring for sick family members or selecting and arranging for appointments with medical and/or nonmedical practitioners.

Not all lay advice comes from existing networks, however. Sometimes people seek out new sources of advice or create a new network of lay advisers. A person with Parkinson's disease, for example, may look for a group of fellow sufferers, whose advice on some matters may be more valued than that of longtime friends or even doctors who have not experienced the disease themselves.

One specific form of advice is the lay referral to a source of help (Freidson, 1970: 290). Through lay referrals, the individual learns of many treatment options (which are usually linked with their lay advisers' evaluation of what might be the problem), including a favorite (or least favorite) doctor; the type of specialist to try; less orthodox practitioners, such as an herbalist or acupuncturist; self-help health groups; and alternative healing groups, such as a psychic healing circle, prayer group, or meditation center.

A study of Puerto Ricans in a small northeastern city, for example, found that sick persons with effective networks of kin and fictive kin (*compadrazgo*) received much concrete assistance in selecting and negotiating entry to both institutional health resources (e.g., prenatal care programs) and noninstitutional help (e.g., *espiritistas*—spiritual healers). The study concluded that such kin networks should be viewed as health educators because of their role in teaching members where to seek help, how to select among available help resources, and how to deal with bureaucratic and other roadblocks to getting help (Schensul and Schensul, 1982).

Social interaction with family, friends, and acquaintances often plays an important part in the decision to seek help. One study of the decision to take a health problem to a clinic found that the individual rarely sought help at the physically sickest point. Rather, the nature of symptoms themselves appeared to be less significant than social interaction in prompting the decision to see a doctor:

> For our patients the symptoms were "really" there, but their perception differed considerably. There *is* a sense in which they sought help because they could not stand it any longer. But what they could not stand was more likely to be a situation or a perceived implication of a symptom rather than any worsening of the symptom *per se* (Zola, 1983: 118).

For example, a person might be motivated to seek help after a friend's description of some serious disease that could possibly be related to her symptoms; symptoms that were formerly not worrisome then become significant, even though she had experienced no change in the symptoms themselves. Similar factors are probably involved in the decision to seek nonmedical forms of help. Thus the motivation to do something about a health problem often results from social interaction that heightens the significance imputed to the symptoms.

People do not always seek help mainly to *cure* a health problem. For example, a person might go to a *shiatsu* (Japanese acupressure) therapist for pain relief but not accept the diagnostic interpretations the therapist gives. Some people consult medical doctors for diagnoses more to rule out feared serious outcomes than actually to treat the symptoms. Similarly, some people want the medical diagnosis but distrust the medical treatment (especially certain drugs or surgery). One middle-class American woman said, "I still think they give you too much medication, which I accept gratefully and then don't take" (quoted in McGuire, 1988). We have too little data on what patients actually hope to accomplish by consulting medical and nonmedical health experts, but probably much of what professionals call noncompliance (discussed further in this chapter) is due to the fact that the doctors' orders are not necessarily what laypeople want when they seek professional help.

THE HIDDEN HEALTH CARE SYSTEM

Far too often, when people speak of the health care system, they refer only to the professionalized, institution-oriented *illness care* system of doctors and other professional health workers, hospitals, clinics, insurance companies, pharmaceutical companies, and government agencies. This form of care is important, because it is complex and powerful. It also has extensive economic significance, as discussed in Chapter 12. There is, however, another highly important system of health care.

Home and Family Care

The **hidden health care system** refers to all the laypersons who are often the real *primary* health care providers (Levin and Idler, 1981).[1] The vast majority of efforts to maintain health take place in the home and other private spheres of action, including diet, rest, recreational exercise and relaxation, hygiene, adequate shelter, avoidance of dangerous substances, and prevention of accidents and injuries (Pratt, 1976).

Likewise, most health care takes place in the home, and is either self-administered or given by members of the family. Virtually all care of minor illnesses occurs outside the formal health care system. Imagine how many people in any given day may be taking care of themselves or someone else who is miserable with such illnesses as chicken pox, a bad head cold, or stomach flu! Even for health problems that have been treated in the formal system, most of the actual care is done at home: giving medications, tending a person restricted to bed, changing dressings, and monitoring symptoms. Furthermore, throughout the society enormous amounts of energy and time are also required to care for persons with chronic illnesses, disabilities, and mental retardation, and those who are dying. A 1979 survey (Feller, 1983) found an estimated 4.9 million adults with chronic health problems who lived in the community rather than in institutions such as nursing homes or hospitals, but required help for everyday activities such as walking, bathing, dressing, preparing meals, and eating. In addition to these nonmedical forms of health care, an estimated 1.3 million people received

---

[1] This usage differs from the common one in the literature, where "primary providers" refers to general practitioners, pediatricians, and other medical doctors or nurse practitioners who, in contrast to specialists, are supposed to be the first to evaluate patients' needs.

some form of medical or nursing treatments (e.g., injections or physical therapy) at home. Older adults accounted for the vast majority of persons needing home care, and the rates of persons needing assistance increased dramatically for those over age eighty-five. The "graying" of modern societies, described in Chapter 2, results in a larger proportion of members surviving to an age at which they need long-term care for chronic health problems.

Even in nations with large government expenditures for health care, the formal health care system is predicated upon the expectation that most care will be given at home. Indeed, the transfer of even part of these services (for example, complete care of all victims of Alzheimer's disease or AIDS) to the formal sphere would probably swamp the system. Informal health care, which provides care at little or no cost to the government or insurers, has thus remained a part of the domestic economy.

There are several health-related benefits to self- and home-treatment, especially compared with treatment of the same problems in a formal—usually institutional—setting. Those who participate in the care of their own illness are more likely to experience a sense of independence, mastery, self-confidence, and control than those who are the passive recipients of care. A number of studies show the benefits of self-care, especially in treatment of chronic illnesses such as diabetes, hemophilia, and kidney disease (see Levin and Idler, 1981: 79–80).

Home care of illness and injury is typically more personal than formal or institutional care, although personal ties can be problematic, since care givers can have negative as well as positive feelings for the sick person. Home care is also likely to involve more nurturance than perfunctory tending, although the actual care too varies from home to home. Another advantage of home care is greater continuity; the patient will not have to face an unfamiliar shift of nurses or a new specialist. Finally, home care is usually not as isolating as institutional care. Persons whose chronic illnesses are cared for at home may participate, perhaps in a limited way, in the "normal" worlds of the household, school, community, and even work.

For most of us, the idea of home care raises cozy images of our comfortable room, surrounded by our favorite home entertainments, with Mom bringing us whatever we want for comfort: home-cooked special foods, a hot-water bottle, or a soothing drink. This image is, however, not the reality for many sick persons. For instance, what is the reality of home care for the widowed elderly person living alone in a bare furnished room, or the single mother who is seriously ill?

Nor are all families loving sources of nurturing care. Many families offer their members—especially children and elderly dependents—daily lives of negligence or outright abuse (Steinmetz, 1978; Straus et al., 1980). Indeed, the very health-related problems for which they need care may exacerbate these victims' abuse by other family members. Constant demand for help negotiating stairs or bathrooms, for example, might drive a tired care giver "over the edge" to abuse or neglect. Some long-term or arduous care tasks can also strain the emotional and physical resources of even a well-intentioned family.

Just as persons with disabilities need special enabling environments, so too is the optimum setting for recuperation or the management of chronic illness one that is enabling. Much home care, like many institutional settings, is disabling. For example, a person with a debilitating chronic illness may require assistance with treatments (e.g., dialysis or injections), the management of routine activities (e.g., bathing or fixing meals), and transportation (e.g., climbing stairs or riding to a friend's apartment). Like institutional care, home care given by families, volunteers, or paid workers sometimes subordinates the sick person's needs to other household goals, such as keeping to a certain schedule. Home care sometimes increases sick people's dependency rather than enabling them to manage on their own as much as possible.

U.S. health care policies have barely begun to explore (much less fund) a vast range of physical and social arrangements that would support such enabling environments as noninstitutional collective living situations, copatienting, adequate services to sick persons living independently, barrier-free physical settings for chronically ill persons, and well-trained and well-paid institutional and home health workers. Satisfactory funding for home care of the disabled, the chronically ill, or people recuperating from accidents or acute illnesses needs to include the full range of help needed. Most existing programs are oriented to the treatment of acute conditions and fund only skilled nurses and certified therapists; however, some people might need homemaker help with grocery shopping, child care, or personal care, services not covered by most insurance unless the person is institutionalized (Soldo, 1985). Even in communities where home health support services are available, there is enormous variation in the degree to which individuals are eligible for the help they need at costs they can afford.

Women's Roles

When people speak of home care, they typically mean care by a *woman* (e.g., wife or mother), an assumption that becomes particularly problematic in light of women's changing roles within the larger society. The assumption that it is the wife-mother who should care for the family's sick results in real restrictions upon women's opportunities in the public sphere, especially the world of work. Mothers, far more often than fathers, nurse sick children. Employed mothers reported three times as many hours of work lost due to family (primarily children's) illnesses compared to employed fathers (Carpenter, 1980). Missing work to care for a child who has a sore throat is not a mere inconvenience; it may also seriously reduce a woman's job opportunities. The world of work assumes key participants will not be taking off time to care for dependents; anyone (female or male) who takes home responsibilities more seriously than work risks losing promotion opportunities or even the job itself.

Furthermore, the care-giving role requires many women to forgo paid jobs to care for a chronically disabled relative. Although there may also be some rewards for such duties, caring for some homebound sick persons can be a twenty-four-hour-a-day responsibility, leaving little time for personal needs. One study found that 40 percent of the women in households that included older parents requiring care spent the equivalent time of a full-time job providing that care (Newman, 1976). A report issued by the Older Women's League noted that women spend an average of seventeen years caring for children and eighteen years assisting aged parents. Some 35 percent of the persons giving care to the elderly are themselves older than sixty-five (cited in the *New York Times,* May 13, 1989; see also Lewin, 1989).

Few families can afford many of the time- or labor-saving arrangements that might relieve care givers' burdens; domestic help, day care, or elevators, and hydraulic lifts, for example, are expensive. Where they exist, some community nursing and social service agencies and volunteer groups do help families with certain of these needed resources. For example, in the United States the hospice movement provides support services for some families of persons who choose to die at home rather than in the hospital. Other support available in some areas include adult day care centers, hot meal delivery services, and visiting physical therapists. Especially in the United States, however, very few of the costs of home health care are provided under the terms of health insurance or government medical programs, and many Americans lack adequate insurance coverage to pay even for available services (see, for example, an analysis of policies and resources for family care of elderly and disabled persons by Moroney, 1980).

The assumption that the health and illness care role belongs to the wife-mother is so pervasive that media and health education programs assume that women will rearrange their lives to provide for the health of their families. One British health education project published a pamphlet urging measures women should take to prevent their husbands from having heart attacks. It recommended, for example, that

> The sensible wife will first decide whether her husband should lose weight, and then plan his menu accordingly. Pressure and pace at work, family responsibilities and general worries can be controlled to some extent by the man himself. . . . But perhaps more important is the tolerance and understanding of his wife. Let your husband talk about his worries, and whenever possible

take the work from him—draft letters, pay bills, arrange for the plumber to come yourself (quoted in Graham, 1985).

In efforts to contain rising medical costs, the notions of community care and home health provision have become attractive government policy emphases (discussed further in Chapter 12). Earlier discharge from hospitals, for example, means that recuperating patients return home needing more extensive lay nursing care for longer periods. New technologies make possible the home administration of some fairly sophisticated therapies, such as kidney dialysis and intravenous feeding and medicating. The cost savings of performing these procedures at home is considerable. For example, in 1988 kidney dialysis in a hospital or clinic cost about $2,000 per month, compared with $1,200 per month for home dialysis; feeding by the tube cost about $23,800 a month in a hospital, but only $6,000 a month at home (Findlay, 1988). These procedures are not usually done by the sick person without help, however. In addition to requiring visits from skilled nurses who teach the procedures, supervise home treatment, and monitor the sick person's condition, much home care involves the extensive commitment of family members. As several studies have documented, "community" care is typically given by relatives, not the whole community or even the neighborhood. Furthermore, care by relatives typically means care by female kin. One British study of community care concluded " 'most carers are women and . . . most women will at some time in their lives become carers' " (quoted in Graham, 1985: 44).

This policy shift toward home care is developing precisely at a time when women are beginning to achieve somewhat greater equity in educational and occupational opportunities. Not only are women workers less eager to take on such additional care burdens, but the larger proportion of women in the work force also results in fewer (women) volunteers available for neighborhood assistance to those who need help at home. The policy shift also comes as nurses and other health care workers are struggling to achieve greater recognition (and pay) for the work they do (Brown, 1983).

Although moving more care of the sick to the home superficially appears to be demedicalization, note that it is not the *doctors'* tasks or fees that are being reduced by earlier release from the hospital, but rather the more "menial" tasks of care, which are being transferred to the family or family-paid workers. Whereas previously these tasks would have been done in the hospital by low-paid nurses' aides and practical nurses (LPNs), they are now transferred to unpaid relatives, who are sometimes assisted by very low-paid home health workers; all are women typically (see Fine, 1988). On the other hand, it is nurses—not doctors—who usually make the home visits and monitor acute episodes of the home-bound sick. The nature of professional home nursing does appear to be a move away from a highly medicalized model, partly because it emphasizes teaching the sick person and family to care for themselves.[2] One community health nurse noted that her work was unlike that of doctors or hospital nurses, because she works with the patient in the physical and social context of the family and home life, emphasizing the personal caring aspect of nursing. She added, "In a holistic sense, community health nurses are healers."

The policy move to community-based health care has *not* usually reduced physician control and potential income, however. The home birth movement, for example, has been vigorously suppressed. In the United States, although some physicians have supported the practice of out-of-hospital births, professional organizations such as the American College of Obstetricians and Gynecologists have vigorously opposed it. Certification for trained midwives is available only to registered nurses who have taken extra training, but even these certified nurse-midwives have been severely restricted in their attempts to practice independent of physician control and have had great difficulty obtaining malpractice insurance. The virtual monopoly of obstetricians and hospitals has thus been preserved (Levin and Idler, 1981: 83–103; Romalis, 1985).

Mutual Aid

Self-help and mutual aid groups are another form of hidden health care. These voluntary associations offer *reciprocal* help, usually among persons with similar health needs. The mutual quality of this aid is the key feature distinguishing these groups from professional health care. Members exchange roles as provider and receiver of health and illness care (see Caplan and Killilea, 1976; Levin and Idler, 1981; Levin et al., 1976; Katz and Bender, 1976; Katz, 1979, Katz and Levin, 1980). Examples include support groups such as those for persons with certain diseases (e.g., epilepsy and Parkinson's disease) or disabling conditions (e.g., chronic pain), or who have undergone certain operations (e.g., mastectomies or colostomies) or other traumatic experiences (e.g., the suicide of loved one or rape). Some communities also have volunteer health help that is more one-sided, such as volunteer ambulance and emergency squads.

Self-help groups typically offer their members much mutual social support, concrete suggestions about how to manage the many day-to-day problems, information about their condition and various therapeutic possibilities, and advice about dealing with family, friends, and medical profes-

---

[2]The work of community health nurses (including many nurse-practitioners and nurse-midwives) is comparable to that of their predecessors, public health nurses, who since the 1920s enjoyed greater professional autonomy and respect in their work than did hospital- or office-based nurses (see Melosh, 1982: 113–157). Physicians, however, have perceived them as professional competitors and have often fought to prevent laws that would permit these nurses to work independently. Since nurse-practitioners can provide primary care, comparable to physicians', for about 80 percent of the patients in ambulatory clinics, there are many possibilities for status and role conflicts between the two gender-stratified occupations (Little, 1982; see also Lurie, 1981).

sionals (cf. Morgan et al., 1984; Droge et al., 1986). One aim is to break the isolation of those whose regular networks may not include anyone in a similar situation. As one member explained, " 'In the beginning one is truly cut off, one feels completely different from everyone else. . . . The healthy cannot understand the sick, one really belongs to a world apart' " (quoted in Herzlich and Pierret, 1987: 220).

Mutual help groups appear to be feature of lay health care especially in the United States, where they mesh with cultural values and historical experience of mutual and self-reliance (see Risse et al., 1977). The movement is also widespread in northern Europe and growing rapidly throughout Europe (World Health Organization, 1981). While not specifically organized as self-help groups, similar functions are also performed by healing cults in many traditional societies. For example, in rural Turkey a traditional form of reciprocity is *dertleşmek,* in which neighbors express and share their joys, sorrows, and problems. The therapeutic value of *dertleşmek* has been demonstrated among Turkish immigrant women in Belgium (Devisch and Gailly, 1985).

There is considerable diversity in the social organization of these groups, with many of the long-term groups imitating professional, bureaucratic healthcare organizations, yet many others remaining adamantly loosely organized lay groups. Some are formed at lay initiative; others have been created by helping professions for their clients. Thus there is a difference in the degree of independence of power experienced, for example, by a group of chronically ill persons who organize to do something for themselves and each other, as compared with a therapy group organized by the outreach staff of a hospital.

Mutual help groups also vary greatly in the degree to which they have assumed any political agenda or recognized any of the political issues implicit in self-care or mutual aid. The Independent Living Movement for persons with disabilities and chronic illnesses and the Women's Health Movement have taken a politically activist stance (see Ruzek, 1979; Crewe and Zola, 1983; Doyal, 1983; Tudiver, 1986).

Assuming self-care and mutual responsibility in the face of illness, however, also have *implicit* political consequences, because the sick persons take an active and often knowledgeable role in the treatment of their own sickness. They often consider their proficiency in treating their particular illness to be superior to that of the professionals (cf. Herzlich and Pierret, 1987: 217–218). For example, diabetics who must give themselves frequent injections and persons with renal (kidney) failure who may perform their dialysis at home often distrust having those services performed in hospital. People who have had long experience managing their chronic illness or disability often gain considerable expertise about their condition, and are more likely to expect doctors and other medical personnel to share power with them.

Our recognition of this hidden health care system helps us to understand better the full range of activities people engage in to keep well or to treat illnesses. Not all outside help is professional medical care. Beyond the lay help of home, neighborhood, and mutual aid groups, there are a number of nonmedical healing alternatives that people may seek.

ALTERNATIVE HEALING SYSTEMS

People's belief systems inform their decisions as to when they need help and which kinds of help are appropriate. Even in modern Western societies, where biomedicine is the dominant medical paradigm, people may use several healing systems simultaneously with biomedicine. A study (McGuire, 1988) of middle-class Americans who used various alternative, spiritual healing approaches (e.g., Christian faith healing, psychic healing, and Eastern or occult healing) found that virtually all adherents used both biomedical *and* alternative systems. Furthermore, their beliefs shaped how they combined these various approaches. For example, one man had his broken arm x-rayed and set in a cast by medical professionals at the hospital, but followed this treatment with frequent prayers at home and in his religious group. He believed that the prayers resulted in faster and more effective healing. Adherents of the various alternative healing approaches felt that medical doctors were not necessarily the best source of help for such problems as chronic pain and illness, because they treat the symptoms, not the cause. These adherents believed that the "real" causes of such illnesses were spiritual (or the socioemotional by-products of spiritual problems). Thus by definition modern medicine alone was not a sufficient source of help (McGuire, 1988).

Even people who are not consciously using alternative belief systems seek different sources of healing help, depending upon how they understand or express their problems. Someone with back pain, for example, might consult a pharmacist, massage therapist, orthopedist, physiatrist, or chiropractor, depending upon how the person interpreted the pain, its seriousness, and its possible causes. For many people, seeking help for health or illness includes several options in addition to orthodox medical care.

Nonallopathic Practitioners

One longstanding alternative source of health-related help is a professional practitioner from a formal healing system other than allopathy. Although **allopathy** is only one approach to doctoring, as described in Chapter 10, it has attained a virtual monopoly of medical education, licensing, and practice in the United States and Canada. It is also the dominant form of medicine practiced in most of Europe, although some nonallopathic approaches have greater legitimacy and freedom there than in North America. Medical systems that dissent from the dominant one have often been called sects, being seen as analogous to religious sects that dissent from the established church (see Jones, 1985). These medical systems are based upon completely different, competing paradigms of illness causation and cure.

Probably the best-known alternatives in the United States are two nineteenth-century challenges to allopathy: chiropractic and osteopathy, therapeutic systems based on the idea that malalignments of the musculo-skeletal system also produce problems in the neuro-endocrine system. Osteopathy has become largely subordinated within regular (allopathic) medical practice and licensing. Until the 1980s, chiropractic was actively suppressed by the AMA and licensing legislation. Although it has since gained greater legitimacy and recognition (e.g., chiropractic treatment is now covered by much health insurance), chiropractic is still viewed by many (or most) medical practitioners as an unacceptable alternative to diagnosis and treatment by a medical doctor (Wardwell, 1983; see also Albrecht and Levy, 1982; Baer, 1984, 1987; Coburn and Biggs, 1986).

There are few studies on how patients combine the use of both chiropractic and medical doctors. Apparently some persons use the chiropractor as their main physician, turning to medical doctors occasionally if referred by the chiropractor or if they believe they need medication (which chiropractors cannot prescribe). Others use medical doctors as their primary physician, seeking chiropractors when the malady is something medical doctors do not treat effectively. Relatively few medical doctors reciprocate in referring patients to chiropractors. Indeed, until 1979 the AMA forbade its members to make such referrals (*New York Times*, 1979).

Homeopathy, a holistic form of pharmacological therapeutics developed in the early nineteenth century (Kaufman, 1971), is now more common in Europe and Latin America than in the United States. In England, for example, homeopathic physicians are licensed to practice and are reimbursed under the National Health Service. The homeopathic movement also encourages laypersons to self-treat certain illnesses and to learn to use some of the homeopathic medicines (Coulter, 1984).

Like homeopathy, naturopathy utilizes presumably milder medicines, primarily herbs. One form of naturopathy, Thompsonism, was influential in the United States in the eighteenth and nineteenth centuries because it was linked with the rising tide of political populism and the needs for lay modes of healing in frontier and other rural communities (Cassedy, 1977; Numbers, 1977). The various natural health movements were generally suppressed in the United States, but in some European countries, such as Germany, these practices were more acceptable as a complement to biomedicine (Maretzki and Seidler, 1985; Roth, 1976). Contemporary versions of naturopathy as well as homeopathy appear to be increasingly used in the United States and Britain, perhaps as a result of dissatisfaction with the dominant, allopathic medical system (Taylor, 1984).

Another extant nineteenth-century alternative to allopathy is hydrotherapy, which utilizes water (e.g., baths, mineral water, and mud) for treatments. There are few sociological studies of the extent of use of these alternative therapeutic systems, but evidence suggests that they are used in conjunction with biomedicine, although without the knowledge of the patients' medical doctors. One German study found that an estimated 30 to 40 percent of patients of medical doctors also consulted such nonallopathic practitioners as homeopaths, naturopaths, and hydrotherapists (Haehn, 1980).

Some traditional Oriental medical practices have recently been introduced into Western societies.[3] The paradigms of illness and healing of such therapies as acupressure, acupuncture, and Oriental herbal medicine are very different from those of Western biomedicine. Acupressure, or *shiatsu*, is generally administered like a massage, so it is not in direct competition with licensed medicine, but neither is it typically covered by medical insurance. Acupuncture, which involves the insertion of needles, is under tighter legal control. In most of the United States nonphysician acupuncturists are required to work under the supervision of licensed doctors, although some states have made allowances for licensing nonphysician acupuncturists (who, ironically, are often better trained as acupuncturists than physicians who took relatively brief training in the method). Patients who utilize acupuncture alongside regular medical treatment often do not tell their own physicians for fear of alienating them (Kotarba, 1975).

Because these alternative medical systems are in direct competition with allopathic medicine, political and legal maneuvers regarding their practice have concrete economic effects. Like allopathic medicine, these alternatives are organized as professional practices, with their own body of knowledge, training and certification standards, code of ethics, and organizations (see the review of literature in Cassidy et al., 1985). Like biomedicine, they rely largely upon learned diagnostic and therapeutic techniques, which do not require the patient to understand or agree with the underlying paradigm in order to be effectively treated.

Indigenous Healers and Healing Groups

The acceptance of an underlying belief system is more likely to be a feature of **indigenous healing**, or native, folk, or popular practices for health and healing. Anthropologists have documented a vast array of such systems around the globe. The early literature, however, generally assumed

---

[3]Professionalized practice is also a feature of other Asian medical traditions, such as Ayurvedic and Yunani medicine, but these have not been extensively "borrowed" by Westerners (see Kleinman et al., 1978; Leslie, 1976).

that as societies became modernized and Westernized, they would shed these "primitive" beliefs and practices and substitute the biomedical system, but this expectation has not been borne out (Kleinman, 1984).

Furthermore, indigenous healing has remained widespread in modern industrialized societies. Social scientists once interpreted these beliefs and practices as remnants of peasant, old-country traditions or as characteristic of uneducated, lower-class persons who could not afford modern medical treatment. Although there appear to be different healing systems operating in the various subcultures of modern societies, indigenous healing beliefs and practices are in fact relatively widespread among educated, fully acculturated, and economically secure persons (McGuire, 1988; see also Wagner, 1983; Westley, 1983).

The sheer diversity of indigenous health and healing beliefs and practices makes it very difficult to generalize about these alternative options. Some indigenous practices are conducted by healers—lay specialists who have particular knowledge and/or spiritual or natural "gifts" for healing. Other indigenous healing is done by the sick person or nonspecialists in the group. In the United States, for example, indigenous healing approaches include those of spiritual healers, mediums, shamans, herbalists, lay midwives, fire doctors (for burn pain), bone setters, leg lengtheners, astrologists and spiritual advisers, and occult healers. Indigenous healing also includes a wide variety of meditation approaches, prayer, spiritual exercises, massage and other "body work," exercise disciplines, and martial arts.

Although most indigenous healing occurs outside orthodox medical practice and is generally denigrated by the medical establishment, a number of medical doctors have incorporated some of these alternative practices into their treatment of patients. One study of these physicians found that their personal web of experiences, including religion and spirituality or their own illness or pain experiences, led them to integrate alternative approaches with mainstream medical practices. It concluded that dissension among physicians may be greater than the professional organizations would like to acknowledge, and that many so-called mainstream physicians hold views about health and healing and behave in ways that deviate from mainstream medical norms (Goldstein et al., 1987).

One small fringe of indigenous *and* orthodox medical practice includes what has been called "quackery," or fraudulent healing, usually for financial gain. Much labeling of quackery has been the effort of the medical profession to suppress any competition to its professional dominance. For example, the AMA funds a Bureau of Investigation to trace "quacks" and aid in their legal control and prosecution (Young, 1967). This effort also polices the AMA's ranks, since many "quacks" are medical doctors who deviate from acceptable professional standards (Roebuck and Hunter, 1975; Young, 1967).

Because indigenous healing, by contrast, is loosely organized, there are no clear-cut boundaries for acceptable practice. To the extent that indigenous healers are members of an established community in which they work, however, ordinary social control is operative. Someone who is believed to be pretending to heal and exploiting neighbors' needs in time of trouble would almost certainly be punished. When indigenous healing occurs more anonymously (e.g., by a traveling healer or advertised nostrums), there is greater potential for deliberately fake healing. Most indigenous healing, however, is comparatively sincere; it is practiced by people—healers and patients alike—who, to some degree, share a belief system in which that approach to healing is plausible and indeed advisable.

Some of these alternative approaches are systematized by recognized movements; others are developed by independent healers, often drawing eclectically from a wide range of Western and non-Western traditions. The various spiritual healing approaches are generally based upon a larger religious belief system. For example, healing done in pentecostal prayer groups is not an isolated activity of the group but an expression of the groups' larger belief that God acts directly in believers' everyday lives in response to their prayer and faith.

Spiritual healing is rather widespread, even in modern Western societies. Obvious examples include Christian faith healing, Christian Science and other New Thought healing, psychic healing, and healing approaches imported from various Eastern spiritual traditions such as Zen and Tibetan Buddhism and Jainism (Braden, 1963; Csordas and Cross, 1976; Johnson et al., 1986; McGuire, 1982; 1988; Moody, 1974; Nudelman, 1976; Poloma, 1985; Skultans, 1974; Tipton, 1982; Wagner, 1983; Westley, 1983).

Ethnic and other subcultural belief systems inform the indigenous healing practices of most ethnic groups in the United States (and elsewhere). The healing actions of such persons as the Mexican-American *curanderos*, Navaho singers, Puerto Rican *espiritistos*, Hawaiian *kahunas*, Eskimo shamans, or Haitian voodoo healers are based upon complex systems of ideas about illness and power (Garrison, 1977; Gill, 1981; Harwood, 1977; Hill, 1973; Kiev, 1968; Murphy, 1964; Scott, 1974; Snow, 1974; Snyder, 1983; Trotter and Chavira, 1981; Vogel, 1970).

The Effectiveness of Indigenous Healing

The foremost reason why people use indigenous healing is that it *makes sense* to them. Indigenous healing beliefs are plausible, especially to people who grew up in a culture or subculture in which they were common. Indigenous healing "works" partly by fitting into people's understandings of their world and how it operates. Young (1976: 8) pointed out that therapies are considered efficacious not merely when they are a means of curing sickness,

Box 9-1   One American Healer[4]

Marge is a forty-eight-year-old pediatric nurse employed full-time in a large hospital in a suburban community. She is successful in her career, with the appropriate advanced degrees and experience for high level positions, although she has not chosen to leave active nursing for administration. Her husband is a senior partner in a law firm in a nearby city. The couple has four grown children. . . .

Marge is involved . . . in several groups using alternative healing. She personally utilizes some Eastern methods . . . but she does not teach these methods nor is she affiliated with a group in which Eastern spirituality is a focus. As a nurse, she has used Therapeutic Touch for about three years. She uses her psychic healing methods to "get in touch with" the pain and suffering of the children in her ward; patients do not need to know that she is "sending" them healing energies. Privately, she has been practicing psychic healing for about six years; her methods are eclectic and she tries new "modalities" as she learns about them, discarding some approaches, keeping others. Her main support group is a psychic healing circle that meets each week in members' homes. . . . When she seeks healing for herself, she usually turns to the members of this group. In addition, she attends the monthly or weekly meetings of three regional holistic health and metaphysical societies. These meetings are important sources of new ideas and techniques. She has also taken numerous workshops and short courses on various alternative methods: foot reflexology, rebirthing, and crystal and color healing.

Marge does healing almost any time, any place and with anyone—including many people who do not know she is "sending" them healing energy. Marge described working on healing herself and others even while doing the dishes or in the elevator at work. Sometimes she engaged in it deliberately; other times, she felt, it was simply a part of her being. She stated: "I believe that in every moment of my life I release energy to those around me. I think everybody needs it every moment. . . . I feel that whoever makes connection with me or I make connection with them, I'm using my energy to heal."

She is also a good example of the general lack of clear financial motivation on the part of many "expert" alternative healers. She charges private clients only a nominal fee (from $15 to $30, depending upon ability to pay) for a thirty-to-ninety-minute session, and she earns about $100 to $150 (depending upon the number of registrants) for teaching a day-long workshop. These services are, however, occasional and minor sources of income for Marge. Her professional salary, combined with that of her husband, supports a high standard of living; Marge views her paid work as healer as a sideline, done mainly as a service.

Source: From *Ritual Healing in Suburban America* by Meredith B. McGuire with the assistance of Debra Kantor. Copyright © 1988, by Rutgers, The State University. Reprinted with permission of Rutgers University Press.

---

[4]This is a composite portrait to protect the identity of the actual healers studied.

"equally important, [when] they are a means by which specific, named ¿nds of sickness are defined and given culturally recognizable forms".

Indigenous healing forms and transforms the illness experience. It utilizes symbols and ritual action, meaningful to believers or members of that culture, that can produce change on several levels: social, bodily, and emotional.[5] A number of studies of symbolic healing suggest that just as mind, body, and society are linked in illness causation, so too are they (potentially at least) part of the healing process (Csordas, 1983; Devisch, 1987; Dow, 1986; McGuire, 1983; Moerman, 1979).

The therapeutic practices themselves also make sense to members of the subcultural group. To an outsider, the Vermont folk remedy of a honey-vinegar mixture may seem nonsensical and repulsive. To persons raised in that rural New England subculture, however, it may be a plausible and appealing way of conceptualizing problems of health and illness; the remedy invokes images of benign nature, living "near to the soil," and being in harmony with the laws of nature by which health is maintained and produced (Atkinson, 1978).

In summarizing several outcome studies, which generally evaluate the results of healing efforts in terms of Western medical as well as indigenous standards, Kleinman (1984: 150) observed, "These studies document three things: that folk healers are frequently effective, that there are limits to their efficacy, and that, while toxicities of folk healing are infrequent, they do occur."[6]

This summary, along with Kleinman's caution that each form of healing has to be viewed in its own social context, probably also applies not only to folk healers but to the full range of alternative healing practices in modern Western societies.

---

[5]Biomedicine also uses symbols of power to enhance its effectiveness. For example, a pill may symbolize medical power to cure inside the body (Pellegrino, 1976). Surgery, lab tests, and diet regimens may likewise be used as ritual symbols (cf. Posner, 1977). Medical costumes and settings (e.g., stethoscopes and white uniforms) symbolize professional expertise. Such symbols increase trust and expectancy and, indirectly, may increase healing effectiveness (Frank, 1973). Much of what is called the placebo effect may in fact be related to symbolic healing (Moerman, 1983).

[6]We need to keep in mind that the *exact* same generalizations could be made about healing by medical doctors: They are frequently effective, their efficacy is limited, and some treatments are dangerous or iatrogenic. This evaluation does not mean, however, that one should not consult a doctor, but it does imply we should be cautious about naive assumptions that medical treatment is necessarily beneficial or safe. Likewise, we should avoid romantic notions that folk healing is necessarily beneficial or safe. The effort to evaluate or compare the effectiveness of folk healing with medical healing is greatly complicated by the fact that because they typically operate with totally different paradigms, their notions of what constitutes a "successful" healing are very different. While there is much overlap in what problems they consider to need healing, folk and medical healing usually have very different goals. Thus efforts to compare them or to evaluate one by the terms of the other are greatly confounded.

ADHERENCE TO THERAPEUTIC RECOMMENDATIONS

Part of the health-seeking process is whether and how the sick person follows the recommended therapeutic procedures. For example, is a recommended diet followed? Are prescriptions filled and medicines taken? A medical doctor's recommendations may not be the only course of action to which a sick person would adhere; the advice of a lay consultant, an herbalist, a massage therapist, or spiritual healer might also be considered. Some sick persons deliberately seek several opinions—medical or otherwise—and therefore obtain several therapeutic recommendations. Adherence thus implies actively choosing which advice to follow.

Some formulations of the sick role have included following the doctor's orders as a role expectation (see Chapter 6). Many doctors, likewise, consider it a patient's duty to comply with their therapeutic regimen. The very notion of patient compliance implies a power relationship: The doctor is treated as authoritative and powerful, the patient as powerless and appropriately obedient (Chrisman, 1977; Stimson, 1974).

A number of studies show that health care professionals greatly underestimate the amount of patients' nonadherence to medical regimens (see the review of literature in DiMatteo and Friedman, 1982: 35–57; Kasl, 1975; Stimson, 1974). Since patients do not want to alienate their doctors, they often hide their nonadherence to the doctors' recommendations and the extent of their search for other opinions. Many patients, especially those dealing with chronic illnesses, develop their own strategies for managing their illness. Such strategies include the selective use of biomedical approaches, but often also involve other therapeutic approaches, advice from more than one doctor, and/or their tailoring of the doctor's advice. From the patients' point of view, such noncompliant health-seeking behavior is rational, and it preserves for them some element of control (Herzlich and Pierret, 1987; see also Alexander, 1982).

Rather than conceptualizing the sick person's role in terms of degree of compliance with doctors' orders, it is useful to understand the meaning of medications and other therapies from the perspective of the sick person. One study found that many people with epilepsy modify and self-regulate their use of prescribed medications in an attempt to assert a degree of control over their condition (Conrad, 1985; see also Trostle et al., 1983). In a similar assertion of control, hemodialysis patients from a wide range of educational and ethnic backgrounds utilized nonprescribed treatments (e.g., special diets and exercises, religious and folk healing, herbal treatments, massage, and acupuncture) without the knowledge of their medical doctors (Snyder, 1983).

Noting the extent of nonadherence to doctor's recommendations, Zola (1983: 217) argued that to "take one's medicine" is in no sense the "natural thing" for patients to do. If anything, a safer working assumption is that most patients regard much of their medical treatment as unwanted, intrusive, disruptive, and the manner in which it is given presumptuous.

The patient is engaged in an ongoing process of evaluation of recommended therapies; whether the recommendation is medically correct is only one, sometimes minor criterion in this evaluation. Other criteria include such matters as: Does the doctor appear to understand my illness correctly? Do the doctor's methods of diagnosis, interpersonal style, and treatment meet my expectations of competent? Is there a safer, more pleasant, or less drastic alternative (especially to surgery and powerful medications)? Does it feel like this therapy is working? When dissatisfied, patients may try to modify the treatment either by negotiating with their doctor or by modifying the plan by themselves (i.e., noncompliance). Both approaches represent patients' attempt to assert some control (Hayes-Bautista, 1976).

Much patient nonadherence can be traced to difficulties of understanding and communication in the doctor-patient interaction (Svarstad, 1976), as described further in Chapter 10. Part of the "problem," however, is due to important differences in the perspectives and goals of doctors and their patients. The doctor's focus is typically upon curing or managing the specific disease presented by the patient. Laypersons, by contrast, are more likely to have a broader notion of health and illness and to be concerned with all aspects of their life, not merely one health problem, no matter how serious. For example, a patient may feel that the depression experienced as a side effect of blood pressure medicine is so debilitating that continuing the medication is not worth the price (cf. Twaddle, 1981b).

Often the decision not to follow the doctor's recommended course of action (or not to seek professional help in the first place) is due to a discrepancy between the layperson's and the professional's understandings of the sickness. For example, in rural Appalachian culture there is a common belief that the purpose of medical treatment is to cure sickness. There is a profound suspicion of medical practitioners, especially in their treatment of chronic illnesses (such as coal miners' black lung disease), because they charge fees and require repeated visits but cannot actually cure the disease. Lay conceptions of black lung in particular hold the progressive deterioration to be an inevitable, irreversible consequence of working in the mines. Thus health care programs designed to ameliorate some effects of the disease have not had much success in attracting participants or generating adherence to regimens of exercise and diet (Friedl, 1982).

A Massachusetts study of sufferers of specific chronic illnesses found that primary care physicians and nurse practitioners showed very limited knowledge of their patients' conceptions of these illnesses. While professionals were more likely to know the beliefs of college-educated patients than those of less-educated patients, overall they understood the lay explanatory models used by less than half of the patients in the study (Helman, 1985). This lack of shared understanding of the nature of the illness is likely to lead to considerable nonadherence to doctors' orders and to dissatisfaction on the part of both medical professionals and their patients.

Adherence to any therapeutic regimen is likely to require some effort. The sheer logistics of putting all recommendations into effect are enormous, especially for chronic illness, for which the therapeutic regimen must last a lifetime and is likely to become more demanding as the condition deteriorates. Health seeking is an active process throughout, but the active participation of the sick person is especially evident when it comes to choosing and putting some or all therapeutic advice into effect.

SUMMARY

The process by which people seek health is an active one. Both preventive care and the treatment of problems involve numerous decisions about the body and its needs. Self-treatment is far more common than treatment by professionals, medical or nonmedical. In addition to professional medical care, there is a vast hidden health care system providing advice, preventive and therapeutic care, emotional and practical support, and guidance in the search for professional care.

Orthodox Western biomedicine is only one of several healing systems available in most societies. Other options include nonallopathic practitioners, and various indigenous healers and healing groups. The individual, then, has a range of health-seeking options. Even after consulting outside help, the individual also chooses which advice or therapeutic regimens to accept and put into practice.

RECOMMENDED READINGS

Articles

Noel J. Chrisman, "The health-seeking process: An approach to the natural history of illness," *Culture, Medicine, and Psychiatry* 1, 1977: 351–377.

Hilary Graham, "Providers, negotiators, and mediators: Women as the hidden carers," pp. 25–52 in E. Lewin and V. Olesen, eds., *Women, Health, and Healing: Toward a New Perspective.* New York: Tavistock, 1985.

Books

Alan Harwood, *Rx: Spiritist as Needed: A Study of a Puerto Rican Community Mental Health Resource.* New York: Wiley, 1977. This highly readable ethnography describes the beliefs and practices underlying the use of Puerto Rican spiritual healers in a U.S. urban environment.

Lily M. Hoffman, *The Politics of Knowledge: Activist Movements in Medicine and Planning*. Ithaca: State University of New York Press, 1989. The author presents case studies of activist movements that challenged the occupational self-interest of professions, especially the medical profession.

Lowell S. Levin and Ellen L. Idler, *The Hidden Health Care System: Mediating Structures and Medicine*. Cambridge, MA: Ballinger, 1981. A highly readable synthesis of the literature on the role of families, self-care, religious groups, community groups, and mutual aid in the larger system of health care.

Meredith B. McGuire, with the assistance of Debra Kantor, *Ritual Healing in Suburban America*. New Brunswick, NJ: Rutgers University Press, 1988. This study describes the beliefs and practices of middle-class, educated, suburbanites who use various nonmedical healing alternatives (such as faith healing, meditation, psychic healing, acupressure, and massage) in addition to medical treatment.

Chapter Nine

The Social Construction of Medical Knowledge

Our culture and social structure shape the way we understand and interpret our bodies, illness, and disease as well as whether or how we perceive illness. This chapter examines how what we know about illnesses is socially constructed, used, and changed.

A sociological approach to knowledge about illness differs from the biomedical approach in that it does not assume the objective existence of what medicine categorizes as disease.[1] The sociologist does not take for granted that disease entities exist in nature and await "discovery." This perspective does not mean that people's health conditions have no objective foundation. People do experience real pain, sickness, and death. This approach does, however, mean that laypersons' and professionals' *ideas* about illness are **social constructions**, or the result of human activity. Therefore, no matter how empirically precise these ideas are, they are always open to the influence of social factors in their production, transmission, and development. The very fact that medical ideas are bound by assumptions implicit in a language and a culture's rules for producing knowledge means they are always delimited in their representation of the real world (see Young, 1978).

MEDICAL IDEAS AND SOCIAL FORCES

These ideas about body, health, and disease are nonetheless very powerful in shaping a society's medical reality. The knowledge held by any given culture or group is the product of its social history. Western medicine's knowledge of its disease categories is a social product, as is the knowledge of diseases in other medical systems, such as Ayurvedic medicine in Asia and *curanderismo* in Latin America.

In Chapter 8 we described lay conceptions of health, illness, and the body. By contrast, formal medical knowledge in Western societies is typically highly specialized and based upon bioscientific theories and categories of thought. The contemporary medical paradigm represents a major historical change in how the body is viewed. Scientific **paradigms** are frameworks of formal knowledge that members of a given scientific community share, mainly due to having undergone similar educations and professional initiations; to sharing a common professional language, rules of evidence, and conceptual schemes; and to relying on the same professional literature and communication of the same scientific community (Kuhn, 1970: 176). These paradigms are rather like lenses; the world viewed through one paradigm looks very different from the world viewed through another. We

---

[1]Any social constructionist approach to knowledge must recognize how sociological ideas are in turn influenced by social processes and historical developments.

shall examine briefly the recent history of current medical paradigms and how they have come to have such powerful impact upon the practice of medicine and the development of the medical profession.

Although Western medical practice is based upon scientific knowledge, the practitioners themselves are not typically scientists. The scientist's objective is to gather empirical data, and to analyze, interpret, and generalize from these findings. Scientists are not necessarily concerned with the practical application of scientific knowledge. By contrast, the practitioner's goals is more pragmatic: to deal with the specific conditions of individual patients or clients. What the practitioner needs to know is likewise more practical. The only portion of medical knowledge relevant to doctors is that which relates to conditions they are most likely to encounter in clinical practice. Much medical knowledge is thus often "recipe knowledge," or "knowledge limited to pragmatic competence in routine performances" (Berger and Luckmann, 1967: 42). For example, pediatricians' use of immunizations does not require their detailed understanding of the latest scientific theories about the operations of the body's immune system (although their medical education typically introduced this subject). Rather, they rely upon "recipe knowledge" of which immunizations are recommended for children, at which ages, and with what common side-effects and contraindications. They also rely upon knowledge of where to turn when a situation is no longer routine.

A person's access to or possession of a valued form of knowledge can be an important factor in determining one's power and prestige in any society. For example, if the knowledge of how to make a valued ritual potion is held only by the women of a particular family, then their knowledge is the basis of some power or honor. Knowledge is unevenly distributed in a society, often along lines of gender, social class, age, ethnicity, and the division of labor (Berger and Luckmann, 1967: 76–81). Access to and possession of specialized, formal knowledge, such as medical knowledge, is particularly uneven. Because very few people in modern societies possess advanced medical knowledge or technical skills, being able to control such knowledge is the basis of rewards (e.g., high fees), power, and privilege. People who control specialized knowledge are thus in a position to limit the access of others to that knowledge (e.g., by controlling professional school admissions and discouraging laypersons from gaining knowledge). The social distribution of knowledge both reflects and shapes social distinctions of power and prestige.

"Discovering" Disease: A Historical Example

Many diseases that were diagnosed frequently in the past either are not commonly found today or are no longer recognized as diseases. Similarly, some conditions diagnosed as disease nowadays may very well cease to fit any disease category in the future. The forces shaping the "discovery" of disease categories are not purely objective, scientific factors; rather, value judgments, economic considerations, and other social concerns frequently enter the process. For instance, a famous physician during the American Revolution identified a disease he called "revolutiona," which was characterized by presumably irrational opposition to the "natural rule" of the English monarch (Conrad and Schneider, 1980: 49). In the 1850s, the classification of "diseases of the Negro race" included "drapetomania," which caused slaves to run away from their masters, and "dysaethesia aethiopis," which accounted for laggard work habits among slaves (see Cartwright, 1851). Disease categories thus have political uses, and those on whom they are imposed may suffer serious consequences.

A prime example of changing medical definitions is a disease, prevalent in the latter half of of the nineteenth century and the first part of the twentieth century, that had the following characteristics:

> It retards the growth, impairs the mental faculties and reduces the victim to a lamentable state. The person afflicted seeks solitude, and does not wish to enjoy the society of his friends; he is troubled with headache, wakefulness and restlessness at night, pain in various parts of the body, indolence, melancholy, loss of memory, weakness in the back and generative organs, variable appetite, cowardice, inability to look a person in the face, lack of confidence in his own abilities.
>
> When the evil has been pursued for several years, there will be an irritable condition of the system; sudden flushes of heat over the face; the countenance becomes pale and clammy; the eyes have a dull, sheepish look; the hair becomes dry and split at the ends; sometimes there is a pain over the region of the heart; shortness of breath; palpitation of the heart . . . ; the sleep is disturbed; there is constipation; cough; irritation of the throat; finally, the whole man becomes a wreck, physically, morally and mentally.
>
> Some of the consequences of [this disease] are epilepsy, apoplexy, paralysis, premature old age, involuntary discharge of seminal fluid, which generally occurs during sleep, or after urinating, or when evacuating the bowels. Among females, besides these other consequences, we have hysteria, menstrual derangement, catalepsy and strange nervous symptoms (Stout, 1885: 333–334).

This serious disease was onanism, better known as masturbation. The fact that the doctor writing this description of symptoms slips easily into referring to it as an "evil" alerts us to the strong moral connotations that this disease label carried. This supposedly scientific medical category thus clearly reflected the moral and social judgments of the doctors who applied it (cf. Engelhardt, 1978).

What functions did the identification of masturbation as a disease serve? For the distraught parents of a moody teenager, the label explained a wide range of behaviors. It is less likely that the young person experienced much relief at having this diagnosis applied to symptoms such as acne, poor appetite, or split ends. Another important function was to establish this "disease" as within the proper jurisdiction of the medical profession. The author of the above description concluded emphatically that "the treatment of this disease should be undertaken only by a skillful physician" (Stout, 1885: 334).

Applying the category of disease to masturbation implied etiological explanations. The **etiology** of an illness is a set of ideas about its causality in general or about the origins of a particular illness episode. Like all ideas, they are human constructions that change over time. Early etiological theories of masturbation implicated the loss of seminal fluid, whereas later theories emphasized the overstimulation of the nerves, which led to general debility. Several authorities held that all sexual activity was potentially debilitating, but that masturbation was especially injurious because it was "unnatural" and thus more likely to disturb the nerve tone (Engelhardt, 1978: 15–17). The diagnosis of masturbation as a disease syndrome is no longer common; indeed, in some medical and lay conceptions it is now considered to be quite normal and healthy.

Identifying a person's problems as the disease of masturbation subsequently implied a particular course of therapy in accordance with etiological ideas about the disease. Therapies were supposed to first, eliminate the practice and, second, calm the nerves and rebuild the person's sapped strength. Some of the more tolerant therapies included hard work, a simple diet, tonics, cold baths, sedatives and narcotics such as opium, and alternative sexual outlets such as prostitutes or mistresses (Engelhardt, 1978: 19). If these therapies were not successful, more drastic measures were often recommended, such as restraining devices, acid burns and rings inserted in the foreskin to make masturbation painful, circumcision (of males and females), clitoridectomy (surgical removal of the clitoris), vasectomy, acupuncture of the prostate or testicles, and even castration (Engelhardt, 1978; Barker-Benfield, 1975). Such a seriously debilitating disease required serious measures, including drastic surgery.

Those symptoms once clustered and classified as signs of the insidious disease of masturbation may still exist (e.g., some teenagers still have acne, split ends, and dull, sheepish looks), but the characteristics are no longer classified as a disease. Conversely, new classificaionts, such as premenstrual syndrome, have been defined into existence as a disease. Such new categories both justify medical control and legitimate the expense of medical care for that disease. For example, in the United States socially constructed disease categories are the only basis for most insurance reimbursement. The process by which symptoms are selectively clustered and defined as disease is a social process and reflects cultural assumptions and power relationships (see Johnson, 1987).

Science as a Social Product

With its emphasis upon a scientific model, biomedicine has developed increasingly complex **nosologies** or typologies of diseases. The medical model held that each particular disease could be characterized by a specific pathological configuration and attributed to a definite, unique cause. Thus medicine has emphasized the classification and description of all diseases. The movement toward ever more precise differentiations of medical nosologies and etiologies is based upon the assumption of **disease specificity**—the medical belief that each disease or syndrome has characteristic qualities and causes that are specific to that category of disease. This assumption has led to a focus on the individual rather than the social and contextual locus of sickness (Cassell, 1986; see also Dingwall, 1976: 50).

Medical ideas are the product of social processes and are continually changing. All scientific work involves the social construction of facts and interpretive schemes (Latour and Woolgar, 1979: 243; Berger and Luckmann, 1967: 60–72). Modern medical science strives to be as empirically neutral as possible, for example, by conducting blind experiments in which neither administrator nor subject knows whether a substance being given is the experimental substance or an inert control substance. Nevertheless, much medical research cannot be readily conducted neutrally, because— among other reasons—live human bodies are not readily detached from the persons who inhabit them. Thus neither the scientific observers nor the objects of scientific observation can have their influential social characteristics and attitudes eradicated.

Social, economic, and political factors greatly influence the scientific discovery of new diagnostic categories. Funding for research is largely dependent upon what is socially defined as a serious problem at the moment. For example, a disease syndrome known as GRID (Gay-Related Immune Deficiency) received relatively little medical attention or research funding, but when the same syndrome was later considered to be a national threat to the heterosexual population and redefined as AIDS (Acquired Immune Deficiency Syndrome), enormous increases in research funding enabled scientists to identify several variants of the syndrome and to describe some of the complex ways it can damage the body (see Shilts, 1987). Funding for research on what is now recognized as a serious international health problem was thus significantly delayed due to the politics surrounding a stigmatized illness.

Often the development of new disease categories is connected with the assertion of a new occupational specialization. Considerable professional prestige is attached to "discovering" and describing a "new" disease or syndrome. Finding new diseases is thus an active process; medicine is consciously oriented to creating disease categories where previously there were none (Freidson, 1970: 252). The case of menopause as a medical syndrome illustrates this process.

Creation of Medical "Problems": The Case of Menopause

Social and economic considerations promote the search for new diseases. For example, menopause, the period of women's lives in which menstruation naturally ceases, is now indexed in the *International Classification of Diseases* (1989: 524–525). While menopause is a normal biological process, in the last fifty years, it has come to be seen as a medical problem in the United States and many other Western societies. The Western biomedical literature generally treats menopause as an estrogen deficiency disease or ovarian dysfunction that produces various physical and emotional problems (see Bell, 1987; McCrea, 1983). There is, however, considerable cross-cultural variation in its biophysical, social, and emotional concomitants.

In our culture, symptoms such as hot flashes, headaches, dizziness, fatigue, anxiety, insomnia, irritability, depression, and general emotional problems are typically associated with menopause. Cross-cultural data suggest, however, that women's responses to the cessation of menstruation may be connected to the patterns of their roles. For example, in Islamic and many African societies, menopause brings relative freedom from many of the restrictions of women's lives: They are no longer required to be secluded, veiled, and restricted in their male company. These women experience few of the physiological and psychological symptoms attributed to menopause in Western societies (Townsend and Carbone, 1980). Menopause is thus a good example of how social meanings influence individuals' physical experiences and perceptions of their own bodies.

The Western medical construction of menopause, however, ignores these social meanings, reducing the experience to a set of biochemical processes presumed to characterize all female bodies, regardless of cultural or socioeconomic factors. Medical knowledge often becomes detached and independent of the research upon which it is based. Thus limitations in the original research are not taken into account in the accumulated stock of knowledge. For example, the medical construction of menopause is based in part on clinical studies with small numbers of subjects, typically drawn from patient populations—women whose menopause was surgically induced (e.g., through oophorectomy) or whose problems with menopause had already been medically defined as severe enough to warrant treatment. There are severe methodological limitations to such studies, and cautious researchers know not to generalize too extensively from them to the general populace. Unfortunately, once in the medical literature, these ideas are treated as facts that are presumably generalizable to all women (Kaufert, 1988). Part of the reason for this misuse of medical knowledge is that the medical construction of menopause meshes with physicians' assumptions about bodies and diseases. Thus to define and treat a normal process as a disease fits the medical model, and the idea that menopause is a disease implies a concrete medical course of action.

In the United States, the definition of menopause as a deficiency disease resulted from the professional efforts of a small, elite segment of the American medical profession during the 1930s and 1940s. A study of the medical literature during this transition shows that this process involved both the "discovery" of a theory of etiology of this "disease" and the development of pharmacologic methods of treatment. Using the paradigms of sex endocrinology, doctors attributed menopause to the deficiency of hormones (in particular, estrogen) regularly produced by the woman's body before cessation of menstruation. The development of an inexpensive synthetic estrogen replacement, DES (diethylstilbestrol), subsequently made the medical management of this "disease" possible (Bell, 1987).

Although these specialists acknowledged that most menopausal women (a common estimate was 85 percent) experienced few or no problems, the efficacy of DES created the possibility of treating *all* menopausal women. Indeed, despite growing criticism and concern over the safety of estrogen replacement therapy (some studies had linked it to cancer and some other serious conditions), by 1975 estrogens had become the fifth most frequently prescribed drug in the United States. A survey done the same year found that an estimated 51 percent of women had taken estrogen for at least three months, with a median use of ten years (see Kaufert and McKinlay, 1985; McCrea, 1983). In 1975 one gynecologist stated:

> I think of the menopause as a deficiency disease like diabetes. Most women develop some symptoms *whether they are aware of them or not,* so I prescribe estrogens for virtually all menopausal women for an indefinite period (quoted in Brody, 1975: 55 [emphasis added]).

In the mid-1970s the scientific literature firmly began to implicate estrogen therapy in iatrogenic diseases, (i.e., those caused by medical treatment). Debates over the curbing of estrogen replacement therapy involved conflicts between the pharmaceutical companies and the Food and Drug Administration, which ruled in 1976 that the industry must prepare a warning on the risks of estrogen for insertion in packages. Subsequently, estrogen use declined dramatically.

The conflict generated a debate within the medical profession itself, highlighting the differences in perspective between biomedical researchers and physicians in clinical practice (Kaufert and McKinlay, 1985). The definition of menopause as a deficiency disease resulted from the efforts of a small elite of specialists, together with the development of a disease etiology that lent itself to medical management and the promotion of a pharmacological agent that could be used in the treatment of the newly created disease.

Denial of Medical "Problems": Tardive Dyskinesia

Despite the general disposition to find new diseases and syndromes, the medical profession sometimes *resists* accepting new disease categories. Social and political factors also account for some contraints against medical "discovery." Tardive dyskinesia is a seriously debilitating, often irreversible disorder of the central nervous system, characterized by a variety of involuntary movements, most notably of the lips, jaw, and tongue. It is a "new" disorder partly because it is a pervasive, iatrogenic side effect of antipsychotic (neuroleptic) drugs, such as chlorpromazine, which came onto the market in the 1950s. In the 1960s and 1970s, the prevalence of tardive dyskinesia increased because neuroleptic drugs were being prescribed more frequently and in higher doses. Even after the syndrome had been identified and named in 1960, many clinicians did not accept or use the diagnostic category (Brown and Funk, 1986: 116–124).

One significant factor in this resistance was that acknowledging the existence and pervasiveness of tardive dyskinesia hurt the economic and political interests of many clinicians. The institutional and professional mandate to control the deviant behaviors of patients often superseded concerns for the drugs' physical risks for patients. The researchers and others who called attention to tardive dyskinesia were generally identified with the National Institute of Mental Health, medical schools, and research institutes, whereas the clinicians who dealt with patients with the syndrome were working in mental hospitals and private psychiatric practice.

Many clinicians simply did not *observe* the disease, even in patients with obvious symptoms. The professional self-interest of these psychiatrists was involved; they relied heavily upon pharmacological methods in their claims for efficacy in the treatment of psychoses, and their claims for recognition and remuneration as medical professionals were linked with their emphasis upon biopsychiatry and psychopharmacology. Since the patients were generally already defined as mentally ill, their complaints could be readily discounted and their overt symptoms attributed to other problems, such as brain disorders (Brown and Funk, 1986). The economic and political interests of these physicians prevented them from recognizing the disease they were creating.

IDEAS AND IDEOLOGIES

Despite the supposed value-neutrality and objectivity of "scientific" medicine, the knowledge produced, held, and used by its practitioners is, with considerable regularity, connected to their personal social location and the larger social situation of medical institutions in that society. In particular, social stratification (by criteria such as social class, age, political power, gender, and race) appears to be closely correlated with ideas about the body, health, illness, and healing. Thus medical ideas often reflect or serve as ideology.

Ideology is a system of ideas that explains and legitimates the actions and interests of a specific sector (i.e., class) of society. For example, when the coal mining industry was in conflict with coal miners' representatives over black lung disease, the medical ideology of the industry promoted a very narrow definition of the disease, thereby diminishing the industry's legal responsibility toward the victims and its social responsibility for prevention of the syndrome (see Smith, 1981, 1987).

Ideas about health and illness frequently serve as legitimations for the interests of one group over another. A **legitimation** is any form of socially established explanation that is given to justify a course of action (see Berger and Luckmann, 1967: 92–128). In Chapter 6, we examined how ideas of health and illness legitimate the larger social order. Here we shall focus on legitimations for the interests of certain social groups in the stratification system.

In Western industrialized societies, the medical profession has organized itself, as is described further below, specifically to promote its interests. Different professional interests pertain to other health-related occupations, such as nurses, pharmacists, x-ray technicians, midwives, and physical therapists. Incorporated into their ideas about health and healing are legitimations for their occupational statuses and income. Their knowledge about illness simultaneously legitimates their professional domain.

Other interests served by medical legitimation include those of the health-related industries: pharmaceutical industries, biotechnological industries, hospitals, nursing homes, and the medical, life, and disability insurance companies. Medical legitimations are especially important for various agencies of social control, such as the courts, mental hospitals, prisons, hospitals, and schools; this role will be discussed further below. Ideas about health and illness are also used to legitimate the interests of such parties as employers, workers, producers, consumers, polluters, environmentalists, and the military.

Ideology influences actions subtly, most often without the actors' awareness. It is incorporated in the language and rituals of everyday interaction, and thus comes to be taken for granted and unnoticed or unexamined (cf. Emerson, 1970; Fisher, 1986). For example, the language used in referring to a patient as "the broken hip in room 305" depersonalizes the ill person, transforming her into a "case" that can be "managed" more readily by a professional team. Even matters of professional dress (such as a uniform, clipboard, and stethoscope) subtly symbolize status differences.

Ideological aspects of thought and practice often go unnoticed because they are often self-confirming. Since ideology shapes people's expectations and what they consider to be evidence, it often produces evidence that confirms those expectations. If, for example, I expect old people to be befuddled, my observations of them are likely to confirm my expectation. Indeed, if an individual protests that he is not befuddled, I may interpret his protestations as further evidence that he is so confused that he cannot see the validity of my judgment. Also, when I treat him as befuddled, he may come to act that way and further confirm my prejudgment. The "evidence" that confirms my expectation is a self-fulfilling prophecy.

Although interest groups tend to be attracted to ideas and practices that mesh with their particular interests, the concept of ideology does not adequately predict any given individual's behavior. We should avoid using this term in any simplistic or deterministic sense. Material interests are not the only motivating force for individuals; for example, spiritual or altruistic motives might lead people to work for conditions that are not in their personal interest. Interest theories, however, suggest that in general people tend to hold ideas and engage in practices that serve or at least do not conflict with their own interests.

Some examples of medical practice in Western industrialized societies show the influence of ideological elements, but there are also ideological aspects to healing practices in other cultures as well. The following examples illustrate some ways that interests influence ideas of health and illness, medical research, and individual diagnosis and treatments in Western bioscientific medicine.

Medicalization

Medicalization is the process of legitimating medical control over an area of life, typically by asserting and establishing the primacy of a medical interpretation of that area (see Conrad and Schneider, 1980; Illich, 1975; Zola, 1983). The process of medicalization is illustrated by the medical treatment of pregnancy and childbirth, as doctors took over a substantial business previously done primarily by midwives.

With the medicalization of childbirth, aspects of women's reproductive lives that are not pathological were brought under the canopy definition of illness. Medical education for the new specialization of obstetrics and gynecology fostered the notion that the events of childbearing—pregnancy, labor and delivery, and puerperium (the period immediately following childbirth)—could best be understood in purely physical and pathological terms (Hahn, 1987). The medical profession persuaded the public and the regulators of health care that women needed doctors to manage their pregnancies and childbirth. There is extensive evidence, however, that initial medicalization was linked more with doctors' professional interests than with the patients' well-being. Indeed, when medical control over childbirth was first being consolidated, doctors and hospitals had abysmal records, especially for spreading infection to both mothers and babies (Oakley, 1984; Wertz and Wertz, 1977).

The interests of other groups also influence medical ideas and practice. Various industries often exert great pressure and economic influence on medical research. For example, the tobacco industry has spent very large sums of money trying to fight any authoritative medical conclusion that smoking is a health hazard. Manufacturers of products requiring government approval as being safe for sale also have considerable interests vested in the outcomes of research on their products.

Corporate Interests

A good example of how ideology figures into the definition of, diagnosis of, and response to illness can be seen in ideas about occupational health hazards. In recent years chemical companies, unions, workers' rights groups, medical authorities, and several government agencies have been involved in a growing confrontation over issues of the genetic protection of workers and their offspring. One episode occurred in 1979, when the Department of Labor cited and fined American Cyanamid for requiring women to be sterilized to keep their jobs at the company's lead pigments manufacturing operations in West Virginia. Numerous chemicals central to the manufacture of paints, pesticides, herbicides, plastics, and heavy metals have been strongly implicated in reproductive damage. Sterility, miscarriages, and birth defects have been identified with workers' exposure to these chemicals. The policy outcomes rest on several health-related ideas and issues, such as: Are these reproductive problems merely multiple coincidences? Are women more at risk than men (who also contribute genetic material to their offspring)? Are these reproductive problems only one manifestation of health threats (such as cancer) that might affect all workers? (Rawls, 1980; see also Henifin and Bertin, 1984; Marshall, 1987).

The companies that manufacture such products often sponsor research on these medical issues. In the mid-1960s Dow Chemical Company supported research on cytogenetics, a branch of genetics that focuses on changes in chromosomes. The company's medical director believed that unusual changes in chromosomes, such as breakage and other mutations, might be forewarnings of cancer and birth defects. His studies showed connections between such chromosomal changes and worker exposure to certain toxic chemicals. The medical director and his research associates eventually quit their positions at Dow, asserting that the company was suppressing the damaging research results and refusing to implement policies to inform workers of their existing health conditions or future risks (Severo, 1980). The event of a company's medical director confronting the industry is somewhat uncommon, because doctors who are employed or supported by an industry experience inherent constraints against identifying or diagnosing illnesses caused by that industry.

Captive Professionals

The company doctor is a good example of what Daniels (1969) called "**captive professionals**," or those whose presumed professional autonomy is compromised by organizational pressures from the bureaucracies that employ them. Daniels's study noted that psychiatrists practicing in the armed services accommodated their professional judgments to the military's manpower needs and values. Whereas psychiatrists working for mental hospitals tended to diagnose patients as mentally ill (in accordance with the expectations of the employer institutions), psychiatrists working for the military (where sickness reduced active manpower) tended to deny soldiers' claims of illness (Daniels, 1969, 1972; cf. Rosenhan, 1973). The diagnoses made by both of these "captive professionals" served to legitimate administrative decisions of the bureaucracies that employed them (cf. Ingleby, 1982: 136–137).

Similarly, many medical personnel employed by industry are "captive professionals." One Canadian study found that company doctors exhibited a "lack of sympathy with or intolerance of workers' attitudes towards health and safety in the workplace," and often perceived workers' health concerns as "fashions" or unreasonable fears. Rather than press the company to engineer changes in the production process or to initiate expensive monitoring programs, these doctors often emphasized workers' use of protective equipment and the screening and exclusion of supposedly "hyper-susceptible" workers (Walters, 1982). Although the corporate physician is potentially in a position to influence improved occupational health for employees, the professional's employer—not the individual worker—is still the "client," so ethical ambiguity and conflicting pressures are inherent in the structure of the job (Walsh, 1987).

While some professionals' organizational situation makes them clearly vulnerable or "captive" to their employers' interests, all professionals are likely to be influenced by their identification with certain class or status interests. Source of income indirectly affects medical decisions and doctor-patient relationships. For example, there is a tendency for doctors employed by industry not to diagnose occupational diseases, whereas doctors employed by unions or workers' health clinics tend to diagnose such diseases frequently (Lewin, 1987a). Similarly, in countries such as England, where doctors are paid a set salary, regardless of the treatments they recommend, kidney failure is more likely to be treated with home dialysis or transplants, whereas in the United States where some physicians can make considerably more money by offering in-clinic dialysis, this treatment is the foremost recommended therapy (Simmons and Marine, 1984; see also

Kutner, 1982; Riska, 1985). Surgeons in fee-for-service practice are likewise more likely to urge patients to undergo experimental surgery, such as coronary by-pass, whereas those employed by prepaid health plans are much less likely to decide to perform such operations (Millman, 1976: 238–239). And doctors who have mastered a particular surgical procedure are less likely to recommend it for patients than doctors who are eager to practice that procedure (Scully, 1980: 195–196).

Whose Interests Are Served?

While ideologies legitimate certain interests over others, they are often accepted by people whose interests are not necessarily served by those ideas. Ideological elements are often subtly diffused in a society through popular culture, educational institutions, mass media, and commercial advertising. For example, whose interests were served by the turn-of-the-century glorification of women's domesticity? Throughout the first half of this century, this ideal was meshed with popular ideas and fears of bacterial contagion to create much more work for housewives, who were taught in school and in women's magazines that they should be occupied with "scientific cleaning" and buying numerous products to protect their families from these dangerous invisible agents (Ehrenreich and English, 1978: 127–164). Interest groups exert power to shape ideology and to have it accepted and disseminated through channels such as the mass media and public education (Berger and Luckmann, 1967: 119–124).

Ideologies are not peculiar to medicine under capitalism and absent under other social and economic arrangements. *All* medical systems embody ideologies, but the nature of these ideologies varies according to the structure of that society. In capitalist societies, the treatment of health and healing as commodities to be bought and sold under market conditions produces certain economic benefits for various individual and corporate interests. Medical systems in noncapitalist societies, however, also utilize ideologies to legitimate and promote the interests of certain groups, such as state bureaucracies, dominant ethnic or tribal groups, or patriarchal powers.

Reification: Diseases and Bodies as Objects

Ideas that serve as ideologies often come into use subtly, frequently without explicit intention or awareness that the ideas have ideological uses. One such set of ideas are contemporary medical conceptions of the nature of disease and of the body. The product of this development is the notion that diseases are discrete, identifiable (or potentially identifiable) entities— in short, objects. The body is likewise treated as an object, separate from the person who inhabits it.

This conception illustrates the process of reification and its ideological functions. **Reification** is the "apprehension of human phenomena as if they were things," or something other than human products (Berger and Luckmann, 1967: 89). Reified reality confronts people as something outside themselves, as a nonhuman object. Institutions, social roles, norms, and other social processes are often reified; they come to assume a greater-than-human authority and inevitability. Reification thus entails a certain amount of mystification, as the human roots of phenomena are veiled (see Taussig, 1980).

Reification of disease means conveniently "forgetting" the social processes by which the concept of disease is produced. It means denying the social meanings embodied in symptoms, diagnoses, and therapy, and in the very experience of illness itself. Reification of the body results in an even greater dehumanization because of the close connection between the body and the identity of the individual. For example, an anesthetized body lying on a gurney before surgery on its testicles is medically no more than an object with a pathological entity (disease) in its tissues (things) that must therefore be surgically removed. To the person himself, however, that body and those testicles are an important part of who he is—his very self.

Reification creeps pervasively into the practice of bioscientific medicine because the guise of the scientific process masks the human factors involved in the creation of medical knowledge, as illustrated earlier in this chapter. It also occurs when any individual practitioner fails to acknowledge that a diagnosis or medical disposition is a human creation. The diagnostician constructs a disease identification from an assortment of ambiguous signs and symptoms elicited by human processes, and interpreted in the context of a human evaluation of the patient's social and psychological—as well as physical—condition.

Diagnoses are the product of social interaction, yet rarely does a physician accept authorship of a disease identification. Rather, the disease comes to be seen as a feature or property of the patient (Taussig, 1980). For example, the complex process by which a physician applies the diagnostic label "diabetes" to a patient's condition is forgotten, and the diabetes is treated as an objective thing that the patient "has." The reified disease identification often assumes primacy; if it conflicts with the patient's subjective illness experience, the objectified disease-thing is often treated as more real than the sick person's feelings. To the extent that patients internalize this image of their bodies and diseases, the reified reality shapes even their self-perception and experience.

One of the ideological functions of the reification of disease and the body is an emphasis upon individualistic rather than social or political responses to disease. In the above example of workers' health risks in a chemical factory, the location of disease as a property of individual bodies led to an emphasis on finding which individuals were more likely to be susceptible to work-place toxins. It promoted the idea that those who were identified as being at risk should be counseled to change jobs, rather than reducing the exposure of all workers or eliminating the industrial processes that required the use of toxic substances. Reification transforms occupational disease into a thing that befalls some individuals instead of the result of specific human decisions affecting workers' health.

The emphasis upon disease as an object that occurs within an individual also produces a tendency to locate responsibility for illness in the individual. It is thus one form of **blaming the victim** (Ryan, 1971), a type of legitimation that argues that the victim rather than the agent of a misfortune (e.g., rape, homelessness, or family abuse) was actually responsible for the occurrence. In the case of illness, the sick person is assumed to be responsible for having taken health risks, such as accepting a hazardous job, failing to use seat belts, or moving to an area with polluted water. As described in Chapter 4 the individual is often held accountable for unhealthy lifestyle choices, such as smoking, drinking, poor eating habits, and lack of exercise. The individual's emotional style and characteristic response to stress are also blamed (Crawford, 1977; see also Sontag, 1978).

Such attention to the individual as the locus of disease often results in inattention to the sick person's whole situation. Even extremely caring physicians can lose sight of the sociostructural roots of patients' suffering by focusing upon an utterly individualized image of disease. For example, one study of doctor-patient communication noted the extent to which the patient's larger social predicament (e.g., an extremely stressful workplace) was generally ignored or reduced to individualistic treatments, such as recommendation of tranquilizers or a vacation (Waitzkin, 1984).

Instead of examining the work conditions that create stress, attention is focused on how adequately the individual responds to stress. Instead of looking at the marital, family, or work pressures of a compulsive overeater or smoker, emphasis is placed upon the individual's will power to control personal behavior. And when the individual is unable to comply with doctors' orders to get more rest and exercise, the facts that she is a single parent of four young children and works full-time in a stressful, subsistence-level job are considered barely relevant; she is viewed as responsible for her own health. This approach to disease as a condition of the sick individual thus depoliticizes illness causation (McKinlay, 1986). By contrast, adequate social policies for prevention require an awareness of the social causes of illness and the social contexts of the sick person.

THE DEVELOPMENT OF MODERN BIOMEDICINE

We sometimes view the present nature of medical practice as a cultural given. When we think of medical care, our ready mental images include doctors, hospitals, nurses, medical laboratories, operating rooms, x-rays, hypodermic needles, and pills. The institutions, occupations, and technologies that we identify with medical care are, however, the peculiar result of specific political, economic, and social interactions. The history of modern medicine shows that many alternative courses were possible, and that the particular form that medical knowledge and practice have taken in this society made certain medical advances possible but also limited the field by cutting off other potentially fruitful approaches to health and healing.

The paradigm of modern scientific medicine incorporates a number of assumptions about the nature of the body and disease that are discussed below. Ideas do not just "happen," however, but rather are produced, accepted, and transmitted in a political and social context. The elevation of this particular paradigm to become *the* medical mode for understanding disease and the body occurred in connection with the political process by which the medical profession gained dominance relative to other social authorities and healers.

Professional Dominance

In the nineteenth century, most medical doctors were barely considered professionals. Their credentials were relatively easy to achieve (or fake), their body of medical knowledge was skimpy, their tools for diagnosis and therapy were primitive and often dangerous, and their abilities to heal were not particularly impressive. There were several competing kinds of physicians, each with very different ideas about the causes and treatments of sickness. Furthermore, physicians were only a small percentage of the total number of persons practicing various healing arts, who included, among others, midwives, bone setters, nurses, pharmacists, barbers (who performed minor surgery), herbalists, and folk and religious healers.

Within just a few decades, however, in the early part of the twentieth century medical doctors had achieved virtually total professional dominance. In the process described below, they had successfully eliminated, coopted, or subordinated all competing health professionals, and had acquired a state-legitimated monopoly over the health care market in the United States. While medicine enjoys similar professional preeminence in other nations, it lacks the degree of state-legitimated dominance over the entire health care system that characterizes the American situation (cf. Berlant, 1975; Coburn et al., 1983; Freidson, 1970; Herzlich and Pierret, 1987; Ramsey, 1977; Schepers, 1985; Willis, 1983).

A profession is a service occupation characterized by legitimate control over the market for its services and over a body of specialized knowledge or expertise. The **professionalization** of medicine as an occupation is thus a sociopolitical movement organized to achieve a "monopoly of opportunities in a market of services or labor and, inseparably, monopoly of status and work privileges" (Larson, 1979: 609). For medicine to achieve professional status, three main developments were necessary: (1) achieving standardization and cohesion within the profession; (2) convincing the state at various levels to grant a monopoly, for example, by requiring medical licenses to engage in healing practices; and (3) gaining public respect and persuading the public to accept the profession's definitions of what problems properly should be brought to it for service.

One definitive characteristic of a developed profession is its autonomy, which is an organizational product of its ability to dominate its area of expertise in the division of labor. In the case of the medical profession, autonomy is evidenced by doctors' legal protection from encroachment by other occupations. A second factor in medical autonomy is the profession's control over the production and application of medical knowledge and skill, especially the training and licensing of physicians. A third indication of medicine's status as a developed profession is its presumed self-regulation with a code of ethics (Freidson, 1970).

In 1847, the American Medical Association (AMA) was established as a professional organization for physicians from the medical belief system dubbed *allopathy*, which was characterized by "heroic" and invasive treatments such as bloodletting, purging, blistering, vomiting, and medicating with powerful drugs (e.g., opium) and poisons (e.g., mercury and arsenic). Allopathic physicians called themselves "regular" or orthodox physicians, but the public was, understandably, attracted to some of the less dangerous forms of medicine practiced by competing approaches such as homeopathy, naturopathy, and hydropathy.

The initial program of the AMA was relatively straightforward: to create internal professional cohesion and standardization by controlling the requirements for medical degrees and by enacting a code of ethics that would exclude "irregular" practitioners from the ranks. These efforts were aimed primarily at reducing the influence of the chief competitors, homeopathic physicians, who had organized the American Institute for Homeopathy in 1844. Between 1850 and 1880, the two camps became increasingly polarized, as the AMA censured members who continued to have dealings with the "enemy." For example, in 1878 the local medical society expelled a Connecticut doctor for having consulted with a homeopathic physician—his wife. "Regular" physicians lost considerable ground in the latter half of the nineteenth century, while homeopathy gained as much public respect and legal considerations as allopathy. "Regular" practitioners accounted for nearly 90 percent of all doctors, but the proportion of "irregular" physicians increased in the mid-1900s. For the latter half of the century, "irregulars" commanded approximately one-fifth of the market (Starr, 1982: 88–99).

The AMA and the "irregular" physicians cooperated, however, in their political efforts to have states enact licensing laws, because they shared a common interest in eliminating competition from persons who had not attended any form of medical school, such as midwives, ministers, pharmacists, and folk healers. The AMA has, from its outset, been especially interested in exposing and prosecuting what it calls "quackery," which is practically defined as all forms of medicating or healing outside the profession's control. A related campaign successfully eliminated much competition from patent medicine manufacturers and eventually subordinated the practice of pharmacy to medical control. Licensing legislation began to specify the quality of the medical education required, and some states set up boards of medical examiners, initially making allowances for various "irregular" forms of professional training alongside the "regular." The courts and legislatures had begun to grant professional prerogatives to thus-approved doctors. Gradually, "regular" medicine coopted and absorbed most "irregular" physicians, but rejected and actively opposed later organized alternatives such as chiropractic and Christian Science (Starr, 1982: 99–112; see also Baer, 1984; Wardwell, 1972).

Scientization of Medicine and Medical Training

The most dramatic change in the medical profession's dominance occurred after the turn of the century. The adoption of "scientific" medicine and the insistence upon standards of rigorous medical education were central strategies in the professionalization process. Science and education did not, however, characterize the actual practice of "regular" medicine at that time. In fact, scientific training was available to only a small elite of physicians, mainly researchers and educators, who had the money to study in Europe (Berliner, 1976).

Control of medical education was critical to a monopoly in the market. In the early 1900s, practicing physicians made relatively poor incomes; one comparison suggests that they earned less than an ordinary mechanic of the day (Berliner, 1976: 584). There appeared to be a growing oversupply of physicians relative to the market of paying clients. Licensing laws had not resulted in fewer physicians but merely more medical schools. While the national population grew between 1870 and 1910 by 138 percent, the number of physicians increased by 153 percent. Many professional leaders objected not only to the numbers of new physicians these medical schools were graduating but also to the fact that they had recruited "undesirable" students: women, blacks, immigrants, and working-class persons. Advocates of reforming medical education believed that medicine could not become a respected profession if its ranks included such lowly elements. Shortly after the turn of the century, the AMA underwent a major internal organization and subsequently made such "reform" its primary focus (Starr, 1982: 112–117).

After a preliminary review of medical colleges, the AMA invited an outside group, the Carnegie Foundation, to conduct a thorough investigation of the approximately 160 medical colleges in the United States and Canada. The resulting report in 1910 was devastating to many medical education programs (Flexner, 1910). The report's foremost objection was to the lack of medical science in the curriculum and training experiences. It recommended that the great majority of medical schools should be closed; that the first-rate schools should be strengthened on the model of Johns Hopkins (which had a singularly science-oriented program); and that a few medium-quality schools should be greatly improved to meet the upper standard. With the support of state legislatures and many universities themselves, the governing body of AMA subsequently became the de facto national accrediting agency for medical schools. The report's recommendations were dramatically supported by funding from numerous philanthropic foundations. By 1934 the nine largest foundations in the U.S. had given over $154 million to implement reforms (Berliner, 1975).[2]

These "reforms" of medical education had exactly the kind of effects the AMA wanted: increased internal cohesion of the profession and increased control of the market. Not only had the supply of licensed physicians been dramatically cut, but the homogeneity of the professions had also been assured by greatly limiting access to medical education for women, blacks, Jews, and all who could not afford the newly required four years of college and four full-time years of medical school. The declining numbers of new physicians adversely affected the poor and rural areas. Flexner had expected that the new highly trained graduates would disperse throughout the country, but in practice they gravitated to the wealthiest regions. The increased cost of their medical education reduced the likelihood that they would accept the modest incomes of practices in small towns and rural areas (Starr, 1982: 123–127). There were likewise fewer doctors for blacks. Due to widespread discrimination and segregation, blacks received treatment mainly from black physicians, but the "reforms" dramatically reduced their numbers (Starr, 1982: 124). Only two of the seven medical schools for blacks survived the "reforms." Since the medical colleges run by "irregular" physicians had been somewhat more open to interracial admissions, their disproportionate demise also reduced opportunities for blacks to become doctors.

In the latter part of the nineteenth century, considerable numbers of women had entered medical practice. In the decade from 1880 to 1890, women doubled their proportional representation of all doctors in the United States (from 2.8 to 5.6 percent); seventeen medical colleges for women were founded in that period. After considerable struggle, women

[2]The conspicuous role of the capitalist philanthropies, notably the Rockefeller Foundation (which gave some $66 million to just nine medical schools in the aftermath of Flexner's report), has led some to suggest a direct affinity between capitalist classes and the type of medicine they chose to support (see Brown, 1979; and the critique in Starr, 1982: 228). Even if there were no deliberate collusion, it is true that the outcome was a version of medicine that necessitated extensive expenditures on pharmaceuticals, medical technology, and capital-intensive hospitals, as described further in Chapter 12.

began to be admitted to elite medical schools after 1890, and by 1893–94 women constituted 10 percent or more of the student body at nineteen of the coeducational schools (Starr, 1982: 117).

Women's acceptance into coeducational settings was far from smooth, however; they experienced considerable harassment from male professors and students (Morantz-Sanchez, 1985). Many physicians believed that women's menstrual cycles made them incapable of professional work. For example, one doctor declared that the " 'periodical infirmity of their sex . . . in every case . . . unfits them for any responsible effort of mind . . . [and that during their menstrual] condition, neither life nor limb submitted to them would be as safe as at other times' " (quoted in Wertz and Wertz, 1979: 57). After the turn of the century, women were increasingly excluded from the profession of medicine. All but three of the seventeen women's medical colleges closed, and coeducational medical colleges maintained quotas that, until the 1960s, limited women to about 5 percent of admissions (Starr, 1982: 124).

Because they were excluded from mainstream medicine, some women turned to the less prestigious area of public health, such as campaigns for better hygiene, nutrition, and mother-and-child health care. The medical profession often opposed these efforts, which it perceived as threats to its dominance and as competition for health expenditures. For example, female public health advocates campaigned for the Sheppard-Towner Act of 1921, which provided health care for mothers and infants until 1929, when the AMA pressured Congress not to renew funding (Morantz-Sanchez, 1985).

Professional Autonomy and Control

By the 1930s, the medical profession had achieved significant autonomy. It controlled the recruitment and training of new physicians, including the length and content of medical education, as well as the examination and licensing by which new doctors could be admitted to practice. The profession defined (and regularly expanded) the scope of its work, specified its own standards of practice, and maintained the right to enforce them (Freidson, 1970).

The prerogative to define the scope of medical work is connected with the process of *medicalization* by which increasing numbers of areas of life were brought under medicine's purview and control. Childbirth, alcoholism, obesity, infant feeding formulas, and menopause are just a few of the areas that previously were not defined as properly "medical" matters but, through the medical profession's influence, were redefined as issues needing doctors' attention, regardless of whether the medical approach was more effective than nonmedical. Other efforts to expand their markets included the campaign to persuade well persons get an annual checkup.

In defining the scope of its work, the medical profession also eliminated much of its competition. Some professional competitors, such as homeopathists and osteopaths, were coopted; others, such as pharmacists, nurses, anesthetists, and x-ray technicians, were subordinated; whereas still others, such as midwives, clergy, and barber-surgeons, were outrightly driven from legitimate practice (Gritzer, 1981). The AMA also worked to limit public health authorities severely; medical professional interests campaigned (usually successfully) against public dispensaries, the compulsory reporting of tuberculosis, municipal laboratories and vaccination programs, the provision of health services in the public schools, and national public health programs, which were all viewed as competitors in the provision of services and as threats to the profession's autonomous authority over its domain. By controlling licensing, the access to facilities (e.g., hospitals and labs), access to other physicians as backups, and the legitimacy of third-party reimbursement, the medical profession greatly reduced its competition (Dolan, 1980).

The medical profession rapidly consolidated its control over the conditions of its work as the organization of hospitals specifically reflects. In recent years, however, the profession may have lost some of its control in many institutional settings, such as the new for-profit hospital corporations described in Chapter 11. Because of its market monopoly, the medical profession also asserted its control over the terms of its remuneration. American medicine is organized on a fee-for-service basis in which, rather than receiving a set salary, most doctors charge each patient a fee for each service performed. The profession's model of the ideal economic relationship was one of direct payment by the patient-receiver to the health care provider. The rise in importance of third-party payment from the government, insurance companies, labor unions, or fraternal organizations, who paid part or all of some patients' medical fees, represented an intrusion and danger to medical dominance. As Starr (1982: 235) observed, "to be the intermediary in the costs of sickness is a strategic role that confers social and political as well as strictly economic gains." Over the years the medical profession has vehemently asserted its interests in campaigns against national health insurance, Social Security health benefits, Blue Cross and Blue Shield, prepaid health plans, Medicare, and Medicaid. As shown in Chapter 11, the role of third parties has nevertheless increased, resulting in some regulation and limitation of medical practice and payments.

Modernization and Medical Practice

The features of modern medicine are in many ways the products of the broader process of modernization, which has similarly shaped other institutional spheres, such as industry, education, and communications. The specific historical development of the medical profession also contributed to certain structural features of modern medicine.

Several aspects of modernization apply to the development of medicine. One is the trend toward **institutional differentiation**, in which various institutional spheres in society become separated from each other, as each comes to perform specialized functions. Differentiation resulted in the separation of healing functions from the institutions of religion and the family. A second aspect of modernization is **rationalization**, the application of criteria of functional rationality to many aspects of social and economic life. When applied to the division of labor, rationalization promoted bureaucratic forms of organization and an emphasis upon efficiency, standardization, and instrumental criteria for decision making. The structure of the modern hospital reflects this rational principle of organization.

Rational ways of knowing emphasized the use of empirical evidence to explain natural phenomena without reference to nonnatural categories of thought. Weber (1958: 139) observed that this led to the "disenchantment" of the world, meaning that phenomena once held in awe or reverence were stripped of their special qualities and became ordinary. The human body itself has been thus "disenchanted." For example, the modern view of the body contrasts strongly with the medieval notion that the body should not be dissected lest it be unfit for reuniting with the soul in resurrection. Bodies that are considered spiritual temples must be respected; bodies that are disenchanted entities require no special reverence. The key feature of the rationalization process is not so much the particular explanations of phenomena but the belief that all phenomena can be rationally explained. A by-product of this belief is an increased emphasis upon technology and technique by which rational knowledge can presumably be translated into control. Modern societies particularly value rational mastery. For example, we believe that if we can explain what causes a disease, then it is only a matter of time before we can develop a technology or technique for healing or even preventing the disease.

While the process of rationalization occurred in all modernizing medical systems, an additional feature in capitalist societies was **commodification,** or the process by which such qualities as health, beauty, and fitness are transformed into objects that can be bought and sold in the marketplace. Not only material objects such as pharmaceuticals and prosthetic devices but also the entire range of health services become commodities to be bought and sold. Commodification encourages both the sick and the well to become avid consumers of the nebulous product known as health.

Although these aspects of contemporary Western medical systems are linked with the larger process of modernization, many of the specific characteristics of modern medicine are the products of the historical-political struggle for professional dominance and the assumptions implicit in the biomedical belief system described below. Indeed, it is entirely likely that if different factions and competitors had won those early battles for legitimacy and a share of the medical market, we would today have an entirely different model of medical knowledge, of what constitutes health and health care, and of what it means to be a doctor.

Assumptions of the Biomedical Model

The present system of medical knowledge is based upon a number of assumptions about the body, disease, and ways of knowing. While many of these assumptions have a long history, they do not necessarily produce better medical care. They also deflect attention from nonmedical measures for promoting health, such as nutrition and public health, and as the last part of this chapter illustrates, contribute to serious problems in doctor-patient communication.

Mind-Body Dualism.   The medical model assumes a clear dichotomy between the mind and the body; physical diseases are presumed to be located within the body (Engel, 1977; see also Gordon, 1988; Kirmayer, 1988). The medical model also holds that the body can be understood and treated in isolation from other aspects of the person inhabiting it (Hahn and Kleinman, 1983).

The philosophical foundations for this split may go back to Descartes's division of the person into mind and body, or *res cogitans* and *res extensa*. The practical foundations, however, probably lie in medicine's shift to an emphasis upon clinical observation (toward the end of the eighteenth century) and pathological anatomy (beginning in the nineteenth century). Foucault (1973) demonstrated that medicine shifted its ways of viewing the body and developed a "clinical gaze." Previously, physicians "saw" the body indirectly, mainly through patients' descriptions of their experience of a malady. By contrast, the "clinical gaze" emphasized direct clinical observation and physical examinations; technological developments, such as the invention of the stethoscope in 1819, gave physicians access to direct (and presumably more objective) clinical knowledge than previously could be gained only indirectly. Foucault noted that the way the body is viewed has profound political implications. The ascending medical perspective saw the body as docile—something physicians could observe, manipulate, transform and improve (see also Armstrong, 1983). Increasingly sophisticated pathological anatomy meant that diseases were conceptualized in terms of alterations in tissues that were visible upon opening the body, such as during autopsy. This mode of conceptualizing disease had a profound effect in splitting body from mind in the practice of clinical medicine (Sullivan, 1986: 344–345).

Physical Reductionism.   The medical model not only dichotomizes body and mind, but also assumes that illness can be reduced to disordered bodily (biochemical or neurophysiological) functions. This physical reductionism, however, excludes social, psychological, and behavioral dimensions of illness (Engel, 1977). The result of this reductionism, together with medicine's mind-body dualism, is that disease is localized in the *individual* body. Such conceptions prevent the medical model from conceiving of the *social* body, or how aspects of the individual's social or emotional life might impinge upon physical health. As described in Chapter 3, another result is medicine's general inattention to social conditions that contribute to illness or could aid in healing (Bologh, 1981).

Specific Etiology.   A related assumption of the biomedical model is what Dubos (1959:130–135) called the "doctrine of specific etiology," or the belief that each disease is caused by a specific, potentially identifiable agent. It developed from the nineteenth-century work of Pasteur and Koch, who demonstrated that the introduction of specific virulent microorganisms (germs) into the body produced specific diseases. One primary focus of scientific medicine became the identification of these specific agents and their causal link to specific diseases. The doctrine of specific etiology was later extended beyond infectious diseases and applied to other diseases, such as deficiency diseases in which the specific etiology was not an intrusive microorganism but the lack of a necessary element, such as vitamin or hormone.

Dubos noted that while the doctrine of specific etiology has led to important theoretical and practical achievements, it has rarely provided a complete account of the causation of disease. He asked why, although infectious agents are nearly ubiquitous, only some people get sick some of the time. Accordingly, an adequate understanding of an illness etiology must include broader factors, such as nutrition, stress, and metabolic states, that affect the individual's susceptibility to infection. As noted in Chapter 2, the search for specific illness-producing agents worked relatively well in dealing with infectious diseases but is too simplistic to explain the causes of complex, chronic illnesses. Also, as Dubos (1959) observed, this approach often results in a quest for a medicinal "magic bullet" to "shoot and kill" the disease, producing an overreliance on pharmaceuticals in the "armamentarium" (stock of weapons) of the modern physician.

The Machine Metaphor.   One of the oldest Western images for understanding the body is a comparison with the functioning of a machine. Accordingly, disease is the malfunctioning of some constituent mechanism (e.g., a "breakdown" of the heart). Other cultures use other metaphors; for example, ancient Egyptian societies used the image of a river, and Chinese tradition refers to the balance of elemental forces (Yin and Yang) of the earth (Osherson and AmaraSingham, 1981). Modern medicine has not only retained the metaphor of the machine but also extended it by developing specializations along the lines of machine parts, emphasizing individual systems or organs to the exclusion of an image of the totality of the body. The machine metaphor further encouraged an instrumentalist approach to the body; the physician could "repair" one part in isolation from the rest (Berliner, 1975).

Regimen and Control.   Partly as a product of the machine metaphor and the quest for mastery, the Western medical model also conceptualizes the body as the proper object of regimen and control, again emphasizing the responsibility of the individual to exercise this control in order to maintain or restore health. Modernizing trends toward rationalization have further encouraged the notion of the standardization of body disciplines, such as diets, exercise programs, etiquette, routines of hygiene, and even sexual activity (Turner, 1984: 157–203).

This brief history shows that the knowledge and practice we know as medicine have their roots in sociopolitical processes. The ideas and assumptions of biomedicine forcefully influence economic and power relationships both within the relationship between practitioner and patient and in institutions (e.g., law) of the larger society. We must remember that these medical realities are socially produced.

SUMMARY

What we know about health, illness, and the body is socially constructed. Both lay and professional medical knowledge are influenced by social, economic, and political factors. The categories and even the very language for describing and understanding diseases are likewise subject to powerful social influences. Diseases and disease syndromes are "discovered" and professionally accepted through concrete social processes; other disease categories are similarly denied, dropped, or disavowed by social processes. Such social influences shape not only ideas but indeed also the experiences of our own and others' bodies and bodily conditions.

The nature of modern medicine is partly determined by the larger process of modernization, especially the extension of rationalization to the body and ways of knowing about and treating the body. In capitalist societies, the additional societal process of the commodification of health and health care has altered the economic meaning of medical services, as health has become an ambiguous product to be bought and consumed.

Medical knowledge sometimes serves ideological purposes, legitimating the interests of certain persons or groups. Ideological aspects of thought and practice are typically very subtle, and often go unnoticed by people who believe and use them. The medicalization of various areas of life and the uses of medicine in service of various institutional goals illustrate some of the ways ideology influences medical ideas and practice. The tendency of bioscientific medicine to treat diseases and bodies as objects masks the social history of ideas of disease and the social processes of finding disease. Reification also leads to a view of disease as a property of the sick person, thus reducing the significance of the social and environmental causes of the disease and the social context of the person's illness.

Many characteristics of the contemporary medical establishment can be traced to political developments in the recent history of the profession. Certain features of modern medicine are the results of the assumptions of the biomedical approach itself, which is characterized by its dichotomization of mind and body, physical reductionism, the doctrine of specific etiology, the machine metaphor for the body, and an emphasis upon bodily regimen and control. These assumptions have concrete implications for the delivery of health care.

RECOMMENDED READINGS

Articles

H. Tristam Englehardt, "The disease of masturbation: Values and the concept of disease," pp. 15–24 in J. W. Leavitt and R. L. Numbers, eds., *Sickness and Health in America.* Madison: University of Wisconsin Press, 1978.

Frances McCrea, "The politics of menopause: The discovery of a deficiency disease," *Social Problems* 13(1), 1983: 111–123.

Bryan S. Turner, "The government of the body: Medical regimens and the rationalization of diet," *British Journal of Sociology* 33(2), 1982: 254–269.

Vivienne Walters, "Company doctors' perceptions of and responses to conflicting pressures from labor and management," *Social Problems* 30(1), 1982: 1–12.

Books

Samuel Butler, *Erewhon.* New York: New American Library, [1901] 1960. A fictional utopia based on dramatically different definitions of health and illness.

Barbara Ehrenreich and Deirdre English, *For Her Own Good: 150 Years of the Experts' Advice to Women.* Garden City, NY: Doubleday, 1978. Locating women's health in the larger context of patriarchal relations, the authors show how women were persuaded by "experts" to accept numerous constraining (and often dangerous) practices in many areas of their lives on the grounds that they were "for their own good."

Eliot Freidson, *Profession of Medicine: A Study of the Sociology of Applied Knowledge.* New York: Dodd, Mead, 1970. This classic study of the structure of medical knowledge and professional autonomy serves as a useful basis for understanding current debates about the status and proper roles of medicine and various other health-related occupations.

Paul Starr, *The Social Transformation of American Medicine.* New York: Basic, 1982. A sweeping history of the medical profession's rise to professional dominance, Starr's interpretation is nonetheless overly idealistic, attributing the success of medical dominance more to American attitudes and values than to the triumph of the economic interests and political maneuvering that he amply documents.

David Sudnow, *Passing On: The Social Organization of Dying.* Englewood Cliffs, NJ: Prentice-Hall, 1967. This sensitive ethnography shows how social organization and interaction in hospital settings produce varying definitions of sickness and even death.

Chapter Ten

Modern Biomedicine: Knowledge and Practice

Social constructions enter the practice of Western medicine through not only the ideas and professional organization of biomedicine, but also the routine social interactions between medical personnel and their patients. Detailed examination of doctor-patient interactions show how professional dominance is maintained at the interpersonal level. Many of the problems of this relationship are due to social-structural factors in medical training and practice. Other very important factors are embedded assumptions of the medical model of disease and treatment. Some of these medical assumptions also make it difficult for physicians and the society as a whole to respond effectively to the emerging dilemmas in modern health care: the proper ends of medical treatment and the limits of medicine.

When people turn to medical professionals for help, they typically enter the patient role. Unlike the sick role, which is defined by broader social expectations (see Chapter 6), the patient role involves primarily the reciprocal expectations and norms held by the doctor and patient.[1] These expectations are emotionally charged; doctors and patients alike are often deeply dissatisfied with the actual situation.

Although each patient negotiates a different relationship with each particular doctor, a number of general social-structural factors shape the doctor-patient relationship. Two factors in particular are at the root of many of the problems in Western medical practice: (1) professional dominance, and (2) rationalization of the body in the medical model. Professional dominance creates and exacerbates social chasms between doctor and patient, while the medical model's rationalization of the body creates enormous discontinuities between medicine's paradigm of disease and curing on the one hand, and patients' experience and understanding of their illness and their needs on the other.

Although individual doctors could do much to overcome these problems in their own work with patients, these two characteristics are thoroughly embedded in the structure of the profession, medical education, hospital and other medical institutional structures, and the organization of medical practice. Without structural change, they will continue to limit the potential for individual change in the doctor-patient relationship. While the issue of patient (or consumer) dissatisfaction is a genuine concern, a more serious problem is that inadequacies in the doctor-patient relationship may gravely impede the very process of healing. The following discussion suggests some of the ways these social-structural factors may diminish the healing effectiveness of medical practitioners.

[1]The role of patient is qualitatively different relative to other professional and nonprofessional workers (such as nurses, technicians, or hospital orderlies), and varies dramatically according to institutional context (such as doctor's office, hospital, patient's home, clinic).

PROFESSIONAL DOMINANCE

The professionalization of medicine produced social distance between the practitioner and the sick person. The doctor is assumed to be the relatively knowledgeable "expert"; the patient, the relatively ignorant recipient of the doctor's professional services. Indeed, typically the patient is limited in ability to judge whether the doctor is using adequate medical knowledge, making competent treatment recommendations, and providing good service.

The greater the **social distance** between two people, the less sensitivity either is likely to have toward the other's problems. Doctors who themselves have had extensive experience in the patient role may be more empathetic toward their own patients (cf. Hahn, 1985a). In addition to the social distance inherent in the expert-layperson dichotomy, physicians are often separated from their patients by other factors: gender, ethnicity, and socioeconomic background. Status differences according to gender often supersede status differences between doctor and patient. Thus, for example, male doctors were rarely interrupted by their patients, whereas female doctors were interrupted somewhat more frequently (West, 1984: 150). Social distance also figures into the hierarchy of hospital and other institutional settings, where a greater social distance among the various levels of staff as well as between staff and patients results in insensitivity to each others' problems (Freidson, 1970: 109–136; see also Gubrium, 1975).

The sick person who wants medical help is in an intrinsically weak position. Power differences between doctor and patient have been further widened by medical control in both the larger arena of politics and law, and the narrower situation of the structure of medical practice. Maintaining a position of professional power serves to legitimate physicians' economic rewards and professional autonomy. For example, when patients are in awe of doctors' knowledge and skill, they are more likely to defer to physicians' judgment and to consider high fees to be reasonable.

Professional power also protects physicians from potentially damaging problems such as therapeutic failure. If a diagnosis is incorrect or a treatment does not work, the distance in knowledge between doctor and patient reduces the likelihood that the patient would be able to evaluate whether the failure was due to the doctor's lack of knowledge or skill. One study found that in a hospital setting doctors and other staff limited information given to patients and their families as a protective device in the management of medical mistakes (Millman, 1976). Sometimes keeping patients ignorant of their condition enables the doctor to manage them more effectively by preventing emotional responses that the physician might find disruptive or unpleasant. While individual doctors do not necessarily consciously engage in these protective legitimations, the very structure of the profession promotes them.

Information Control

One of the foremost ways doctors protect their professional power is by controlling the flow of information to the patient. On the one hand, the doctor cannot possibly, even in a long-term relationship, communicate to the patient everything the expert knows relevant to the limited actual circumstances of the patient's condition. On the other hand, patients need information about their condition: What is wrong with me? How serious is it? What is the expected outcome? What are my treatment options?

The more information patients have, the better able they are to understand their situation, evaluate options (including whether they are getting adequate medical care), and participate in treatment decisions. Such evaluation and decision making is, however, often threatening to the physician's control of the case. As a result, some physicians consider the "good" patient to be one who trustingly accepts the doctor's judgment and obediently complies with doctor's orders, full of unquestioning appreciation of the doctor's ministrations.

Although the doctor-patient relationship is based upon reciprocal role expectations, many doctors cast patients in stereotypical roles that serve to justify information control and doctors' dominant position relative to patients. One such expectation is the notion that patients are generally medically ignorant and childlike, and unable to comprehend explanations of the causes, alternative treatments, and expected outcome of their conditions (Segall and Roberts, 1980; see also Millman, 1976). Several studies have found that the majority of physicians consistently and markedly underestimated their patients' level of comprehension (McKinlay, 1975; Pratt et al., 1957).

Information control involves both information-gathering and information-giving. The doctor controls the medical interaction, deciding how much and which information to seek, and how much and which information to impart to the patient. The rationale and method for this model of a medical encounter are discussed further below. The medical interview and clinical examination consist of many such information-gathering and -giving decisions. Doctors control the information-gathering aspect by framing questions, cutting off patients' statements, ignoring certain patient input as irrelevant, and actively eliciting other input. The doctor decides whether and how extensively to conduct a physical examination, which tests to have done, and what follow-up study is needed; these aspects of a consultation are highly variable, a matter of the doctor's discretion (Fisher, 1983).

The medical interview is a constrained, prestructured form of talk. West (1983) found that patient-initiated questions are "dispreferred." Her detailed analysis of twenty-one medical exchanges showed that only 9 percent of the 773 questions were initiated by patients. The doctors' control of the interviews was further evident in that they did not respond to 13 percent of the relatively few questions put to them by their patients; patient assertiveness thus resulted in *less* response from doctors, whose pervasive dislike of patient-initiated questions was linked with the physicians' reluctance to answer "too many" such questions (West, 1984: 156). Patients sensed that their questioning was not the preferred pattern for the interaction; when they did pose questions, nearly half (46 percent) exhibited some anxiety, such as stutters or nervous giggles. By contrast, the patients answered all but 2 percent of the doctors' questions, which tended to be phrased in a way that limited patients' options for answering (e.g., "Do you feel X, or do you feel Y?").

Information-giving and question-asking exchanges between doctor and patient vary significantly according to social class. A British study of general practitioners' consultations found that patients' social class differences accounted for a significant proportion of the variance in both the information doctors gave in answer to questions and in the explanations volunteered by the doctors. Doctors may misinterpret working-class patients' reticence to ask questions as due to their lack of interest, but this study suggested that such patients' diffidence may be due more to the social distance between them and the doctor, and perhaps also to learned patterns of deference to higher social classes (Pendleton and Bochner, 1980).

Another study of fifty-one general practitioners in southern Wales found a wide range of doctor-patient communication strategies (Comaroff, 1976). Some physicians viewed the interaction as a one-way provision of professional skill in which the patient was passive recipient with nothing of value to contribute. Other doctors had more complex patterns of interaction with patients and were less likely to have a single, simple stereotype of their patients and their input. These data suggest that the differences are not due just to variations in individual doctors' personal need for power, but also to their differing images of their professional role. While related to power, these images are more a matter of ideals and ideologies.

Uncertainty and Control

Information control includes basic communication about diagnosis and treatment. Sometimes, even long after a doctor has a working diagnosis, the patient is not told what the problem may be. Before the enactment of a series of laws in the United States in the 1970s, it was possible for doctors to perform surgery, put patients on medication, and order other treatments without the patients' informed consent. Just what kind and how much information is necessary or desirable is, however, still debated.

Especially in the treatment of potentially fatal or particularly fearsome diseases, such as cancer, many doctors prefer to tell their patients as little as possible. As recently as the 1960s, most physicians routinely withheld from patients diagnosis of feared diseases and prognosis of impending death. One study found that 95 percent of physicians did not disclose a diagnosis of cancer to patients (Oken, 1961; see also Glaser and Strauss, 1968). The same questionnaire, distributed nearly two decades later, found a complete reversal: 90 percent of the physicians claimed they disclosed all information (Novack et al., 1979). But although physicians believe they are giving their patients all relevant information, many patients are dissatisfied with both the amount and the quality of information they receive (McIntosh, 1974). Even for nonfatal illnesses, many doctors do not communicate their full diagnosis or prognosis. Doctors may want to "protect" patients from unpleasant information. This paternalistic approach may simultaneously protect the doctor from dealing with the unpleasant reactions such knowledge might evoke. Giving bad news is very uncomfortable for physicians, as one surgeon explained:

> I really hate this part of the work. I feel terrible . . . always . . . it never seems to get easier. . . . I know it's not my fault . . . I didn't give the patient the disease . . . but I always somehow feel that it is . . . and besides . . . I never really know what to say. They sure never had a course on this part of medicine when I went to school, but let me tell you, I could sure use it now . . . and I usually don't ever get to know these patients who think their lives are in my hands. How am I supposed to deal with it? I hate doing it . . . but I can't avoid it! (quoted in Taylor, 1988).

In response to this stress, physicians adopt complex strategies to routinize the painful task, including telling the truth, professing uncertainty, evading the issue, and dissimulation. One study found that the majority viewed their role as selecting and interpreting information for patients (Taylor, 1988).

Uncertainty is an inherent difficulty for both doctor and patient. While precision, certainty, and control are goals of bioscientific medicine, clinical practice rarely comes close to meeting such goals. Real patients' problems are often complex, and even highly trained physicians cannot know everything about every possible problem. Diagnoses have, at best, only a certain probability of accuracy; straightforward diagnoses of well-known diseases have only a higher probability of accuracy than those of complex, poorly understood diseases. Control in treatment is likewise often elusive; much therapy is a matter of trial and error. Medical training provides some preparation for dealing with clinical uncertainty (Fox, 1957), but routine medical practice often involves judgments whose accuracy and effects are uncertain and—in some cases—unknowable. One physician, describing his experience with medical mistakes, commented:

> Many situations do not lend themselves to a simple determination of whether a mistake has been made. Seriously ill, hospitalized patients, for instance, require of doctors almost continuous decision-making. Although in most

cases no single mistake is obvious, there always seem to be things that could have been done differently or better: administering more of this medication, starting that treatment a little sooner. . . . The fact is that when a patient dies, the physician is left wondering whether the care he provided was inadequate. . . . Medicine is not an exact science; errors are always possible, even in the midst of the humdrum routine of daily care. Was that baby I just sent home with a diagnosis of mild viral fever actually in the early stages of serious meningitis? Will that nine-year-old with stomach cramps whose mother I just lectured about psychosomatic illness end up in the hospital tomorrow with a ruptured appendix? . . . A doctor has to confront the possibility of a mistake with every patient visit (Hilfiker, 1984).

The patient's situation in the face of uncertainty is even more anxiety-producing, because the patient lacks medical expertise. Doctors often prolong patients' uncertainty, even after their own uncertainty about the disease or therapy has been reduced or resolved. Waitzkin and Stoeckle (1972) suggested that physicians may use their control over patient uncertainty to preserve their power and keep their options open. For example, the head of one pediatric ward had a policy of aggressively treating children with leukemia up to the moment of death; no child was ever labeled terminal, no matter how unsuccessful the treatment. The mother of a child who was obviously succumbing asked this doctor, "Is my child critical?," to which the doctor replied, "No." Another member of the staff asked him privately, "Why did you tell her the child is not critical, when we know he has only a few weeks to live?" The doctor's answer: "He is not technically critical until he is on some life-support system. To control information about the child's status further, he ordered that the records not be shown or otherwise divulged to the distraught mother. His opinion was that if the mother knew how near to death her child was, she might refuse the course of chemotherapy he had ordered for the boy.

Doctor-patient negotiations over information vary according to the type of illness. In the course of the long-term treatment of chronic illness, the balance of power is often altered, requiring a renegotiation of the doctor-patient relationship. Patients are likely to become increasingly expert about their specific condition and thus more assertive in challenging their doctors (cf. Calnan, 1984; Herzlich and Pierret, 1987: 212).

Doctor-patient communication is especially problematic in the face of the uncertainty related to diseases such as multiple sclerosis (MS), a gradually debilitating, incurable disease of the nervous system. Because many MS victims are in young adulthood, when serious chronic illness is least expected, doctors at first may not consider the diagnosis. MS creates uncertainty for both the doctor and patient partly because its early symptoms are unclear or elusive. Another reason is that the diagnosis is fearsome to both the sufferer and the doctor because MS is incurable and potentially severely debilitating. Physicians thus frequently fail to diagnose MS correctly or postpone telling their patients of the diagnosis until it is inevitable.

One study suggested that this protective strategy for the doctor can create significant problems for the patient, perhaps leading to iatrogenic emotional difficulties (Stewart and Sullivan, 1982). Lacking physician confirmation that their symptoms were indeed related to a "real" illness, many MS patients were viewed by family, friends, and doctors as hypochondriacs or as "imagining things." As a result many sufferers experienced symptoms of stress that were actually more troublesome than the MS-related symptoms themselves. They lost faith in their doctors, shopped around for others, challenged physicians' diagnoses, and self-diagnosed (actions that typically elicited very negative reactions from physicians). Similarly, a study of interactions in a clinic for chronic illness sufferers showed that a major concern of the patients was to convince others—especially doctors—of the reality of their diseases. This was done by elaborating their illness behavior, but the sicker they behaved, the less likely doctors were to believe them. Likewise, their "doctor shopping" to confirm the fact of their illnesses increased the likelihood that doctors would label them as "crocks" (Alexander, 1982).

One researcher analyzed in detail the transcripts of three such doctor-patient encounters that were marked by tension, ambiguity, and no apparent resolution (Paget, 1983). Without much background about the patient, the reader sees in the transcript an apparently neurotic woman, overly preoccupied with little details of her body's functioning. After these three meetings, her doctor's assessment was that the patient's health was good and that her problem was "nerves." The transcript takes on an entirely different meaning, however, when we realize that the woman had recently had an operation for cancer. Her primary agenda in each of these encounters was clearly to address her fears that her cancer would metastasize or was not fully excised, but those fears *never* once became a topic of discourse. The doctor did not acknowledge that her fears existed or that they might be legitimate; he only heard her seemingly minor complaints about her teeth and her scalp. Indeed, an analysis of the doctor's responses to her input shows that he was not really listening to *any* of her expressions, perhaps because he had already defined them as the product of her "nerves," and therefore medically unreal or unimportant. She too contributed to the ongoing misunderstanding between them by referring only indirectly to the operation in the first encounter and not at all thereafter. She was afraid to express her fears and yet afraid to ignore them. The patient's uncertainty regarding her cancer produced fear, but this unnamed fear led to expressions that the doctor labeled as psychosomatic. His response—disconfirming the reality of her problem—produced further ambiguity, which only exacerbated the woman's fears.

Often such patients come to view physicians as evasive, nonsup-
portive, insensitive, uncaring, or dishonest. One MS patient said:

> I went to seven or eight doctors in less than two years. I'd tell them about my
> pins-and-needles feelings, or my numbness, or my weak arms and they'd all
> do the same thing—nothing. I really got upset with those doctors. They'd
> usually just say that my problems were normal for a woman my age (25) and
> things like that. And I'd get really uptight because they would just give me a
> valium and not try to find out what was really wrong. Some of them thought I
> was going off my rocker. They thought I was imagining the problems. . . .
> One of them just threw up his arms and said he didn't know what was wrong
> with me. Now isn't that some way for a doctor to act. I got so I didn't believe
> any of them. I knew something was wrong and felt they could find out if they
> would just try (quoted in Stewart and Sullivan, 1982: 1401).

In such situations the doctors' inability or unwillingness to communicate a
diagnosis resulted in the patient's suffering and loss of trust in the doctor-
patient relationship.

The Micropolitics of Professional Dominance

When a patient interacts with a doctor, the relationship is not symmet-
rical. In addition to the physician's presumed medical expertise, a number
of microstructural factors increase the relative power of the doctor in the
medical encounter. The professional dominance of doctors is enhanced by
their control over minute parts of their interaction with patients.

Language Use.   Doctors control even seemingly medically irrelevant
aspects of the doctor-patient interaction, such as humorous exchanges and
other sociability (West, 1984: 152; see also Todd, 1983). Several patterns of
language use reflect the subtle ways in which dominance is asserted. For
example, interrupting is an assertion of whose input to the interaction is
more important. Doctors frequently interrupted their patients, whereas
they were seldom interrupted *by* their patients.

Doctors' unilateral use of false-familiar terms increases the gap between doctor and patient. For example, many doctors expect to be addressed deferentially by their title ("Dr. Jones"), but regularly address
patients—regardless of age or other status—by their first names. Another
false-familiar practice is the routine use of the condescending question,
"How are we today?" Likewise, the use of diminutives is a subtle assertion of
doctors' dominance and condescension. For example, one study of doctor-
patient interactions in two gynecological settings (public clinic and private
practice) found that doctors frequently used diminutives in talking to patients. For example, a doctor teaching women to perform breast self-
examinations said, "Just march your little fingers . . ." (Todd, 1983).

The Dossier.   The doctor typically has far more information about the patient than the patient has about the doctor. Such one-sided familiarity serves to remind the patient which party is dominant (Stimson and Webb, 1975). The medical record functions as a third agent, introducing the patient (and personal details about the patient, such as marital status and age) even before the face-to-face interaction. One researcher observed that doctors often appear to be more oriented to the patient's objectified record or chart than to the patient him- or herself (West, 1984: 132–133). Records can indeed take on a reality greater than that expressed by patients themselves. Patients' narratives of their illness experiences often bear little resemblance to the case record (see Kleinman, 1988).

Patients typically lack access to or control over these records. They are prevented from seeing their charts, reading their records, or challenging items of information in their files. Particularly in institutional settings such as hospitals, control over medical records is a form of social control over inmates (Goffman, 1961). In ordinary office practice too, patient records often contain information that is discrediting. For example, a doctor in a group practice may read a colleague's comment that a patient is a constant complainer and accordingly decide not to give that person's current problem serious attention.

Social Organization of Space.   The physical setting of most medical encounters is likewise supportive of the physician's dominance. Medical staff have the uniforms and "props" of authority—white coats, stethoscopes, framed certificates, and complicated equipment. Office and hospital consultations are on doctors' "home field," which is organized to their specifications. For example, rarely is the doctor's office arranged so that doctor and patient are seated in equally important positions; much of the interaction may in fact occur in the examining room with the patient undressed and in an awkward posture. Studies of the uses of space, posture, and gesture demonstrate that such differences are related to power and stratification (Henley, 1977).

Social Control of Time.   Significantly, doctors exert considerable control over the time spent with patients. One useful indicator of relative power in a dyad (i.e., a two-person interrelationship, such as teacher-student or executive-underling) is which party is in a position to make the other wait for access to his or her presumably more precious time. Typically, the patient waits to see the doctor rather than the reverse. In private practice, physicians often overbook patients to assure that every block of office consultation time is filled, but they are more sensitive to the need for customer satisfaction than doctors in clinic or institutional settings, where patients are not free to take their business elsewhere.

The allocation of time spent with patients depends partly upon the expectations and rewards for doctors in a particular institutional setting. One study found that prenatal patients in one hospital experienced different waiting times and received very different amounts of doctor time depending upon whether they were being seen in the obstetrics clinic, family practice clinic, or midwife service. Reflecting different organizational—as well as health care—objectives, residents in obstetrics spent an average of five to ten minutes with a prenatal patient, and expected clinic nurses to do the job of communicating information about pregnancy and delivery. By contrast, midwives spent an average of twenty minutes with patients, and family practice residents spent up to forty-five minutes with patients. The researcher noted that family practice residents were encouraged and rewarded for the time spent with patients, whereas obstetric residents were discouraged from devoting time to "normal" pregnancies and were informally sanctioned if they failed to process their share of the patient work load fast enough (Lazarus, 1988).

One study showed that 73 percent of patients' visits to doctors lasted fifteen minutes or less (Lawrence and McLemore, 1983). Because doctors' goals include the efficient, task-oriented use of this brief time, the interview and examination are directed to gathering information that they believe is directly relevant to fairly routinized diagnostic decision rules (as described below). A British study corroborated the impact of a sense of time constraints on doctor-patient communication. Even when time is actually available for more medical work, doctors narrow the objectives of their routines (and typically uninteresting) practice by thinking not "What can I do for this patient?" but "What can I do for this patient in the next six minutes?" (Horobin and McIntosh, 1983: 328). One physician commented on his tight control of patient interactions:

> The doctor's primary task is to manage his time. If he allows patients to rabbit on about their conditions then the doctor will lose control of time and will spend all his time sitting in a surgery [office consultation] listening to irrelevant rubbish. Effective doctoring is characterized by a 'quick, clean job' (quoted in Byrne and Long, 1976: 93).

In much American practice of medicine, the sense of time constraints is further heightened by the more direct linkage of physicians' income with the number of patients seen and the number of specific medical services provided.

Patients are unlikely to know the criteria by which the doctors are judging their input, and often the information about the problem that the patient wants to give is discarded or interrupted by the doctor. One study found that, on average, doctors cut off patients' descriptions of their complaints within the first eighteen seconds (Beckman and Frankl, 1984). This practice is particularly problematic, because patients only rarely readily reveal the important reasons that triggered their visit (Good and Good, 1982). For example, a patient may start out by presenting a "simple" problem such as a persistent rash, but may have really come to the doctor mainly to obtain reassurance that he does not have heart disease like his brother who recently had a heart attack. If given the time to present all their concerns, patients frequently identify three or four problems, of which the first mentioned is often not the most serious.

Doctors' information-giving time is likewise greatly constricted by the brevity of the ordinary medical encounter. One study found that only about 9 percent of a session was devoted to communicating information about the illness to the patient. If an average session is ten to fifteen minutes, the information-giving part is barely one minute. An analysis of 336 encounters in several outpatient settings showed that doctors spent little time informing their patients, overestimated the time they did spend, and underestimated their patients' interest in obtaining information (Waitzkin, 1985).

THE DOCTOR-PATIENT RELATIONSHIP

Broader structural factors also shape the pattern of miscommunication between doctors and their patients. As described in Chapter 8, patients come to the medical encounter with fundamentally separate (and often irreconcilable) expectations and goals from those of their doctor: What am I doing and why? What are the central facts about my situation? How should we proceed to make sense of this? What is my expected outcome?

Rationalization and the Medical Model

As outlined in Chapter 9, modern biomedicine has developed a conception of disease as separate from the person experiencing it. Rationalized medicine views the body as an object; the body is incidentally inhabited by a person who can potentially help or hinder the task of treating diseases of the body. People cannot, however, simply leave their bodies at the repair shop. While individual doctors may choose to relate to their patients as persons and not just bodies, such an approach is not an essential part of curing in the biomedical model. In many ways, the training and socialization of medical personnel actively discourages them from seeing their patients as whole persons with social, emotional, aesthetic, spiritual, and other health-related facets to their lives.

Medical training emphasizes technical skills in diagnosing and treating pathologies (physiological deviations that constitute or characterize disease). Thus doctors are trained to approach a medical encounter with a patient with the goal of efficient diagnosis of a pathology and active treatment intervention. By contrast, the patient comes to the doctor with a broader, and more often vague, set of goals. The patient's needs may be related to a range of problems, some of which are unrelated or only indirectly related to an identifiable pathology or bodily condition. The patient may be experiencing illness but lack a clinically detectible pathology. The illness may also be a chronic condition in the face of which the doctor's active intervention is not very effective, although the patient may suffer from certain socioemotional aspects of the illness and its management. With a narrow disease-oriented training, doctors are likely to misunderstand completely what these patients need.

Most persons seeking medical help do not need the kind of medical intervention that physicians have been trained to appreciate. In medical school, internships and residencies, the emphasis is upon the "interesting" cases, which are typically acute and dramatic, and thus challenging—but not impossibly so—for the doctors' diagnostic skills. Often too cases are defined as interesting if they offer the chance to practice new surgical techniques; once the doctor has mastered these procedures, such cases become less interesting (Scully, 1980: 166–171). In ordinary office practice, however, such "interesting" cases are proportionately very rare, and doctors are likely to be bored and impatient with the majority of patients' health problems.

One hospital's head midwife, who was involved in training obstetric residents, noted:

> It is a rare medical student who wants to sit with a woman in labor. Residents will even pass on watching normal deliveries. They see people as pathology, as a uterus. I rarely see the art of medicine, the understanding of seeing a patient as a total entity—where she is going, where she has been. I heard a resident say that 'If I never do another normal vaginal delivery, it won't be too soon.' They train for pathology but go into private practice with normal patients. There is more money in it, and it is the least amount of time for the most amount of money (quoted in Lazarus, 1988: 39).

In general practice, which includes most of the work done by general practitioners, pediatricians, family practitioners, internists, and obstetrician-gynecologists, only about 15 percent of consultations are for the kind of acute, major, or life-threatening conditions that are likely to be "interesting." By far the largest proportion of office visits are for seemingly minor, self-limiting conditions or for well-person preventive care; chronic illnesses are the second largest category. Physicians whose medical training was oriented toward "interesting" cases find such routine work far less rewarding. One doctor exclaimed:

> Our skills are absolutely wasted . . . frustration and boredom set in. There are days when you go home and think, 'Have I got to do this for another twenty

years?' You've done a lot of work but you really haven't done anything for anybody. . . . There's no stimulation at all . . . (quoted in Horobin and McIntosh, 1983: 321).

Labeling Patients

Doctors' socialization leads to negative stereotypes of patients. The use of such stereotypes does vary according to the institutional setting; doctors in private practice are less likely than doctors on hospital staff to use pejoratives openly to refer to patients, although they may hold some of the same negative attitudes (cf. Hahn, 1985b). Nevertheless, the values reflected in these attitudes toward patients are encouraged in both the self-selection of doctors and their medical education. Doctors learn that "real" medicine is about pathologies, not patients.

In a U.S. study, 439 family physicians anonymously answered a questionnaire about those patient characteristics to which they responded negatively (Klein et al., 1982). The doctors reacted negatively not only to various social and personal traits of their patients but also to certain medical conditions, especially those for which medical treatment offered little or no likelihood of cure or clear alleviation. The authors suggested that physicians particularly dislike situations, such as emphysema, senility, diabetes, arthritis, psychiatric conditions, and obesity, that challenge their faith in the potency of bioscientific medicine. While they may find a challenging case with a high probability of a dramatic cure "interesting," they dislike conditions, such as back pain, chronic vague pains, headaches, and chronic fatigue, that offer little probability of cure while bringing their competence or diagnostic skills into question. Furthermore, they dislike conditions for which they believe the patient or others are responsible, such as sexual behavior, auto accidents, suicide attempts, and other self-inflicted injuries (Klein et al., 1982; see also Hahn, 1985b; Jeffery, 1979; Roth, 1972; Smith and Zimny, 1988).

One study found the leading common characteristics of patients that doctors label as "gomers" ("*g*et *o*utta *m*y *e*mergency *r*oom") were illnesses and/or personal characteristics that created management difficulties for the hospital staff (Leiderman and Grisso, 1985). Many patients were identified as "gomers" because their conditions defied solution by modern medical intervention. Their deterioration under treatment was thus a source of frustration and ideological doubts for doctors, especially the beginning doctors who typically staffed hospital emergency rooms and clinics.

Many of the other derogatory terms used for patients reflect similar values. A widespread distinction in doctors' stereotyping of patients is between "sick people" and "trolls." The latter term is applied to patients whom doctors believe lack a "real" disease and to those held culpable for the cause of and/or the failure to control their condition. Other derogatory terms for undesirable patients include "albatross," "turkey," and "crock." Medical education encourages compassion for "sick people" but contempt for "trolls." Such negative stereotypes often supersede even the medical model itself in informing the doctor's understanding of a case, thus leading to failed empathy (Stein, 1986).

Contempt for "trolls" is particularly encouraged in the United States by the use of student-doctors to staff emergency rooms and clinics that serve a disproportionate number of these "undesirable" patients compared to fee-for-service private practice. The characteristic contempt is illustrated in this quote from a junior resident in an emergency room:

> At least 40–50 percent are gomers. Some weeks there is nothing but alcohol-induced diseases. The other night on call I met only three people with genuine diseases—having nothing to do with anything they ever did to themselves. I spend hours [with them] and check them everyday, but some guy who comes in with alcoholic pancreatitis—I'll tune him up and fire him out the door, and not give two shakes about him (quoted in Mizrahi, 1986: 102).

Hospital staff generally admitted that they often treated undesirable patients less thoroughly. Sometimes the stereotypes led to misdiagnoses and other medical mistakes (Mizrahi, 1986). For example, a homeless person brought unconscious to the emergency room may be treated as a "gomer" under the assumption that the condition was alcohol-induced, whereas a thorough treatment might discover that the symptoms resulted from a serious neurological problem.

Doctors' negative stereotypes of patients are also based upon social and personal characteristics. Doctors tended to consider "undesirable" those patients whose behavior violated the physicians' personal norms, even those with little or no relevance to health. The largest category of social characteristics (33 percent) eliciting negative responses from doctors included such violations as being dirty, smelly, vulgar, chronically unemployed, promiscuous, homosexual, malingering, or on welfare, Medicaid, or workers' compensation. Doctors' expectations of patients are based largely upon white, middle-class values that are accentuated by the self-selection and professional training processes. Social class differences also appear to figure into some negative stereotypes (Klein et al., 1982).

Doctors' often unrecognized value judgments of patients can result in failed empathy and less adequate care, as illustrated by one resident who admitted that he had detested patients who demanded Vistaril (an anti-anxiety drug often used in pain control) (Stein, 1986). He had viewed them as not legitimately sick but rather as weak, irresponsible, and dependent. Coming from a religious, rural, self-sufficient background, he valued patients who were self-sufficient in their health care and who rarely complained. Until he himself experienced considerable pain from minor surgery (and quickly wrote himself a prescription for Vistaril), he had a strong negative stereotype of patients whose requests for pain medication did not mesh with his personal values.

A study of the medical education process showed how both the structure of medical training and professional ideology work against the development of humanistic doctor-patient relationships.[2] New physicians are taught to avoid interaction with patients, to restrict the time spent with them, and to limit the patient input they listen to in medical interviews (Mizrahi, 1986: 118–119). This study concluded that the very structure of internship and residency teaches doctors to get rid of noninteresting patients. Reflecting both the attitudes of his supervisors and his personal experience with enormous time pressures, one junior resident said, " 'There are different kinds of ideal patients. When you're an intern, the ideal patient is someone you can get out and get out quickly' " (quoted in Mizrahi, 1986: 74–75). Interns and residents, for example, were informally rewarded for quickly and efficiently taking patient histories, and they learned not to bother with inquiring about social aspects of the cases because nobody noticed or appreciated if that were done.

Medical students learned, formally and informally, that what their professors and supervisors really wanted them to do was to narrow their clinical findings efficiently to biophysical data relevant to possible pathology. One senior resident explained:

> I guess I could use the excuse that I don't have the time to do that [deal with patient's social problems]. . . . It would be nice to bullshit with your patients for an hour or so and get a feel for their social situation. . . . It may affect the complaints they present with. . . . If I was Marcus Welby [a former TV physician] and saw one patient per week, maybe I would be more concerned. I doubt it though, because it's really not appealing to me. If I really wanted to do it, I would have majored in social work or psychiatry. What appeals to me is treatment of sick people by diagnosing their diseases and giving medications. *I like good hard facts and physical findings*—things I can deal with on a tangible basis—not some intangible nebulous feeling of what their social situation is (quoted in Mizrahi, 1986: 95 [emphasis added]).

This attitude reflects the medical model's separation of the disease from the socioemotional aspects of the patient's illness; doctors are socialized to view the nonbiophysical aspects as "fuzzy," "soft" facts that are ultimately irrelevant to their essential task.

[2]For more detailed and textured description of the medical education process and its impact on treatment of patients, see Becker et al., 1961; Bloom, 1979; Coombs, 1978; Davis-Floyd, 1987; Groopman, 1987; Konner, 1987; Light, 1980; Merton et al., 1957; Scully, 1980.

TRANSFORMING THE SICK PERSON INTO A CASE

Just as the medical paradigm views the body as separate from the person, so too does the interaction between doctor and patient often involve isolating salient information about the sick body from the sick person him- or herself. One of the effects of most medical encounters is to transform the sick person into a medical case. Drawing from their medical training and the biomedical paradigm for interpreting disease and pathology, physicians use the medical encounter for relatively narrow goals: the efficient eliciting and honing of facts relevant to a medical diagnosis, the precise application of a set of decision rules for proceeding, and active therapeutic intervention. Although their understanding of the medical encounter is informed by rational biomedicine, it is also the product of situational factors, cultural biases, and subjective influences that are often subtly embedded in the doctors' practice of medicine itself (Stein, 1986; see also Mishler, 1984).

Social Influences on Medical Judgments

The process of locating and interpreting medical evidence is always socially mediated. Such medical judgments as the factors that the diagnostician considers relevant, the clues that are thought worth seeking and thus are elicited in conversation and testing, and those that should be overlooked or discarded often entail social as well as biological attributes. For example, doctors treating elderly persons sometimes do not carry out routine tests in physical examinations, because they assume patient problems are due to senility or old age (Glassman, 1980).

Both the patient and the doctor often treat the diagnosis as a conclusion rather than a working hypothesis. Even before the diagnosis is reached, the physician's expectations and hunches may limit the clues examined. A study of medical thinking showed that doctors tended to develop hypotheses very early in an intake interview, often basing their hunches on only the patient's general appearance and one or two presenting complaints (Kassirer and Gorry, 1978). The physician's expectations are often subsequently self-confirming; contradictory clues are neither noticed nor sought (Jones, 1982: 156–161).

Medical evidence is typically ambiguous and multifaceted. In both scientific and other medical systems, the process of reaching a diagnosis is one of pattern forming. Despite extensive diagnostic technologies, the art of diagnosis in modern medicine is highly imprecise. U.S. data on autopsies show that in biomedical terms one out of three diagnoses were erroneous, and that in one out of ten cases the error could have contributed to the patient's death (*New York Times*, 1987a; see also Altman, 1988b; Sullivan, 1983). To form a pattern, one must actively select pieces of evidence to cluster into an understanding. This process necessarily entails deciding which pieces of information to include and which to exclude (see Locker, 1981).

Similarly, in the interpretation of evidence and treatment decisions nonphysical elements, such as the emotional or social situation of the ill person, become part of the pattern.[3] Often the person creating the pattern is not aware of these elements; instead moral judgments and ideological assumptions enter the process under the guise of objective physical observations. For example, in examining x-rays of workers' lungs for symptoms of asbestosis, company physicians saw very different patterns than did doctors not connected with the industry (Brodeur, 1974: 174).

There is no necessary connection between the many diagnoses and possible treatments. Numerous, sometimes contradictory treatment options exist in any single medical system, and social factors influence which one the doctor recommends. Individual practitioners differ in the *decision rules* that they follow in choosing certain treatments for the same condition. (Decision rules are a form of knowledge that provides a set of minimally acceptable criteria for selecting a mode of treatment, such as surgery or medication.) A British study of ear, nose, and throat specialists revealed that widely varying decision rules determine whether an adenotonsil-lectomy should be performed. Some relied heavily on a physical examination (and practitioners disagreed over what to look for in the examination); others attached no significance to examination findings and relied instead on the case history. Some recommended surgery only when several signs were present on examination; others considered the existence of only one sign sufficient (Bloor, 1976).

Social judgments also enter into physicians' decision rules. Often the therapy proposed by a doctor varies greatly from patient to patient, even when the same biophysical conditions are present. When recommending hysterectomies (surgical removal of the uterus, resulting in sterility), physicians often included in their decision rules such factors as the woman's age, ethnicity, poverty, marital status, and whether she was on welfare, had had multiple abortions, and had already had children (Fisher, 1986). Thus a more serious biophysical condition in a twenty-five-year-old white woman with no children might be less likely to be treated with a hysterectomy than a less serious condition in a thirty-five-year-old black woman with four children.

Judgments of social worth also enter into medical decisions. Studies of treatment decisions and other actions in hospital emergency services show that the young are treated as being more valuable than the old and that welfare cases are treated as being less worthy than those not on welfare. Especially disvalued persons, such as those labeled "drunks" and "PIDs"

---

[3]This is not a criticism; effective treatment probably should take the sick person's entire situation into consideration. The issue here is the extent to which uncritical assumption and ideological biases often enter the process and are treated as part of "objective" reality, without the participants' awareness.

(women with pelvic inflammatory diseases, often assumed to be due to promiscuity), are given even less prompt and considerate treatment (Roth, 1972; see also Sudnow, 1967).

An appreciation of the social construction of ideas of illness, together with an awareness of the flexible processes by which these ideas are applied in diagnosis and therapy, helps explain how cases are constructed. Medical decision making is powerfully influenced by social assumptions that are often implicit and unacknowledged. The creation of a medical case shows that not only medical knowledge but also medical practice is a social construction.

Depersonalization of the Patient

Patients also bring an understanding—sometimes fragmented and contradictory—of the nature of their illness. They enter the medical encounter with an array of important social, emotional, and situational concerns. Drawing from cultural models, the patients have some interpretation of their own illness. Furthermore, they are likely to be struggling with problems of meaning, at least in the instance of feared, serious illness, including: Why me? Who is responsible? Why this disease? What will this do to my identity and my future?

Serious miscommunication and depersonalization occur when the doctor disconfirms or ignores patient concerns and understandings. Box 10.1 illustrates a gravely flawed exchange between doctor and patient. The doctor, intent only upon his biophysical assessment, has failed to hear the person, ignoring or interrupting her attempts to explain her illness. In conducting the interview and writing this report, the doctor is using the technically correct forms he learned in his training. However, in the medical record he produces, the patient is dehumanized and transformed into a reified, thing-like case, very unlike the person who, as revealed in the transcript, speaks eloquently of her commitments, fears, stresses, economic and social problems.

In transforming Mrs. Flowers into a medical case, the doctor reduces her to her hypertension, her noncompliance with the medical regimen, her early signs of heart failure, and her medications. The doctor, following the technically correct approach to interviewing and treating, has completely missed the person with her complex social, psychological, and economic problems. His control of the interview consistently constrains Mrs. Flowers's presentation of her concerns; she is frequently ignored or interrupted when talking about the very matters that brought her to see the doctor. The doctor permits her to speak about her physical complaints, but disallows her psychological or social problems. The interview elicits only facts about her biophysical diseases and medical treatment. Even though Mrs. Flowers's human suffering is very much a part of her chronic illness, it is relegated to a perfunctory referral to a social worker (Kleinman, 1988: 134–136).

BOX 10.1   The Creation of a Medical Case

Background: Mrs. Flowers is returning to the clinic, where she had previously been treated for her hypertension. She is thirty-nine years old, black, the mother of five children. She lives with four of her children, her mother, and two grandchildren in an inner-city ghetto. She works at present as a waitress in a restaurant, but periodically she has been unemployed and on welfare. She has been married twice, but both of her husbands have deserted her. As a result, she is a single head of household. Mrs. Flowers is an active member of the local Baptist church, which has been an important source of support to her and her family for many years. She is also a member of a community action group.

In the household of eight, she is the only wage earner. Her mother, Mildred, is fifty-nine and partially paralyzed owing to a stroke that was the result of long-standing and poorly controlled hypertension. Her oldest daughter, Matty, the unmarried nineteen-year-old mother of two small children, is at present unemployed and pregnant; in the past, she has had a drug problem. Mrs. Flowers's fifteen-year-old daughter, Marcia, is also pregnant. Their eighteen-year-old brother, J. D., is in prison. Teddy, a twelve-year-old, has had problems with truancy and minor delinquency. Amelia, eleven, the baby of the family, is said by her mother to be an angel.

A year ago, Mrs. Flowers's long-time male companion, Eddie Johnson, was killed in a barroom brawl. Recently, Mrs. Flowers has been increasingly upset by memories of Eddie Johnson, by concern for how prison will affect J. D., and by fears that Teddy will get involved with drugs like his older brother and sister before him. She is also concerned about her mother's worsening disability, which includes what she fears may be early signs of dementia.

Dr. Richards: Hello, Mrs. Flowers.
Mrs. Flowers: I ain't feelin' too well today, Doc Richards.
Dr. Richards: What seems to be wrong?
Mrs. Flowers: Um, I don't know. Maybe it's that pressure of mine. I been gettin' headaches and havin' trouble sleeping.
Dr. Richards: Your hypertension is a bit worse, but not all that bad, considering what it's been in the past. You been taking your medicines as you ought to?
Mrs. Flowers: Sometimes I do. But sometimes when I don't have no pressure, I don't take it.
Dr. Richards: Gee whiz, Mrs. Flowers, I told you if you don't take it regularly you could get real sick like your Mom. You got to take the pills every day. And what about salt? You been eating salt again?
Mrs. Flowers: It's hard to cook for the family without salt. I don't have time to cook just for me. At lunch, I'm in the restaurant and Charlie, he's the chef, he puts lotsa salt in everythin'.
Dr. Richards: Well, now this is a real problem. Salt restriction, I mean a low-salt diet, is essential for your problem.
Mrs. Flowers: I know, I know. I mean to do all these things, but I just plain forget sometimes. I got so much else goin' on and it all seems to affect the pressure. I got two pregnant daughters at home and my mother is doin' much worse. I think she may be senile. And then I worries about J. D., and here comes Teddy with the same problems startin' up. I—

Dr. Richards: Have you any shortness of breath?

Mrs. Flowers: No.

Dr. Richards: Any chest pain?

Mrs. Flowers: No.

Dr. Richards: Swelling in your feet?

Mrs. Flowers: The feet do get a little swollen, but then I'm on them all day long at the restaurant—

Dr. Richards: You said you had headaches?

Mrs. Flowers: Sometimes I think my life is one big headache. These here ain't too bad. I've had 'em for a long time, years. But in recent weeks they been badder than before. You see, a year ago last Sunday, Eddie Johnson, my friend, you know. Uh huh, well, he died. And—

Dr. Richards: Are the headaches in the same place as before?

Mrs. Flowers: Yeah, same place, same feelin', on'y more often. But, you see, Eddie Johnson had always told me not to bother about—

Dr. Richards: Have you had any difficulty with your vision?

Mrs. Flowers: No.

Dr. Richards: Any nausea?

Mrs. Flowers: No. Well when I drank the pickle juice, there was some.

Dr. Richards: Pickle juice? You've been drinking pickle juice? That's got a great deal of salt. It's a real danger for you, for your hypertension.

Mrs. Flowers: But I have felt pressure this week and my mother told me maybe I need it because I got high blood and—

Dr. Richards: Oh, no. Not pickle juice. Mrs. Flowers, you can't drink that for any reason. It just isn't good. Don't you understand? It's got lots of salt, and salt is bad for your hypertension.

Mrs. Flowers: Uh huh. OK.

Dr. Richards: Any other problems?

Mrs. Flowers: My sleep ain't been too good, doc. I think it's because—

Dr. Richards: Is it trouble getting to sleep?

Mrs. Flowers: Yeah, and gettin' up real early in the mornin'. I been dreamin' about Eddie Johnson. Doin' a lot of rememberin' and cryin'. I been feelin' real lonely. I don't know—

Dr. Richards: Any other problems? I mean bodily problems?

Mrs. Flowers: No, 'cept for tired feelin', but that's been there for years. Dr. Richards, you think worryin' and missin' somebody can give you headaches?

Dr. Richards: I don't know. If they are tension headaches, it might. But you haven't had other problems like dizziness, weakness, fatigue?

Mrs. Flowers: That's what I'm sayin'! The tired feelin', it's been there some time. And the pressure makes it worse. But I wanted to ask you about worries. I got me a mess o' worries. And I been feelin' all down, as if I just couldn't handle it anymore. The money is a real problem now.

Dr. Richards: Well, I will have to ask Mrs. Ma, the social worker to talk to you about the financial aspect. She might be able to help. Right now why don't we do a physical exam and see how you're doing?

Mrs. Flowers: I ain't doin' well. Even I can tell you that. There's too much pressure and it's makin' *my pressure* bad. And I been feelin' real sad for myself.

Dr. Richards: Well, we'll soon see how things are going.

After completing the physical examination, Dr. Richards wrote the following note in the medical record:

April 14, 1980

39 year old Black female with hypertension on hydrochlorothiazide 100 mgs. daily and aldomet 2 grams daily. Blood pressure now 160/105, has been 170/80–110/120 for several months, alternating with 150–/95 when taking meds regularly. Has evidence of mild congestive heart failure. No other problems.

Impression: (1) Hypertension, poorly controlled
            (2) Noncompliance contributing to (1)
            (3) Congestive heart failure—mild
            (1) Change aldomet to apresoline.
            (2) Send to dietician to enforce lower salt diet
            (3) Social work consult because of financial questions
            (4) See in 3 days, regularly until blood pressure has come
                 down and stabilized.

Signed: Dr. Staunton Richards

Dr. Richards also sent a terse note for a consultation to the dietician, which read: "39 year old Black woman with poorly controlled hypertension who does not comply with low salt diet. Please help plan 2 gram sodium diet, and explain to her again relationship of salt intake to her disease and that she must stop eating high salt foods and cooking with salt."

Source: The Illness Narratives: Suffering, Healing, and the Human Condition, by Arthur Kleinman, M.D. Copyright © 1988 by Basic Books, Inc. Reprinted by permission of Basic Books, Inc., Publishers.

The disease orientation of the medical model and the doctor's professional distance from the patient combine to turn the complex person into a rationalized case with its biophysical parts neatly separated from its social, emotional, spiritual, and economic elements. In this situation, the doctor is also so culturally distant from the patient that he is ignorant of the ideas and social practices that inform her own understanding of her situation. For example, she refers to her "high blood"—a folk illness in lower-class black American subculture. Since "high blood" is believed to result from blood rising to the head, her consumption of pickle juice makes sense as folk remedy, because it is believed to thin or "cut" the blood. Cultural and social factors, such as the limitations posed by her job, make it unlikely that the sick woman would actually follow the difficult instructions for managing her serious illnesses. Rather than understanding these factors, the doctor views what he labels her "noncompliance" as a moral failing. She is not a "good" patient because she does not do what he tells her to do to control her biophysical condition (Kleinman, 1988: 135–136).

An interesting contrast is the inner-city clinic experience of a young black internist from a middle-class background; her understanding of a patient like Mrs. Flowers is remarkably different:

The more I see, the more appalled I am at how ignorant I have been, insensitive to the social, economic, and political causes of disease. . . . Today I saw an obese hypertensive mother of six. No husband. No family support. No job. Nothing. A world of brutalizing violence and poverty and drugs and teenage pregnancies and—and just plain mind-numbing crises, one after another after another. What can I do? What good is it to recommend a low salt diet, to admonish her about control of her pressure? She is under such real outer pressure, what does the inner pressure matter? What is killing her is her world, not her body. In fact, her body is the product of her world. She is a hugely overweight, misshapen hulk who is a survivor of circumstances and lack of resources and cruel messages to consume and get ahead impossible for her to hear and not feel rage at the limits of her world. Hey, what she needs is not medicine but a social revolution (quoted in Kleinman, 1988: 216–217).

In learning the medical model and the specific techniques of clinical practice, doctors are trained to transform the patient into a case. A study of case presentations—a standard training method in which interns, residents, and fellows in a teaching hospital present formal case studies to their superiors—found that the standard discourse depersonalized patients, referring to them as objects: their disease, their treatment procedure, or a shorthand term for their health status (Anspach, 1988). For example, a pregnant woman is transformed into a "Gravida III, Para I, AbI, black female at 32 weeks gestation" (Anspach, 1988: 363). Furthermore, by using the passive voice and referring to technological procedures, doctors' case presentations also failed to acknowledge the *human* agency in observing or treating. For example, they state, "He was put on phenobarb," rather than "I decided to put him on phenobarb," or "The arteriogram showed that this AVM was fed . . . ," instead of "I requested an arteriogram and interpreted its findings to mean . . ." (Anspach, 1988: 366–368).

The very language and interviewing techniques of the standard doctor-patient interaction result in losing sight of the patient as person and the patient's concerns. For example, physicians recode the patients' expressions into medical terminology, which becomes a shorthand for their medical condition and glosses over possibly relevant nonphysical aspects of the patients' description of their problems (see Mishler, 1984). In the example above, Mrs. Flowers's expressions are transformed into "hypertension, poorly controlled," "noncompliance," and "mild congestive heart failure." In recoding the language for conceptualizing the problem, the patient's perspective is obscured (Cicourel, 1983: 238).

Likewise, the structure of the medical interview leads to inadequate doctor-patient communication and truncated, distorted understandings of the patient's problem. Doctors are trained to use a set of formulas for conducting interviews with patients. One such formula is a "decision tree," a sequence of small decisions that culminate in a diagnosis and treatment plan. Accordingly, doctors elicit information from patients that enables them to narrow the range of possible medical problems down to smaller and smaller "branches." While they are talking with patients, doctors are simultaneously mentally testing hypotheses. Thus doctors experience patient input that is not immediately relevant to the part of the decision tree they are then considering as disruptive to their line of thought. Similarly, doctors are trained to proceed in the interview by reviewing each of the bodily systems (respiratory system, circulatory system, and so on), often in a verbal check-list format. This routine device guarantees a certain thoroughness, but doctors often become irritated by the "disruption" of a patient who introduces a question or a point relevant to some area of concern other than the immediate item on the check list (West, 1984; see also Waitzkin, 1989a).

Thus the typical patterns of doctor-patient communication produce a case, a reified representation of a sickness in which the sick *person* is remote or absent. Often subsequent interaction between the patient and doctor as well as other medical staff is based upon this representation, rather than upon any fresh input from the sick person. Such depersonalization results when the focal object of doctors' work is the medical case.

THE ENDS OF MODERN MEDICINE: MORAL DILEMMA AND SOCIAL POLICIES

Implicit in the medical model of disease and curing are a number of assumptions about life and death and the proper ends of medical intervention. These assumptions are so deeply embedded that rarely are they acknowledged, much less examined. They have contributed to major contemporary problems for medical personnel and for society as a whole about how to deal with death and dying, life and potential life, and "normal" and "abnormal" life. In short, should the foremost goal of medicine be preserving and extending life for all patients?

The Medical Model and the Conquest of Death

Comaroff (1984) suggested that the biomedical model's interventionist stance against disease, which is defined as the disruption of the body's organic functioning, led to the acceptance of the conquest of death as a major goal of medicine. While acknowledging that ultimately all persons will die, the medical model makes it difficult and sometimes impossible to *decide* that any given person shall be allowed to die (cf. Kleiman, 1985; Muller and Koenig, 1988). The focus on the conquest of death also reduces medicine's attention to other needs, such as ameliorating suffering or making mundane improvements in the sick (or dying) person's quality of life.

Contemporary medical dilemmas are in part the result of biomedicine's very successes. Modern technologies enable doctors to prolong lives, even though often they cannot actually cure the disease. For example, the technology of dialysis allows persons with otherwise fatal kidney failure to live three or more years longer. Technological developments enable neonatal intensive care units to reduce the rate of respiratory distress syndrome among undersized infants who would have surely died soon after birth in earlier decades. Other technologies simulate virtually every organic function, artificially supplying the body with breath, food, water, immune responses, heartbeat, excretion, and blood cleansing. Similarly, the extremely expensive technology of organ transplantation extends some lives, often for many years.

Whereas in the recent past people expected that death was inevitable and would occur at its appointed time, now they expect medicine to intervene to prevent death and to prolong life. Indeed, in promulgating the successes of scientific medicine, the profession itself may have raised people's expectations unrealistically high. The idea that medicine can and should intervene to prolong life is consonant with both the medical model and physicians' professional ideologies. Doctors want to assert their control over sickness and the loss of life; many physicians view the death of a patient as a failure. The expectation that the goal of medicine is to prevent death has many negative consequences, however.

Our culture is profoundly uncomfortable with death and dying. It does little to prepare people for their own and others' deaths (Kearl, 1989; see also Elias, 1985). Ariès (1974) documented the historical development of modern taboos about death. Accordingly, as society failed to provide a consensus about how to die a "good death," it segregated sickness and death from normal social interaction. Medical institutions perform the latent function of segregating the unpleasantness of sickness and dying, while aspiring to the manifest function of curing.

Death and dying have become medicalized partly because of expectations that medicine will be able to intervene in the process, and partly because many people are relieved to have their family members' dying supervised by medical personnel in a hospital setting. Death is perhaps less threatening if it is thus removed, sterilized, and routinized. At the same time, however, the dying process is partly cut off from the very institutions of society most likely to be able to provide meaning in the face of death: religion and the family. Some alternative arrangements for dying, such as the hospice movement, encourage demedicalizing and rehumanizing the process.

Nevertheless, to choose an alternative arrangement for dying requires that alternatives be available, affordable, and legally allowed; that doctors and family members be aware and consciously accept that the patient is dying; and that there be mechanisms for dying persons to consider their options and express their intentions regarding death. Many social structures and attitudes in our society make it difficult for people to die with dignity. The specter of an unavoidable, overmedicalized end is not unrealistic: Medical technology makes possible keeping the body "alive" with respirators, feeding tubes, intravenous hydration and antibiotics, heart resuscitators, and the like, long after the person in the body has lost the ability to consider or express a desire to live or die.

The Technological Imperative

Another cultural value that makes it difficult to decide to let nature take its course and allow death to happen is the **technological imperative**, a prevalent idea in most Western societies (especially the United States) that urges that if we have the technological capability to do something, then we should do it. The technological imperative implies that action in the form of the use of an available technology is always preferable to inaction. Indeed, once a technology becomes available, its use becomes almost inexorably routinized and considered standard. The failure to apply this standard care—no matter how inappropriate for the individual patient—would be reprehensible (Koenig, 1988). The technological imperative is deeply embedded in many institutional responses to health crises. For example, most hospitals have created (and thus need to use) several high-technology wards, such as coronary and neonatal intensive care units, deliberately equipped and staffed to provide maximum multiple technological responses to patients' conditions. Similarly, much health insurance gives priority to high-tech medicine (such as treatment in a coronary care unit) over low-tech or nontechnological responses (such as home care with the help of a visiting health aide and nurse).

In arguing that the proper goal of medicine should not be the unquestioned prolongation of life, the ethicist Callahan (1987: 173) wrote that "the existence of medical technologies capable of extending the lives of the elderly who have lived out a natural life span creates no presumption whatever that the technologies must be used for that purpose." Similar but perhaps more difficult questions need to be posed about the uses of technology for prolonging the lives of persons who have not lived out a natural life span (see Crane, 1975; Hilfiker, 1983). What medical intervention should be used, for example, for an accident victim left in a persistent vegetative state, for a medically unsalvageable patient, such as a person with cancer of the esophagus who subsequently has a heart attack, or for an irreparably damaged newborn, such as an infant with anencephaly (congenital lack of a brain) or myelomeningocele (which in severe cases produces paraplegia, the lack of urinary control, and brain damage)?

There are also serious ethical questions about the use of medical responses that themselves cause pain or other suffering. For example, under what conditions should a patient or a patient's family be allowed to refuse a prescribed treatment, such as chemotherapy or surgery? The technological imperative has considerable legal support in many states; patients and their families must go to court to assert (and sometimes lose) the right to decide to refuse treatment or life supports. Other legal and ethical rights are also uncertain. Does a person have the right to obtain a particular treatment, even if it will not cure or even provide certain benefits for that individual? For example, does every person with kidney failure have the right to a transplant?

Because they underlie legal and social policies, such ethical issues are matters for the entire society as well as individual practitioners, patients, and families to consider. These issues are difficult for the courts, in part because the courts have increasingly deferred to the medical profession itself as the proper authority on matters of defining life and death. As noted in Chapter 6, the medicalization of moral authority has undermined the authority of other institutions, such as religion and the family.

On issues such as these, however, there is no technical (i.e., purely medical) answer. The boundaries of life and death are blurred, and biomedicine is incapable of clearly delineating them for the courts in purely technical terms, as illustrated by the ambiguities of court cases involving the abortion of second trimester fetuses and the passive euthanasia of patients in a persistent vegetative state. As Callahan (1987: 179) observed, "The 'sanctity of life' has to be the sanctity of personhood, not merely the possession of a body." Moral and legal rights adhere to *persons*, but there are no neat biomedical criteria to distinguish when or whether a body is a person. The choice of such criteria must come from outside scientific medicine, although they may include medically measurable determinants, such as brain death.

Policy Implications

Our society must come to terms with these issues in order to develop sensible social policies: How shall we pay for the care needed by the sick and dying? Toward what ends shall we train doctors and other medical personnel? How shall we allocate our society's research funding? What kinds of institutional support are required to fulfill our health care goals; for example, should society's focus be on high-tech hospital care, or is more societal support needed for other institutional settings, such as public health programs, real homes for the aged, or home health aides. Such policy decisions regularly require difficult choices, since no society can possibly meet every need of all citizens and thus must set its priorities.

These policy decisions have been thrust on us by the burgeoning costs of high-tech medicine; by the medicalization of birthing, dying, and other areas of life; and by the increasing numbers and proportions of the popula- tion who are old and very old. For example, both the physician and hospital portions of Medicare payments are rising dramatically and threaten to deplete those funds. About 25 to 35 percent of Medicare expenditures each year pay for the medical costs of only 5 to 6 percent of the enrollees—those in their last year of life (Lubitz and Priboda, 1984; Scitovsky and Capron, 1986).

In another example, as recently as fifteen years ago babies born very prematurely died shortly after birth. Now many of these babies live, although a substantial proportion suffer handicaps and chronic illnesses. The main factors in their survival are the new technologies in neonatal wards and intensive nursing. These are very expensive services; the necessary three or four months of hospitalization may cost $90,000 or more. In many parts of the United States the rates of premature birth are rising (French, 1989). Because of the burgeoning cost of such care, even though it is medically effective for many babies, society must examine whether this expenditure is the best use for its moneys (see Guillemin and Holmstom, 1986). Might it not be better to spend health care dollars on public health programs that could prevent premature births such as prenatal care and nutrition programs for women of childbearing age?

Similar allocation questions also apply to decisions about who shall receive high-priced organ transplants and other expensive surgery. What proportion of the nation's health care resources should go to care for the elderly and the dying? What priorities should be given to heroic interventions (such as by-pass surgery) compared to palliative efforts (such as pain relief) or to simple care and nursing? The United States operates with a de facto system of rationing health care: The wealthy buy whatever they want; the middle classes buy what their insurance allows and have the option to deplete their other resources to buy more; and the poor get whatever the state and Medicaid systems, public hospitals, and Medicare (if they are elderly) offer. This form of rationing results in enormous inequities (Fein, 1986; Gill and Ingman, 1986). The nation needs to confront the ethical issues that have been only implicit in its health care system and must ask: What are our priorities, and is this the kind of nation we really want to be?

SUMMARY

Modern biomedical forms of knowledge and practice are the particular result of social, political, and economic processes. The accomplishment of professional dominance by medical doctors in this century gives them both preeminence in the medical division of labor and control over the definitions of health, illness, and healing practices.

Medical professional dominance also creates problems for the treatment of the sick. The layperson-expert gap and other sources of social distance often result in poor communication and failed empathy. Doctor-patient relationships may reflect other social distance, such as that produced by gender and class stratification. Much interaction between doctor and patient serves to protect the power of the physician, which often directly disempowers the patient. Both the socialization of physicians and the social structure of medical practice promote patterns of doctor-patient interaction that disrupt real communication and lead to unsatisfactory treatment.

Assumptions implicit in the medical model have made it difficult for doctors and laypersons to admit to the limits of modern medicine and to consider setting different goals for its practice. By focusing on the conquest of death, medicine overemphasizes an interventionist approach to treatment and has difficulty coming to terms with death and dying. Not only do doctors and their patients need to reconsider the proper ends of medicine, but society as a whole is also confronted with massive ethical, legal, and policy issues about health care and medical treatment.

RECOMMENDED READINGS

Books

Daniel Callahan, *Setting Limits: Medical Goals in an Aging Society*. New York: Simon and Schuster, 1987. Callahan outlines the ethical problems posed by the medicalization of aging and dying, together with the burgeoning proportion of society in the old and very old age brackets. In the context of alternative ideas about the proper role of the elderly, he proposes carefully considered guidelines for setting limits for health care expenditures on persons who have lived a full life span.

Barbara Ehrenreich and Deirdre English, *Witches, Midwives, and Nurses: A History of Women Healers*. Old Westbury, NY: The Feminist Press, 1973. A brief historical treatise on how, in the process of medical professional domination, traditional women healers were driven out or subordinated.

Marcia Millman, *The Unkindest Cut: Life in the Backrooms of Medicine*. New York: William Morrow, 1976. A highly readable ethnography of hospital surgical units, with special attention to the social management of medical "mistakes."

Terry Mizrahi, *Getting Rid of Patients: Contradictions in the Socialization of Physicians*. New Brunswick, NJ: Rutgers University Press, 1986. Mizrahi has studied various stages in the training of physicians with a particular emphasis upon what they learned (formally and informally) about how to deal with patients; the serious contradictions in values imparted have important implications for the care of patients.

Articles

Eric J. Cassell, "The nature of suffering and the goals of medicine," *New England Journal of Medicine* 306, 1982: 639–645.

Jean Comaroff, "Medicine, time, and the perception of death," *Listening* 19(2), 1984: 155–169.

Chapter Eleven

Stratification and Power in Health Care Systems

There is enormous variety in how societies respond to the health needs of their members. Economic and social structural arrangements determine how a society cares for members' sick bodies, frail elderly bodies, disabled bodies, infant bodies—the well-being of all its members. This analysis shows the importance of social power in shaping these economic and social structural arrangements. Each society's political economy creates its health care system's goals and policies for achieving those goals.

A health care system is the "aggregate of commitments or resources which any national society 'invests' in the health concern" (Field, 1973:763). As a system, all parts mutually influence each other, for better or for worse. Changes in one part of the system result in changes in another part. The U.S. health care system includes, for example, patients and other recipients of care; patients' families; doctors and many other providers of care; hospitals, nursing homes, clinics, and other institutional settings for care; insurers and others who pay for health care goods and services; industries that produce the many goods utilized in health care; and levels of government that are not only a major source of insurance but also a source of regulations, research funding, public health programs, and health-related policies.

U.S. PROBLEMS IN COMPARATIVE PERSPECTIVE

In this society health care has been equated with medical care, and most data in Chapters 11 and 12 refer only to medical care, its organization, and its costs. Our social policies have not conceptualized—much less accommodated—a total health care system. The development and possible effectiveness of social policy are ultimately a political process in which powerful interest groups vie to define the agenda. The present emphasis upon medical care of disease is itself the political product of relative muscle of various interest groups; any attempt to set a broader agenda for the health of the nation would almost certainly be contested by interest groups benefiting from the status quo.

International comparisons suggest that there are four broad types of health care systems in industrial societies. The U.S. system, exemplifying the first type, is a laissez-faire, commodified arrangement resulting in a diverse and relatively uncoordinated, loosely or unplanned mixture of many different institutional programs for the provision of health services. Profit is a significant motivating factor for many of the system's health service providers, institutions, insurers, and producers of products and technologies; health care is *sold* in an economic marketplace. The medical profession enjoys large amounts of autonomy in regulating its affairs and conditions of work. The second type, a national health insurance system, is similar, except that *all* citizens are insured by third parties (e.g., a government agency or a labor union) that have a significant degree of regulatory control over practitioners and health-related institutions. The Canadian system exemplifies this model. The British National Health Service (NHS) is a prime example of the third type, a health service system, in which most facilities are owned by the nation and most physicians (whether in private practice or on hospital staff) are paid from state moneys. Physicians have relatively large amounts of professional autonomy, although the state has greater control over salaries and institutional arrangements than in laissez-faire or insurance systems. Socialized health systems, such as those in the U.S.S.R. and Eastern Europe, are characterized by yet greater control by the state, which owns and manages all health facilities and employs almost all health personnel (see Field, 1973).

In the United States the power of competing interest groups, together with the ideology of free market competition, has resulted in an amazingly complex, unwieldy and expensive health care system that many suggest is now in crisis. Health care expenditures have been growing dramatically—much faster than other expenses in the Consumer Price Index. Figure 11.1 shows the increased proportion of the total U.S. gross national product (GNP) consumed by health care costs. In 1987 these expenditures amounted to more than $2,130 per person (Malcolm, 1988). Furthermore, these figures include only expenditures for formal health care (e.g., doctors, hospitals, pharmaceuticals, and medical supplies); they do not include most costs of informal care (e.g., assistance with daily living for persons with chronic

FIGURE 11.1   U.S. Health Care Expenditures as a Percentage of Gross National Product. (*Sources:* Department of Health and Human Services. *Health, United States. 1983.* Washington, DC: U.S. Government Printing Office, 1984. 1987 figures from Andrew H. Malcolm, "In health care policy, the latest word is fiscal," *New York Times,* October 23, 1988.)

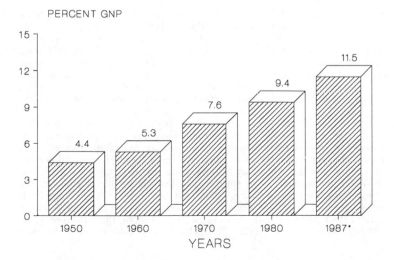

illness) or most health maintenance expenses (e.g., nutrition, pollution control, and accident prevention).

Despite these increased expenditures, the vast majority of Americans are dissatisfied with the health care system in this country. Public opinion polls show that 89 percent of Americans consider their system to need fundamental change, compared to 42 percent of Canadians and 69 percent of the British. The survey found that under the American system, a much larger proportion of citizens are faced with financial barriers to receiving health care than in Britain or Canada, and that substantial numbers are either not covered by health insurance or severely underinsured (Hevesi, 1989). The United States and the Republic of South Africa are the only industrialized nations without some form of comprehensive health care system for *all* citizens (Roemer, 1985). Dissatisfaction with the British health care system, by contrast, is due mainly to the fact that the government has seriously underfunded the NHS, resulting in shortages, understaffing, and growing waiting lists for nonemergency hospital services (Lohr, 1988). Indeed, the Thatcher administration has encouraged competition from for-profit, private health care providers, with the effect of creating a two-tier system: NHS for the poor, middle, and working classes, and private providers for the as-yet small proportion of the upper classes and upper-level employees with private insurance (Clines, 1987).

Comparisons of various health care systems are useful because they show alternative ways of arranging the parts of the system, and they point to areas of success or failure in our system.[1] For example, the Swedish system involves more extensive regulation and control of doctors and hospitals than the U.S. system. It is also more holistic in its concern for health-related issues like nutrition, child care, environmental pollution, and occupational health and safety. The Chinese system incorporates indigenous

[1]The following sources are useful for comparisons among various health care systems, with particular reference to industrialized societies: Altman, 1985; Banta and Kemp, 1982; Burrell and Sheps, 1978; Coburn et al., 1981; Crichton, 1981; Culyer and Jonsson, 1986; Dahlgren and Diderichsen, 1986; Doyal and Pennell, 1981; Evans, 1983; Field, 1976; Gill, 1980; Ham, 1982; Heidenheimer and Elvander, 1980; Hessler and Twaddle, 1982; Kaufman, 1987; Klein, 1983; Leichter, 1979; Light and Schuller, 1986; Marmor, 1982; Marmor et al., 1983a; Maxwell, 1981; Norbeck and Lock, 1987; Numbers, 1982; Raffel, 1984; Rodwin, 1984; Roemer, 1985; Roemer and Roemer, 1981; Sidel and Sidel, 1983; Soderstrom, 1980; Twaddle and Hessler, 1986.

While many commentators treat developing nations' health care issues as utterly different from those of industrialized countries, we would argue that many of the problems are the same: attention to broad social causes of illness and disease, appropriate technology, the most desirable training and deployment of health care workers, effective public health and preventive measures, and maximum utilization of all health-related resources toward a genuinely humane treatment of people in need. Some sources that deal specifically with health care systems of developing countries include Banta, 1986; Donahue, 1986, 1989; Elling, 1981; Good, 1987; Green, 1989; Guttmacher and Garcia, 1975; Heggenhougen et al., 1987; Horn, 1985; Horn, 1969; Low, 1985; McDonald, 1981; Morgan, 1983; Morgan, 1989; Roemer, 1985; Rosenthal, 1987, 1988; Sidel and Sidel, 1982; Simonelli, 1987; Stebbins, 1986; Waitzkin, 1983a.

healing practices and utilizes nonprofessional providers (like the "barefoot doctors", paraprofessionals deployed to rural districts). By contrast, the Kenyan system has devoted huge proportions of national health care expenditures to relatively high technology medicine in a limited number of hospitals. The East German system emphasizes prevention (such as a sizable program for occupational health and safety) and early treatment far more than the U.S. system.

Although Americans spend much more than citizens of other industrialized nations on health care, they do not enjoy generally better health. The United States ranked highest in total private and public spending on health care as a percent of the GNP, but it ranked eighteenth in infant mortality and eighth in life expectancy—far below countries such as Sweden and Canada, which spend considerably less on health care (Sivard, 1987). High expenditures do not guarantee better health because they are at best only indirectly linked with health-promoting or curing practices. For example, two nations may pay the same amount of money for a program of inoculations, but one nation may obtain far fewer inoculations per capita if the profit margins for the materials or provider services are higher in that health care system. Furthermore, health care expenditures are typically only *medical* care cost; these figures do not account for important differences in other health-promoting expenditures, such as nutrition.

As we examine the allocation of resources for health care, we should not assume that all health care spending necessarily benefits health care recipients; in fact some health care procedures and practices are *detrimental* to people's health. For example, some studies show that due to lack of resources, the poor are less likely to be overmedicated or to undergo unnecessary surgery or lab tests (Gould et al., 1989). The poor are not necessarily worse off for not being able to afford coronary by-pass surgery, Caesarian sections, and lots of tranquilizers. The expensive, high tech practices that characterize much of modern medicine produce varying results; some are indeed medical wonders, some are merely satisfactory, and still others are negligible relative to the cost, effort, and sometimes pain they involve. Other results are downright iatrogenic, creating illness rather than healing it. In being denied the benefits of medical treatment, the poor have thus been also spared some of the risks.

The U.S. health care system is the product of a long history of considerable political maneuvering, haggling, and contesting (described briefly in this chapter and the next). This system places a particularly heavy emphasis upon *medical* treatment rather than *health* care. As a corollary, its focus is upon institutional and professional forms of care. Furthermore, the U.S. system—even more so than other capitalist systems—emphasizes the commodification of health and health care; making money is one important driving force in the system (cf. Riska, 1985). The interplay of numerous conflicting interests created the existing system, and the same interests would be exerted vigorously in the face of any effort to change the system. Knowledge of the relative power among these interest groups and their use of different power resources is the key to understanding this system.

The following is a greatly simplified sketch of the various economic interests represented in the U.S. health care system. In this chapter we shall consider the social organization and interests of some of the people involved in receiving or providing health care, especially those whose income is derived from providing such care. In Chapter 12 we shall describe the economic interests of large-scale organizations involved in the system, especially hospitals, medical industries, insurance companies, and government agencies.

Because these interest groups vary dramatically in their relative power, some historical background of that power is helpful. Keep in mind that rapid shifts in the system, in part or whole, can cause descriptive data to become obsolete as new policies, added or reduced economic resources, changed institutional arrangements, and the like produce either ripples or tidal waves of adjustments throughout the entire system. This sketch also suggests the impact of these structural arrangements on the adequacy of health care, especially from the viewpoint of the patients themselves. Certain areas of serious inadequacy suggest particular points of crisis in the system. Can these crises be resolved by adjustments in present arrangements, or is drastic structural change required? If we could build an entirely new system, what might it include?

RECIPIENTS

Although the U.S. system is ostensibly an open market of competing providers, many aspects reduce the market sensitivity of these services and products. As a consumer, the recipient-patient is in an inherently weak position, primarily because medicine has become so sophisticated that the patient typically lacks the expertise to evaluate services (e.g., from the doctor or the hospital) and products (e.g., pharmaceuticals or technological devices). Unlike standardized products, medical services are highly variable. To select a pediatrician or to evaluate the advice of a cardiologist, one cannot simply turn to a *Consumer's Report* rating. While there is much an individual can do to become an informed consumer of medical services, the enormous disparity in expertise between professional and patient places the consumer in a relatively weak position.

The market model also assumes that the consumer is the one making the choices in the marketplace, but in medical care the recipient rarely makes such decisions. Although ideologically the U.S. system emphasizes the patient's freedom to choose doctors, the actual choice may be severely constrained by the limited availability of doctors in a region, by insurance that is limited to certain providers, or by the assignment of a patient without private care to a clinic, military, or other institutional doctor. Whereas in 1984, 85 percent of employees' health insurance allowed the open choice of a provider, by 1988 only 28 percent of insured employees had this choice (Califano, 1989). This dramatic change was mainly due to cost-cutting efforts by employers and insurers. Even the choice of insurance plans is typically marketed not to recipients directly but to their employers.

Furthermore, the recipient's doctor decides in which hospital to place the patient (usually according to where the doctor has privileges to practice). Unlike most other industrialized countries, in the United States the doctor does not relinquish care of (or income from) a patient who is hospitalized. Doctors maintain a relationship with a specific local hospital to which they admit their patients, and they bill their hospitalized patients separately from the hospital bill (Gabel and Redisch, 1979). This arrangement makes the hospital and private practitioner mutually dependent; the patient, however, does not choose.

The doctor is probably the foremost guide of the patient's decisions about health services (Gertman, 1981). The doctor selects the pharmaceuticals and the treatment procedures. The main decisions left to the patient are whether to accept the professional's decisions (and thus "comply") or to seek the services of another doctor or hospital. The value the sick person places on health and life are furthermore difficult to weigh rationally in a market situation. Medical treatment-related decisions are even more complicated by the fact that they often must be made quickly and under stress.

Recipients of medical care are among the least powerful interest groups in the U.S. system. Collectively, some groups of potential patients have wrested benefits from the system, but their successes are related to their political clout (e.g., senior citizens achieving funding of Medicare benefits) and/or their powerful socioeconomic position (e.g., upper-middle-class workers achieving substantial health care benefits from their employers). Less powerful groups of recipients, such as the working poor, have little or no influence against the interests of other parties in the system.

PHYSICIAN-PROVIDERS

The medical "cast of characters," their roles, and their remuneration are the result of numerous historical campaigns, such as medical doctors' achievement of professional dominance (described in Chapter 10). Other occupational groups likewise have asserted their interests in defining their domains, trying to achieve recognition as professions, and attempting to control the conditions of their work and pay. The resulting hierarchy of specialized health care occupations is fluid and changing, but all occupational interest groups utilize whatever resources of power they have to protect their interests. The prestige, power, financial success, and professional autonomy of medical doctors is, however, something of a standard against which other occupational groups measure themselves.

Fee-for-Service Payment

As noted in Chapter 10, medical doctors have achieved a legally recognized monopoly over the provision of most paid health care delivery as well as the training and admission of new personnel. The economic basis of physicians' service is a fee-for-service system in which the doctor typically charges the patient for each service provided at each visit. Technically, this system establishes an economic link between physician-provider and patient-recipient, but few contemporary doctor-patient relationships are so simple, since only about one-fourth of personal health care expenditures are paid directly by patients (Gibson et al., 1984). Various third parties, such as the government or insurance companies, are the source of the vast majority of payments, as discussed below.

Furthermore, although doctors typically bill on a fee-for-service basis, they are not necessarily paid in this way. For example, a doctor in group practice might receive a percentage of the collective receipts. The idea that the mode of payment forges a direct link between provider and consumer is thus more a myth, harking back to the "good old days" of more personal doctor-patient relationships; it also serves as an ideology to support the interests of physician-providers, because the fee-for-service arrangement has allowed them great freedom to set their own terms of remuneration.

In the face of escalating medical costs, many critics are now examining how doctors set their fees. The practice of medicine in the United States is essentially entrepreneurial (i.e., incomes are made in the private business of selling of goods and especially services). What, then, are these services worth? As noted, the market for physicians' services is hardly open and competitive, and few consumers are in a position to barter knowledgeably or with real clout to obtain a "good value." There is considerable evidence that the level of fees is governed primarily by the desired standard of living for physicians (Reinhardt, 1987). Although there has been some erosion in physician income in the 1980s, due primarily to cost-cutting government and insurer regulations, the profession is still exceptionally well paid—in the top 3 percent of all earners in the United States (Pear, 1987b; Altman and Rosenthal, 1990).

Specialists command far greater fees per hour than general practitioners and other doctors engaged in the more labor-intensive primary care. Because the U.S. health care system has no centralized planning or effective controls over the numbers of doctors in the various branches of medicine, there are dramatic and growing imbalances in the supply of specialists. The U.S. Department of Health and Human Services (1980) projected that by the year 2000 there will be an excess of about 150,000 doctors relative to the nation's needs and ability to pay. Despite this overall surplus, there is an expected shortage of family practitioners, which will be greatly outweighed by large surpluses of such specialists as surgeons and obstetricians-gynecologists. Interestingly, the oversupply of specialists has not as yet led to more competitive pricing but instead has tended to increase expenditures by raising the number of medical services recommended for each patient.

There is enormous variation from community to community in the fees charged for the same procedure. For example, a common urological operation would cost as little as $875 in West Virginia or as much as $2,350 in California (Freudenheim, 1988b). While variations in the costs of physician training and practice (e.g., office expenses and malpractice insurance) account for a portion of these dramatic differences in fees, they do not adequately explain them (Reinhardt, 1987). In 1988 the U.S. Justice Department began investigating allegations of price fixing by medical professionals, and federal grand juries in Massachusetts, Arizona, and Georgia were considering criminal indictments on these charges (Gold, 1988; Freudenheim, 1988b). There is a fine and imprecise line between uniform pricing among doctors in a community and illegal price fixing. Nevertheless, doctors who set fees according to "what the market will bear" rarely undercut the "going" rate; rates are thus seldom particularly competitive within a single community. No matter how honest the fee schedule, the patient typically is not able to evaluate its appropriateness.[2]

Fee setting is in a state of flux because there is considerable struggle between the providers and the third-party agencies that pay the bills (Belkin, 1990). For example, in 1988 a study commissioned by the Department of Health and Human Services recommended a complete overhaul of Medicare payments to doctors (Tolchin, 1988a). The study found that the existing fee system overcompensated doctors for invasive procedures such as surgery and diagnostic tests, but did not encourage them to spend time with patients in office visits and other time-consuming medical work.

Many doctors themselves are dissatisfied with how the fee-for-service arrangement has affected their everyday practice of medicine. One thoughtful physician described his realization of how detrimental these economic considerations had become:

[2]This analysis focuses primarily on the economic pressures experienced by all physicians, honest and dishonest alike; illegal behavior is one, extreme response to the opportunities for gain in medical practice. The intervention of third-party payment processes (e.g., Medicare, Medicaid, and insurance companies) and the bureaucratic management of medical economic transactions increase the opportunities for illegal kickbacks and fraudulent billing. Estimates suggest that between 25 and 40 percent of medical claims involve some form of deliberate overcharging (Roth, 1984).

An aged patient had come in to the office and was talking about her aching feet. She not only had several very real physical problems but she was also very lonely and quite hypochondriacal. . . . As she continued to tell me how tired she was, I realized I wasn't listening. I was angry. What she needed was someone to sympathize with her, gently encourage her, and to make some simple suggestions that might alleviate her suffering. I knew from past experience that that kind of listening and empathetic presence would require at least half an hour, but I would only be able to charge $20 for an intermediate call, Medicare would discount the charge significantly, and my half after overhead, would be, maybe, $8. I also knew that if I just stood up, cut the woman off by giving her a prescription for a pain medicine and scheduled her for next month, I could charge the same $20 and move into the next room where another patient was waiting with a small laceration from which I would earn about $30 in perhaps 10 minutes.

As soon as I recognized what I was angry about, I was ashamed. But the truth of my feelings was nonetheless real. . . . I was looking at my interactions with patients more and more as business transactions (Hilfiker, 1986).

These problems show how unsatisfactory the system of highly commodified health service, in which each aspect of care is delivered as a discrete entity, is for both patient and provider.

Clinical Decisions and Economic Considerations

There is considerable evidence that the present fee-for-service arrangement encourages unnecessary and questionable medical procedures, such as laboratory tests and surgery. Doctors and hospitals can add large markups to charges for lab tests. For example, during an office visit a blood sample may be drawn and sent to a mail-order laboratory for several tests. The physician may then add to the patient's bill not only the actual costs of the lab service but also a sizable profit (Reinhardt, 1987). Some estimates suggest that between 20 and 60 percent of these tests are unnecessary, adding nothing to the patient's diagnosis or treatment (Luft, 1983; Pear, 1987a; Califano, 1989).[3]

Likewise, the fee-for-service system indirectly encourages doctors to resort to surgery rather than less invasive treatments. The decision to operate is based upon a number of discretionary choices, perceptions, evaluations, and decision rules that vary considerably among physicians and medical situations. All surgery involves assessing the probability that the operation will improve function, reduce pain, or increase the quality of life as balanced against the risks of complications from the surgery itself. For example, should a precancerous condition of the uterus be

---

[3]Provider profit is hardly the only reason for excessive use of testing. Many tests are ordered as part of "defensive" medicine to protect against a malpractice suit, whereas others are requested by patients to allay fears of certain illnesses.

treated with a hysterectomy if the death rate from hysterectomies is greater than that for uterine cancer (Larned, 1977)? Is a carotid endarterectomy (a controversial operation that clears blockages in the major artery leading to the brain) appropriate if the patient is likely to suffer a stroke from the surgery itself (cf. Wilford, 1988)?

Especially for new and unproven procedures, there is considerable potential for physicians to conduct surgery for reasons that are inappropriate relative to the patient's health and needs. For example, a 1987 study found that only 35 percent of carotid endarterectomies were performed for "clearly appropriate indications" (Chassin et al., 1987). Similarly, critics assert that the U.S. rates of coronary by-passes and Caesarean sections are at least double the appropriate level (cf. Califano, 1989; Shabecoff, 1987a). Compared to other industrialized countries, the United States has exceptionally high rates of surgery without concomitant lower rates of mortality. For example, U.S. surgeons perform coronary by-pass operations at six times the rate in England (where, under the NHS, surgeons' income is not directly related to the number or type of operations performed), and mastectomies three times more frequently (Payer, 1988). We cannot infer that the difference is due only to unnecessary surgery (see Schwartz, 1984), but the socio-economic incentive of fee-for-service is certainly one factor promoting high rates of surgery.[4]

In principle, the physician is an advocate for the patient, representing the patient's interests to insurers, hospital, and other specialists on the case. There is an inherent conflict of interests, however, even for physicians who take their role as advocate seriously, when they are in a position to order for their patients procedures that also happen to be an important source of their own income (cf. Luft, 1983). Physicians' judgment may be also subtly influenced by pressures from their hospital affiliates to fill beds, by their patients' wishes for a "quick fix," or by their own desire to try the latest surgical procedures. Unlike pharmaceutical innovations, surgical innovations are not required to undergo extensive studies for effectiveness or risks. Nor is demonstrated surgical skill a prerequisite for a physician who does operate; any licensed medical doctor can legally perform surgery, regardless of expertise (Millman, 1976; see also Barron, 1989). Studies in comparable U.S. communities have suggested that two important reasons for the wide variation in the number of operations performed are the rate of empty hospital beds and the local supply of surgeons (Evans, 1974; Lewis, 1969; see also Barron, 1989; Roth, 1984).

Even greater potential for conflict of interest is involved when the physician can receive secondary income from the treatment. For example,

----

[4]A possible indicator of the iatrogenic effects of unnecessary medical intervention occurred when, during a 1976 physicians' strike, the Los Angeles mortality rates dropped from an average of 19.8 deaths per 100,000 before the strike to 16.2 during the five-week strike, rising again to 20.4 at the strike's conclusion (*Science News*, 1978).

some physicians own equity in nursing homes to which they subsequently refer patients. Others have invested in laboratories, expensive equipment (e.g., a CT scanner), and paraprofessional staff, all of which are financially successful when used extensively; the temptation for a doctor-owner to overprescribe these services is built into the situation (Miller, 1983). Many physicians have made a substantial investment in office testing equipment that enables them to have the convenience of quick results as well as additional profits. For example, in an advertisement for a urinalysis machine, Akers Medical Technologies told doctors that the equipment offered potential profits of $83,540 per year, assuming fifty tests were performed a day, and that cost of the machine could be recovered in as little as five days (Kramon, 1988b).

The potential for conflict of interest is illustrated in the result of the U.S. program for end-stage renal disease (ESRD), a chronic, debilitating, and often fatal disease of the kidneys. One treatment for ESRD is hemodialysis, which involves such expensive technology that before 1973 the treatment was carefully rationed. In response to a concerted political campaign by well-organized groups of patients and providers, however, in 1972 the U.S. government passed an amendment to Medicare legislation that provided federal reimbursement for ESRD treatments. Even in the first year of the program, the actual costs were many times the projected costs, and since then national expenditures for ESRD treatments have escalated dramatically. One reason is that the legislation lifted barriers preventing people from being dialyzed and encouraging dialysis for all sufferers of ESRD, regardless of their physical ability to benefit from the treatment (Simmons and Marine, 1984). Ironically, the United States, one of the few industrialized nations with no overall policy or the equitable distribution of health care, became the most liberal subsidizer of dialysis for all. By 1977 the rate of dialysis in the United States was nearly double that for Denmark and Sweden, and triple that for England (Riska, 1985).

The other major reason for the dramatic escalation of ESRD therapy costs was that in the United States, unlike other countries, the dominant mode of treatment was in-center dialysis rather than the less expensive home dialysis and kidney transplants (Kutner, 1982). For example, in 1988 kidney dialysis for a single patient in hospital or clinic cost about $9,600 per year more than home dialysis (*U.S. News and World Report*, 1988). Numerous for-profit hemodialysis clinics, with significant capital investment in technology, also actively discourage home dialysis. Similarly, the physician-owners of such clinics may be tempted to place their ESRD patients on dialysis sooner than necessary or not to refer their patients to renal transplant surgeons, since a successful transplant would obviate the need for such treatment (Miller, 1983; Riska, 1985). Regardless of whether physicians are conscious of their economic interests in clinical decisions, the profit connection in the United States results in very different patterns of patient care than in countries where doctors cannot profit from the treatments they recommend.

Malpractice: Economic Burdens and Regulation

The issue of malpractice is related to the socioeconomic basis of provider-recipient relationships. Around the turn of the century, medical societies provided for the mutual defense of members against malpractice suits. Courts deferred to local doctors' judgment as "expert witnesses," which made it virtually impossible for aggrieved patients to get one doctor to testify against another. Furthermore, the medical societies were so successful in protecting their members from suit that they were able to obtain very favorable insurance rates, whereas nonmembers were often unable to obtain insurance at all (Starr, 1982: 111).

In the latter half of the twentieth century, however, the legal and cultural climate changed. Patients became more willing to take doctors to court, partly because of the growing impersonality of economic relationships described above. Rising expectations of the wonders of medical science may also have both enhanced doctors' prestige and remuneration, while creating unrealistic public beliefs about what doctors could accomplish. Simultaneously, courts allowed the wider use of outside experts and cosmopolitan (rather than local) standards of care, while legislation—especially since the 1970s—clarified patients' rights (such as the right to informed consent for procedures). The result has been a dramatic increase in malpractice litigation, increasingly large awards to patient-plaintiffs, and soaring malpractice insurance premiums (the cost of which is generally passed on to the consumer).

The expansion of malpractice litigation has created a number of additional powerful interest groups in the health care arena. Malpractice insurance is typically offered as part of a for-profit insurance industry. Lawyers, courts, and layers of legal paper-processing organizations have likewise become major recipients of the health care dollar. An estimated 60 percent of the billions paid annually for malpractice insurance goes not to aggrieved patients but to the insurance and litigation industries (Califano, 1989). At the same time, however, the expense of litigation prevents the vast majority of injured patients from going to court to obtain *any* compensation (cf. Rosenthal, 1988).

Furthermore, the fear of malpractice suits encourages doctors to practice "defensive" medicine in which clinical decisions are made with an eye to protecting themselves from lawsuits. By practicing defensive medicine, hospital staff often construct a patient's chart as a case record designed more to stand up in court than to describe the patient's actual situation. Communication about the patient then takes place informally, off-the-record, such as by one specialist writing notes to another (Millman, 1976: 145). Defensive medicine also results in unnecessary tests and procedures, costing an estimated $20 billion per year (Califano, 1989). One study estimated that defensive medicine accounts for as much as 15 percent of total physician billings (Freudenheim, 1987a; Reinhardt, 1987). For example, fearing lawsuits if they deliver imperfect babies, obstetricians are more likely to order fetal monitoring during labor and are more likely to perform possibly unnecessary Caesarian sections if the monitor indicates any signs of fetal distress. Another impact of the fear of malpractice suits is that doctors may avoid treating high-risk patients or may shift their practice to a lower-risk specialization; for example, by 1987 more than 12 percent of obstetricians reported that they had left obstetrics and were practicing only gynecology (Tolchin, 1989a).

While the profit incentive of lawyers and insurers in this system is obvious, their influence is an understandable entrepreneurial response to two unmet needs in the U.S. health care system as it has developed. First, the system has had no adequate method of identifying, controlling, or punishing physicians who were incompetent, negligent, or otherwise detrimental to the health of their patients. One of the prerogatives achieved by medical dominance was the right to peer review: Only doctors could effectively sanction malpractice. Historically, however, doctors were very reticent to judge each other. Once a physician passed the initial screening process and obtained a license to practice, fellow doctors were highly unlikely to constrain that practice, much less to take it away. Indeed, typically doctors in a community supported each other, both legally and more subtly. For example, fellow doctors would cover up for incompetent surgeons by doing "ghost" surgery for them. Similarly, although in principle hospitals could refuse staff privileges to doctors whose practices were medically questionable, most relied on local doctors as the source of patients and thus could not afford to alienate them (Millman, 1976: 120–135).

A second reason for the rise in importance of malpractice suits is that the nation provides few other avenues for a family to obtain recompense for the actual costs created by medical mistakes. Iatrogenic medical practices often create years of additional medical expenses as well as the loss of income due to disability, yet the U.S. health care system offers little assistance with such costs. Most patients have no safety net of economic help for serious medical problems. Thus malpractice suits become the last-chance effort to obtain economic relief.

By contrast, in Sweden, where equitable access to health care is a citizen's right, these functions are addressed by the public health system. Their Patient Compensation Fund is publicly financed no-fault insurance that compensates both economic and noneconomic aspects of injury, and settles claims rapidly according to a predetermined schedule. The mere fact of injury is sufficient for compensation; claimants do not have to prove that anyone was at fault. Relatively very few claims are arbitrated beyond this point, and patients are generally satisfied that compensation is equitable and objective. A completely separate mechanism, the Medical Responsibility Board—a freestanding national governmental body—deals with malpractice complaints against physicians. It investigates reported incidents and can employ a range of sanctions, from a reprimand to a recommendation that the National Board of Health and Welfare revoke a physician's license to practice. In 1982, the Responsibility Board's rate of disciplinary actions was 3.3 per 1,000 physicians, compared to an average rate of 2.4 per 1,000 by U.S. disciplinary boards (Rosenthal, 1988).

Corporatization of Medical Production

We still have the image of the doctor as a solo practitioner and independent businessperson, but in fact the trend is toward greater corporatization of health care delivery, as medical production converts to corporate forms of ownership and management, such as incorporated group practice, a health maintenance organization (HMO), or a for-profit hospital corporation (Starr, 1982: 420–449). By 1989 about one-half of U.S. doctors were salaried employees (Altman and Rosenthal, 1990). The projected oversupply of physicians, new patterns of hospital ownership and management, and changes in third-party insurance and government regulation make it likely that yet greater proportions of physicians will be employed in salaried or other somewhat dependent arrangements. Some of these developments are discussed further below.

As a result of these new structural arrangements, health care providers are losing some of the autonomy they gained in their rise to professional dominance (Light and Levine, 1988). Some observers have referred to this as the proletarianization of the medical profession, implying that by being employed in a corporate setting, doctors are being reduced to the status of wage laborers (McKinlay and Archer, 1985; McKinlay and Stoeckle, 1988). However, while corporatization clearly reduces doctors' independence in some areas of their work, their resulting status is not so simple as that of the proletariat relative to the industrial bourgeoisie.

The very rise of the technologically advanced, hospital-based medical practices that enhanced the prestige and authority of the medical profession in the first half of the century has in the second half also produced conditions conducive to the profession's corporate dependence. Modern medicine is capital intensive; few solo practitioners can afford to finance even modest practices. Thus they turn to medical groups, labs, clinics, and hospitals to provide the necessary equipment and support services.

Nevertheless, their relations with their economic sponsors are hardly as disempowering as those faced by the industrial proletariat. Unlike the proletariat, which has only its wage labor to sell, the medical profession retains monopoly control over much needed, complex skill and knowledge

(Navarro, 1988). Also, as Derber (1983, 1984) noted, the proletariat is disempowered by the capitalist employers' consolidation of control over the functions of both production capitalization (i.e., supplying costly facilities for making products) and market mediation (i.e., relationships, such as marketing, by which the product is converted into income). By contrast, while increasingly fewer individual practitioners control these two aspects of their medical production, neither are these two functions usually united in a single employer. Typically the production-capitalization functions reside in what Derber (1984:220) called doctors' "proprietary sponsors" (e.g., hospitals), while the market mediation functions are performed by "market sponsors" (e.g., third-party insurers). While both forms of sponsors place constraints on the conditions of physicians' work, they lack the power enjoyed by capitalist employers over the entire process of production.

Furthermore, the constraints imposed by doctors' sponsors do not reduce all areas of physician control equally. For example, a hospital employer may reduce a physician's control over scheduling and work load, but impose relatively few constraints on the physician's autonomy over technical skills and knowledge (Derber, 1984). The structural situation most threatening to the doctor's professional autonomy is one in which a single agency (such as a for-profit hospital chain) successfully consolidates the production-capitalization functions and the market mediation functions (e.g., by selling its own prepaid insurance to other employers).

The trend toward corporatization has also had an impact on patients as well as professional providers. The corporate interests of hospitals and insurers have thrust considerations of cost effectiveness and profit maximization into the fore. As noted above, today proportionately far fewer patients are free to choose their own providers as compared with a decade ago. Who speaks for the interests of the patient-recipient? As we have described, physician-providers often experience conflicting interests in recommending procedures for their patients; nevertheless, their authority used to be a very powerful source of advocacy on behalf of patients (Mechanic, 1986). If a doctor said, "This patient needs to be hospitalized," that decision was once accepted as authoritative by third-party insurers and hospitals. Physicians' sponsors today, however, are more likely to discourage, question, and even override their professional opinions (cf. Belkin, 1990).

NURSE-PROVIDERS AND OTHER HELPING PROFESSIONALS

As noted in Chapter 10, the rise of the medical profession to professional dominance entailed the subordination, cooptation, or elimination of virtually all competing health care professions. For example, in some countries pharmacists are relatively independent, and can concoct and dispense most medicines without much control by physicians. When patients are simply able to go to the pharmacist for advice and medicine, however, they have much less need to see the doctor. As early as 1906, the AMA's campaign against patent medicines (i.e., proprietary drugs) produced doctors' legal monopoly over the prescription of powerful medicines. Commercial medicine companies had to market their products to doctors rather than to customers (Starr, 1982: 127–134). As a result the nascent profession of pharmacy was subordinated to the medical profession, although many pharmacists do enjoy relative autonomy in their working conditions.

Nonphysician practitioners in the predominantly male professions of dentistry, podiatry, optometry, pharmacy, and chiropractic have also been able to retain relatively independent practices, even while the medical profession exerts its organizational control. Traditionally female health care professions, such as nursing, have not fared so well; they have been kept subordinate in pay, working conditions, educational programs, and bureaucratic organization. The vicissitudes of nursing as an occupation are almost prototypical of the larger historical process of rationalization of health services delivery, which promoted the ever-increasing specialization of tasks interwoven in complex—usually bureaucratic—organizations. The development of nursing and various allied health professions (such as laboratory technology, physical therapy, and radiological technology) is a result of nearly total gender stratification of medical work.

The Development of Nursing

Early nursing was typically private care by an unpaid member of the family or a paid family helper. It was part of the domestic economy and inextricably linked with women's roles. One of the founders of professional nursing, Florence Nightingale, wrote, "Every woman is a nurse" (1860: 3). She also argued that women should not aspire to be doctors because nursing meshed with their "natural" abilities. Nightingale's hospital reforms envisioned genteel nurses competently running hospitals as domestic managers, completely supportive of and dependent on doctors, who were analogous to the male heads of household (cf. Melosh, 1982; Ehrenreich and English, 1973).

Even today, nursing is a predominantly female occupation; in 1980, 95.9 percent of all registered nurses (RNs) were women, but only 13.4 percent of physicians were women. Table 11.1 shows the distribution of women among several health occupations. Thus gender-role expectations figure prominently in the relationships between doctor and nurse (Brown, 1983). The nurse is expected to be deferential, nurturing, and submissive, even while taking an active role in the patient's care. The doctor-nurse "game" consists of a series of strategies, for example, in which the nurse communicates a recommendation without appearing to make a recom-

TABLE 11–1   Selected Health Occupations by Total Employment, Percentage Black and Percentage
Female, 1980

OCCUPATION	TOTAL EMPLOYED	PERCENT BLACK	PERCENT FEMALE
Diagnostic occupations (e.g., M.D., D.O., D.D.S)	643,716	2.8	11.7
Managers in health institutions	108,477	8.6	50.7
Registered nurses	1,266,801	7.5	95.9
Health technologists and technicians	541,509	10.5	73.4
Practical nurses	424,960	17.9	96.6
Health service occupations (e.g., aides and orderlies)	1,726,875	23.4	88.1

Source: U.S. Bureau of the Census, 1980 Census of Population, volume 2, Subject Reports:
Occupation by Industry. U.S. Department of Commerce, Washington, DC: Government Printing
Office, 1984: 1–8.

mending statement, and the physician asks for her recommendation without appearing to be asking for help (Stein, 1967; Hughes, 1988). The
historical emphasis upon "womanly" qualities in nursing has been both an
ideological hindrance to professional recognition and a basis for nurses to
seek a distinctive, caring way of relating to patients in contrast to the impersonality of the bioscientific medical model (Reverby, 1987).

In the early twentieth century, two major developments in medical
care shaped the direction of nursing: the shift to hospital-based care and
the growing emphasis upon scientific medicine. The latter, together with
many technological developments, created the need for highly trained assistance for doctors; the knowledge and skills required of nurses expanded
rapidly. RNs are the single largest group of health care professionals, accounting for about one-fifth of all health workers (Melosh, 1982).

Previously hospitals had been little more than sick wards of the poorhouse, staffed by minimally qualified nurses drawn from the lowest social
classes. Male attendants worked in men's wards and female attendants in
women's wards. Only those who had no family or means of private care
were nursed in hospital settings. In response to the technological developments and public relations campaigns described in Chapter 12, however,
middle- and upper-class persons began to use hospitals for sickness, surgery, and childbirth. As medical and nursing education became hospital-
centered, hospitals became more prestigious and profitable rather than
totally charitable institutions. Their new fee-paying clientele accordingly
expected a much higher standard of care (Melosh, 1982: 15–35; Rosenberg, 1987: 212–236).

Hospitals were expanding rapidly and needed the very kind of disciplined, trained workers they found in nurses; however, the profession was
further subordinated as it lost control over nursing education. Hospital

administrators established nursing schools so that the student nurses would serve the hospital. Student nurses put in sixty- and seventy-hour work-weeks for two or three years of ward service in exchange for their subsistence and a small sum (typically ten dollars a year) for uniforms and books (Rosenberg, 1987: 220–221). The economic disincentives and the structural subordination of nurses made the occupation increasingly unattractive to men. For women, however, nursing was one of the few "respectable" occupations and was considered an appropriate preparation for marriage as well as a source of income.

Along with the growing emphasis upon scientific training of medical doctors in the early decades of the twentieth century, many voices within nursing urged greater professionalization and standardization of training. By mid-century, there was considerable division between those nurses advocating hospital training and those urging higher education (Melosh, 1982: 67–76). At stake was the relatively greater professional independence of nursing as well as ideas about the proper role of the nurse.

Technological developments in medicine also promoted increased specialization in nursing; for example, some upper-echelon nurses specialize for work in the intensive care unit, cardiac unit, or operating room. There has also been a trend toward relegating routine bedside tasks, formerly the role of professional nurses, to lower-paid workers such as licensed practical nurses (LPNs), aides, orderlies, and ward clerks. Although this practice results in considerable cost savings to the hospital administration and somewhat greater professional prestige for RNs, it also means that the RN serves more as a manager than a nurse.

The Socioeconomic Status of "Female" Health Professions

The structural subordination of nursing relative to both physicians and hospital bureaucracies has worked severely against the economic interests of nurses. Recent difficulties in recruiting sufficient nursing staff for hospitals are probably one result of this (Lewin, 1987b). Nurses' wages are low, and between 1971 and 1987 pay raises even failed to keep apace of increases in the cost of living. In 1989 the average salary paid by hospitals for nurses at the top of the pay scale was only $32,160 per year (Tolchin, 1989b), or less than one-third of the average doctor's net income.

Patients and their insurance companies are not generally billed separately for nursing services, as they are for the services of, for example, radiologists, anesthesiologists, and physical therapists. Thus employers of nurses try to keep wages low and to maximize the labor they can extract for those wages. Relative to other professions with comparable years of training, hospital nurses experience several other important occupational disadvantages: unfavorable hours and shift work, high stress, and little opportunity for advancement in status or pay. For example, in 1986 RNs received a maximum salary that was 36.4 percent higher than the starting salary; by comparison, accountants received a 192.7 percent increase, engineers received 183.6 percent, and chemists received 231 percent (Tolchin, 1989b). As doors to other occupations are opening for women, underpaid "women's" professions like nursing have become less attractive.

Predominantly female health care occupations are also characterized by relatively low amounts of professional autonomy. Nurses, medical technologists, dental hygienists, and other auxiliary workers frequently assume many of the less interesting and more time-consuming tasks of hospitals and doctors' offices. These "physician extenders" are able to do as much as 80 percent of the routine tasks of office medical practice; similarly, dental assistants can assume tasks such as cleaning, patient education, and x-ray work that would otherwise account for most of the dentist's time. The amount the doctor or dentist can charge for these services is roughly the same, regardless of whether they are done by the doctor or dentist or delegated to a relatively low-paid assistant.

The medical profession has used its regulatory and educational controls to prevent serious competition from these auxiliary professions (Brown, 1978, 1983). Their control also enables them to suppress the wages paid to other health care professionals. For example, by using the states' Medical Practice Acts to abolish private x-ray laboratories, radiologists (MDs) were able to control the terms of employment of x-ray technicians and technologists, and to prevent them from competing with radiologists' own labs and those of hospitals.

Similarly, the independent practice of medicine by physicians' assistants was made illegal in all states where the licensing boards are controlled by doctors. Since 1971, however, a majority of states have amended their Medical Practice Acts to allow nurses to diagnose some conditions, prescribe some drugs, and perform other medical duties under certain conditions; similarly, since 1978 federal guidelines have allowed direct reimbursement to nurse-practitioners for Medicare patients. Home health care is one area in which nurse-practitioners have been particularly active; they have also served extensively in locations (such as the inner city and remote rural areas) considered undesirable by many physicians. With the predicted surplus of physicians, it remains to be seen whether these less expensive providers will be allowed to continue to practice (Sorkin, 1986).

The tension between physicians and other health care professionals is best illustrated by the competition posed by a new professional classification, the nurse-midwife. Obstetricians have vehemently opposed allowing them to deliver babies. Where they were not successful in preventing nurse-midwives from practicing, physicians often were able to limit the conditions under which they could practice (Brown, 1978). The market for infant deliveries is shrinking, and there is a marked oversupply of obstetricians (U.S. Department of Health and Human Services, 1980). As a surgical specialty, obstetrics has responded to this market condition by greatly increasing the number of Caesarian sections. By contrast, nurse-midwives are trained to help the mother to have her baby naturally; they emphasize a more holistic approach to the mother and child, including both prenatal and early infancy care and education. Their market strategy has been to offer comprehensive services at a much lower cost while appealing to consumers looking for a more satisfying birth experience. Thus far, both groups of providers have been somewhat successful; obstetricians have kept their incomes high, despite fewer deliveries, and nurse-midwives have attracted a growing number of customers while enjoying a greater professional autonomy than most nurses (Little, 1982).

For patients, there is no obvious immediate benefit of these conflicts among health care professionals. For example, giving nurses greater professional recognition and pay may create a happier work force, which may or may not result in better patient care. It may actually increase the professional distance between the nurse and patient. Greater emphasis upon nonphysician providers should be more cost-effective, but the patient will not necessarily realize any financial benefits if the savings go to a hospital chain, insurance company, or group medical practice. Although many of the predominantly female health care professions hold ideals of providing greater caring and patient service compared to the medical profession, the trend toward their specialization and professionalization may promote the further disempowerment of the patient.

NONPROFESSIONAL HEALTH CARE WORKERS

The health industry employs a vast number of nonprofessional workers, such as nursing aides, orderlies, clerks, receptionists, kitchen help, and housekeeping staff. Employment in the health industry reflects patterns of stratification in the larger society. As Table 11.1 shows, the health-related occupations of greatest power, prestige, and wealth are concentrated mainly among white men. Health care work at the bottom of the stratification heap is typically done by black women. Women make up at least 75 percent of all health industry workers, while constituting only about 42 percent of the national workforce. Not only are predominantly female occupations generally low paid, but women also earn less than men in the same job categories. Black workers are overrepresented in the menial and low-status occupations, such as practical nurse or home health aide (Aries and Kennedy, 1986).

Furthermore, women and blacks are concentrated in occupations with the least opportunity for advancement. Especially in hospital settings, there is almost total lack of job mobility, even though various workers can and do perform tasks appropriate to higher echelon workers. The resulting structural inequality promotes conflict, with the technical and managerial elite (doctors and administrators) separated from and opposing the interests of the lower-status workers. Although some of this conflict is muted by the professional ideals of nurses and others, there is a growing pressure for unionization and other collective expressions of worker dissatisfaction (Ehrenreich and Ehrenreich, 1978).

The interests of nonprofessional health workers, like those of nurses and doctors, do not necessarily coincide with the interests of patients. At the same time, however, the health care system's failure to compensate, regulate, and educate its lower-level care givers adequately, has been seriously detrimental to patients. One study of patient abuse in a nursing home noted that the personnel recruited were socially marginal, poorly educated or trained, and generally uncommitted to their work. Their low-paid, low-prestige custodial care of a powerless population of elderly patients promoted neglect and abuse (Stannard, 1973).

Similarly, the U.S. health care system's recent emphasis upon home care has resulted in a new cadre of underpaid, undervalued aides who help the infirm with cooking, cleaning, bathing, dressing, and moving about their homes. By the end of 1987, there were some 50,000 such workers in New York City alone. Most earned less than $7,000 per year (an income at or below the poverty level), and had no job security, no overtime pay, and few or no medical benefits (Iverem, 1988). A 1985 study by the Hunter College School of Social Work (Donovan, 1987) found that 99 percent of these workers were women with a median age of forty-seven; 70 percent were black, 26 percent were Hispanic, and nearly half were immigrants. The typical home health aide was the primary breadwinner for her household, with three to four children to support. Because of their poor remuneration, these women and their families had had no health insurance for 92 percent of their *own* health problems in the previous year.

Thus while federal, state, and private insurers enjoy the cost savings of home care compared with hospitalization, their savings are subsidized by a large number of poor working women. Home health aides are even more disadvantaged than similarly unskilled workers in hospitals, because they have none of the social interaction, reassurance, and prestige associated with working in a medical setting. Further incentives to exploit home health aides exist when the agency employing them operates as a for-profit health industry (Fine, 1988).

In the face of such exploitation and desperate levels of underprivilege, what incentives do workers have to provide excellent care? Untrained workers, with minimal supervision, may even neglect, abuse, or take advantage of their clients. The patients' interests are hardly protected by the system. Patients can request a particular health worker or ask for a change, but with a severe shortage of workers, there is no way to guarantee provision of satisfactory care.

SUMMARY

The social organization of health care services in any health system reflects the stratification and power of various interest groups in that society. Because of the commodified, laissez-faire system in the United States, these interests are particularly obvious as they compete for available resources and control. Social stratification and power are important considerations for understanding the quality of health services; these structural factors strongly influence how people behave. Stratification is related to the social distance between patient and providers and between various levels of health service workers; it is also related to imbalances in the socioeconomic power of recipients and providers.

The stratification and power of these interest groups are also linked to structural incentives and disincentives that affect the quality of health services. Many of the problems of the U.S. health care system can be best understood in light of these powerful socioeconomic structural features, which any attempt to solve the problems of quality, access, and cost must address. In Chapter 12 we shall continue our examination of the socioeconomic interests in U.S. health care with a discussion of the large-scale-organizations that are increasingly powerful in this system.

RECOMMENDED READINGS

Articles

Nancy Aries and Louanne Kennedy, "The health labor force: The effects of change," pp. 196–207 in P. Conrad and R. Kern, eds., *The Sociology of Health and Illness*. New York: St. Martin's Press, 1986.

Doris R. Fine, "Women caregivers and home health workers: Prejudice and inequity in home health care," *Research in the Sociology of Health Care* 7, 1988: 105–117.

John B. McKinlay, "A case for refocusing upstream: The political economy of illness," pp. 484–498 in P. Conrad and R. Kern, eds., *The Sociology of Health and Illness*. New York: St. Martin's Press, 1986.

Howard D. Schwartz, Peggy L. de Wolf, and James K. Skipper, Jr., "Gender, professionalization and occupational anomie: The case of nursing," pp. 559–569 in H. D. Schwartz, ed., *Dominant Issues in Medical Sociology*. New York: Random House, 1987.

Books

John B. McKinlay, ed., *Milbank Quarterly* 66 (supplement 2), 1988. Several excellent essays in this issue examine the changing character of the medical profession in the economic climate of corporatization of medical practice and production.

Susan Reverby, *Ordered to Care: The Dilemma of American Nursing*, 1850–1945. Cambridge: Cambridge University Press, 1987. A thoughtful reexamination of the role of nursing in its economic and organizational setting.

Chapter Twelve

Economic Interests and Power in Health Care

The health care system in the United States is essentially a *medical* care system. As noted in Chapter 11, medical care is not the same as health care. Medical care generally emphasizes acute illness and inadequately addresses other health needs; it emphasizes curative interventions and gives much less attention to prevention, palliation, and basic care. With the development of high technology and specialized medicine, the medical care system has become hospital based and heavily reliant on large, bureaucratic organizations.

The structure and functions of these medical organizations reflect the structure of the larger society. The medical care system is stratified largely according to the class, gender, ethnic, and other divisions in the whole society. In the United States, the medical care system is a major part of the larger system of economic production and consumption; it is structured to allow various interest groups to make significant profits and to control considerable resources in medical production. Although we tend to think of medical care as a small-scale service offered by individual providers, such as those discussed in Chapter 11, in a laissez-faire medical system such as that of the United States medical care is also big business. The powerful interests involved in medical businesses often supersede the interests of both sick people and health care providers. In this chapter we shall offer an overview of some of these large-scale medical care organizations.

As noted in Chapter 11, there is considerable evidence that the American health care system is in crisis. A large proportion of the citizens are not served by the system, and many of those who are served receive insufficient and inferior care. Despite many cost-cutting efforts, the amount spent on health care consumes an enormous proportion of the nation's gross national product, and the costs of most medical treatment continue to spiral upward. Evaluations of health care delivery focus on three criteria: quality, cost, and access. We shall describe some of the social-structural factors that influence these three aspects.

HEALTH CARE INSTITUTIONS

The provision of health care in large-scale institutions, such as hospitals, is a relatively recent phenomenon. In the early nineteenth century, most sick people were treated and nursed in their homes. Almshouse wards were the main form of hospital, nursing home, and insane asylum, offering a modicum of care and custody to indigent persons without a stable home or family members to provide care. These were hardly desirable places to go to get well. They were run as charitable institutions, with utterly paternalistic organization as well as little real curative function (Rosenberg, 1987; Rosner, 1986).

The Development of the Modern Hospital

By the time of the early twentieth century reformation of the medical profession (described in Chapter 9) hospitals too had changed dramatically. Both hospitals and medicine were becoming more rationalized: science oriented, specialized, and bureaucratized. Many towns established community hospitals, which lacked the stigma of the poorhouse wards. The rapid development of new medical "tools," such as antiseptic conditions for surgery, x-rays, and clinical laboratories, provided an important rationale for centering care in hospitals, which could capitalize these facilities and provide the necessary support staff. Thus even in the 1920s hospitals were capital-intensive institutions. Their prestige and growth hinged on the practice of surgery (Rosenberg, 1987: 337–352).

One reason for the increase of middle- and upper-class hospital patients was the growing faith in the efficacy of medicine; another was the concerted advertising by hospitals, depicting well-appointed private rooms and immaculate conditions. An especially important factor was that many physicians urged that their patients be treated in hospitals. In some cases, this insistence was related to the fact that surgeons themselves owned the hospitals in which they practiced; in many other cases, the doctors' insistence was due to the convenience and growing technological advantages of performing procedures in hospital. Income from private patients made community hospitals economically viable. Hospital-admitting privileges became crucial to physicians' careers; hospitals in turn became dependent upon doctors to bring in private patients (Rosenberg, 1987: 237–261). Nursing too was changed from an untrained domestic task to a hospital-oriented and -trained occupation, bringing discipline and efficiency to the care of paying patients. By the 1920s American hospitals were therefore being transformed from charitable enterprises to bureaucratic organizations selling medical commodities in an impersonal marketplace.

The very technology and specialization of tasks that made hospitals plausible sites for the centralized practice of medicine have also been major sources of the spiraling costs leading to the present U.S. health care crisis (for a summary of studies on these cost increases, see McCarthy, 1981). Many powerful forces promote the development and utilization of ever-growing amounts of increasingly sophisticated technologies, which enhance hospital prestige, and attract physicians who will admit the kinds and numbers of patients the hospitals need to be economically successful. Physicians have every incentive to use new technologies both to improve their skills and abilities to treat patients, and to increase the profitability of their practices. The public in general and patients in particular also often promote their utilization by their profound value on full health and their broad faith in scientific medicine to come up with a "technological fix" for every malady (Rushing, 1984).

Although state regulatory agencies have introduced a number of measures to control costs that result from the overutilization of medical technologies, such as requiring a hospital to obtain a Certificate of Need before purchasing certain expensive equipment, most such regulations have failed to reduce costs substantially (Roth, 1984). The proliferation of technologies—from the minor (e.g., blood tests) to the massive (e.g., intensive care units)—have driven up hospital costs not only because they are expensive to acquire and house but also because they necessitate costly specialized support workers. Whereas modernizing capital expenditures in industrial production usually decreases labor costs, technological investments in hospital production generally increase labor expenditures.

Hospital Ownership and Control

Hospitals vary widely in their sources of income and their relationships to their financial sponsors. The three main types are public, private not-for-profit, and private for-profit (or proprietary) hospitals. Public hospitals are funded mainly through the tax revenues of a city, county, state, or national government; their administration is thus linked with that government. Private not-for-profit institutions include community hospitals run by local boards as well as hospitals run by various religious and charitable organizations. Funding is typically a mixture of donations and with patient and third-party payments. Private for-profit hospitals are typically owned and run by either a group of physicians or, increasingly, a business corporation. Funding is usually from patient and third-party payments, although it sometimes comes from direct contract with another organization (such as an employer).

There is a rapidly growing trend in the United States toward the proprietarization and corporatization of health care facilities, such as hospitals, nursing homes, psychiatric hospitals, and free-standing clinics and outpatient surgery centers. *Proprietarization* is the process by which a greater proportion of health care institutions are operated explicitly for profit; *corporatization* is the process by which a relatively small number of investor-owned corporations control a greater concentration of proprietary interests. Between 1977 and 1982, while the total number of U.S. hospitals declined by 2 percent, the number of investor-owned chain hospitals increased by 40 percent (Gray, 1983). Furthermore, this ownership is highly concentrated, with only four firms controlling approximately 70 percent of the more than seven hundred investor-owned hospitals (Berliner and Burlage, 1987).

For-profit hospitals have been highly profitable for investors. For example, in 1980 Humana (one of the largest chains) had a 33.6 percent on return on equity and a 34.4 percent five-year average earning per share, compared to a median for all industries of 16.1 and 14.3 percent, respectively (Sorkin, 1986: 87). Interestingly, one study found that for-profit acute care hospitals are not more efficient than their not-for-profit counterparts, but rather are more expensive to operate; at the same time, however, the study found no evidence that patients admitted to these hospitals were treated less well than those in not-for-profit hospitals (Institute of Medicine, 1986).

The corporatization of health care has involved both horizontal and vertical integration. **Horizontal integration** is the process by which a corporation acquires large numbers of productive facilities, such as hospitals or nursing homes, across widespread markets. For example, in 1984 the Hospital Corporation of America (HCA) was a $4.2 billion concern, owning more than 355 hospitals in the United States, the United Kingdom, and several other countries. HCA typically targeted troubled public and not-for-profit hospitals, particularly Catholic institutions, for acquisition and conversion to for-profit parts of the chain (Salmon, 1985; see also Rosett, 1984). Because these investor-owned chains operate on the stock market, another major way they engage in horizontal integration is by mergers and takeovers. For example, HCA purchased the entire second-largest hospital chain, Hospital Affiliates International (HAI), by issuing $225 million of common stock for a third of the acquisition price (Siegrist, 1983). One brokerage firm predicted that before the end of the century, 80 percent of all U.S. hospitals will be part of chains (cited in Salmon, 1985). These chains are transforming health care into a large-scale, high-stakes industry, described by one editor of the *New England Journal of Medicine* as "the medical-industrial complex" (Relman, 1980).

Vertical integration describes the conglomerate control over several levels of production, such as hospitals, nursing homes, hospital supply companies, pharmaceutical companies, prosthetic supply companies, medical office complexes, and home health care agencies. For example, HCA organized a (subsequently unsuccessful) merger with American Hospital Supply Corporation, the nation's largest medical supplier (Salmon, 1985). Similarly, Caremark, a large home health care chain, was acquired by Baxter Travenol Laboratories, one of the foremost producers of technologies used in home health care. Baxter's Caremark subsequently entered into joint ventures with several hospitals in Cleveland, Chicago, and Boston (Freudenheim, 1988a). Vertically integrated industries have increased capacity to control diverse aspects of the market and to shift resources when one part of the business becomes less profitable.

One particular form of vertical integration portends great structural change in the health care industry. When hospitals are owned by the same corporation as insurers (as in the case of some health maintenance organization [HMO] hospitals), considerable market control is concentrated. For example, Humana operated two community hospitals in Chicago, subsequently purchased a chain of freestanding ambulatory care centers to serve as feeders to the hospitals, and then proposed a new teaching hospital to which the community hospitals would funnel patients—all ideally integrated through the Humana Care Plus, a comprehensive health insurance program (Berliner and Burlage, 1987). As described in Chapter 11, such concentration greatly reduces the autonomy of professionals working in the system. Patients too are severely limited in the options open to them; their weak leverage is further reduced by a very powerful economic system.

Although not-for-profit hospitals do not have market position and dividends to protect, they have increasingly imitated for-profit hospitals in their managerial style and marketing strategies in order to cope with inadequate revenues from unfilled beds and cost-containment regulations. Indeed, many not-for-profit and teaching hospitals have hired for-profit companies to run their operations (Salmon, 1985). Some not-for-profit hospitals have banded together into chains, allowing them economies of scale and managerial efficiency comparable to those of for-profit chains (cf. Light, 1986). Another strategy has been to develop new services or business outlets, such as sports medicine clinics, mobile diagnostic units, outpatient surgery centers, home health care, and even shopping centers, restaurants, and health spas. By diversifying into such unrelated business, not-for-profit hospitals become very like their for-profit counterparts in their operations (Salmon, 1984). The main difference is that not-for-profit hospitals try to plow profits back into hospital improvements, indigent care, or cross-subsidization of an unprofitable partner hospital (Light, 1986).

Hospital Costs and Financing

Payments to hospitals account for the largest single category of national health expenditures, and one that has been notoriously difficult to control. There are four modes of hospital reimbursements. One, characteristic of hospitals operated out of federal, state, or city tax revenues, is the annual budget, which is set in advance and unrelated to the units of service actually delivered. A second form is billing based on "charges" that are set, with no necessary relationship to cost, for each item of service (e.g., use of operating room, each lab test and medication, each day's use of a hospital room). This method of billing, employed since the beginning of private patient use of hospitals, is rapidly disappearing due to political pressure from insurers and government regulatory agencies.

A third, more sophisticated method of billing is retrospective cost reimbursement, by which insurers and hospitals negotiate an agreement about the costs for services provided. This approach forces hospitals to "debundle" charges, making it less likely that they can subsidize an expensive facility by overcharging for other, inexpensive services. A fourth, more recent and complex approach is prospective reimbursement, by which the insurer and/or public agency attempts to predict, on the basis of previous experience and rates of cost increases, the costs for various services in the coming year. The hospital may bill for only that averaged amount, regardless of actual costs. This approach resembles an annual budget arrangement, except that the hospital bills numerous agencies and individuals rather than a single sponsor (McCarthy, 1981).

Financial Constraints.   The diagnosis-related group (DRG) is the most widely known form of prospective reimbursement. DRGs are the basis of payment for all hospital billing in some highly regulated states, such as New Jersey (for an analysis of the political and economic processes producing the New Jersey arrangement, see Morone and Dunham, 1984). In 1983, the federal government also adopted DRGs as a basis for Medicare reimbursements. In this system, each procedure or service that can be provided to a hospital patient is placed in a diagnosis-related category (for example, in New Jersey there are 467 categories), each with a price fixed by computing what similar hospitals had been charging for like cases. The hospital is not paid more if the actual services cost more; if the actual services cost less, the hospital keeps the difference. This plan eliminates the proliferation of hospital procedures and services previously encouraged when hospitals gained from each additional billable service. On the other hand, it places pressures on doctors not to request services that may be beneficial, and it promotes the early discharge of patients—"quicker and sicker."

At the same time, however, shorter hospital stays leave many hospitals underutilized. Concomitant with the decline in hospitalization and the reduction of length of stay promoted by DRGs, hospital occupancy rates dropped from 69.7 percent in 1980 to 56.6 percent in 1985, creating economic difficulties for hospitals with limited other means of raising revenue (Moss, 1987; Tolchin, 1988d). One strategy used by hospitals to compensate for lost revenues was the aggressive promotion of outpatient care, which was encouraged by insurers who expected cost savings relative to inpatient care. Because both hospital and freestanding outpatient services have increased their outpatient costs to the point of nearly equaling the expense of inpatient services, private and federal insurers are now trying to set limits for these services as well (Kramon, 1988b). These developments illustrate the economic and political jockeying for position among powerful elements of the health care system: hospitals, insurers, and government regulators.

Hospitals can remain financially stable—and in some cases even highly profitable—if they can control the mixture of *payers* of their patients' bills. Those in a position to accept proportionately few patients with payers (such as Medicare) that severely restrict the hospital's charges (and no patients without insurance or other means of paying) can be economically comfortable. Overall, however, under the Medicare DRG plan, hospitals received higher per-patient profits than they had under previous cost-cap regulations. In fiscal year 1984–85, 79 percent of hospitals reported profits on their Medicare business; in 1985–86, 80 percent; in 1986–87, 65 percent (Pear, 1988a). The impact on patients is not clear; some of this profitability may be at the expense of needed patient services. The declining profitability since 1986 may result in hospitals' cutbacks in provision of costly services for Medicare patients. Simultaneously the private insurance industry and its customers (i.e., typically patients' employers) are balking at the extent to which they are billed more to compensate for potential hospital income lost for DRG patients.

Problems of Access.   Inner city and rural hospitals, however, do not have the luxury of controlling the mixture of payers, and many of them end up in dire financial straits. The rate of hospital failure in the 1980s was very high. For example, 52 of the 254 counties in Texas have no hospital; in 15 of those 52, the hospitals had closed in 1988 (Belkin, 1988). Some failed hospitals were outmoded and/or substandard, but many were the only ones available to the populace (Reinhold, 1987).

Before the introduction of DRGs, hospitals typically used cross-subsidization to pay for unprofitable services such as emergency rooms. Because emergency rooms are used disproportionately by uninsured and underinsured patients, they are unlikely to generate enough income to cover costs, and in predominantly poor areas they account for massive losses to hospitals. In New York City, for instance, the emergency room was the avenue to hospital admission for half of all patients (French, 1988). DRGs do not take into account the fact that poor people are more likely to be sicker and suffer multiple conditions and complications compared to those who are well-off. Unable to afford primary care, poor persons appear at emergency rooms when they are extremely sick, requiring extensive medical attention. Furthermore, because many poor people lack the resources and safe conditions to be adequately nursed at home, hospitals must keep them longer. Thus stays at inner city hospitals are typically longer than average, but DRG limits are based on average stays (Tolchin, 1988d). Many nonpublic hospitals have responded by eliminating their emergency room services. In Los Angeles, where 27 percent of all non-elderly adults and 30 percent of all children have no health insurance, fifteen hospitals closed or downgraded their emergency rooms between 1986 and 1988; the remaining hospitals were posting multimillion dollar annual losses on their emergency services (Reinhold, 1988).

For-profit hospitals frequently refuse to serve patients who cannot pay or transfer them—often in medically unstable conditions—to public hospitals or those nonprofit hospitals willing to accept indigent patients. This extensive "dumping" of undesirable patients puts an added burden on inner city hospitals, especially the publicly financed hospitals that become the poor's last resort. In Chicago in 1983, after the governor had placed a ceiling on state payments for hospital services to the poor, transfers of patients from private hospitals to the county public hospital increased from an average of 100 per month to 450 per month. A subsequent study found that of 467 patients transferred to Cook County Hospital from private hospitals, 89 percent were black or Hispanic, 81 percent were unemployed, and nearly a fourth were medically endangered by the transfer (Schiff et al., 1986).

In outrage over this and similar instances, Congress outlawed the "dumping" of patients in April 1987. A year later, however, a House Committee report found that federal agencies were not enforcing the regulation and had sanctioned only four hospitals, even though there were 250,000 reported cases of patient dumping (*New York Times,* March 30, 1988; see also Himmelstein et al., 1984). The trend toward proprietarization and corporatization of health care in the United States is closely linked with this underfunding of public care for the poor and underinsured (Whiteis and Salmon, 1987).

For-profit hospitals (and their not-for-profit imitators) also engage in marketing and "demarketing" strategies to maximize their revenues. "Demarketing" is a euphemism for the practice of actively discouraging "undesirable" patients who seek their services. Nonpaying or low-paying patients may be subjected to long waits and inferior facilities compared to paying patients (Berliner, 1983). For example, economically depressed Brownsville, Texas, is served by two hospitals, both owned by for-profit chains. Despite their very low occupancy rates (40 and 50 percent), they regularly turn away all but the most critical emergency cases if patients cannot pay. In addition to these hospitals' concern for profitability, the plight of poor patients is made more desperate by the fact that Texas has one of the least adequate of all state programs of health services for the poor; only those whose income is below 60 percent of the poverty level are covered by Medicaid insurance. The administrator of one Brownsville hospital said, "We ask all the patients for money. . . . We work with the poor patients and tell them we'd be happy to set up a payment program" (quoted in Tolchin, 1988b). Critics charge that the hospitals aggressively intimidate patients into leaving without health care service (Tolchin, 1988b).

A more subtle marketing strategy of profit-oriented hospitals is "cream skimming," or the targeting of a market of highly desirable patients, typically middle- and upper-class persons with good insurance who need treatments that cost the hospital relatively little. Although physicians are still the main source of hospital referrals, more hospitals are engaging in direct advertising and marketing gimmicks to overcome declining occupancy rates. One hospital, for example, advertised refunds to patients who received unsatisfactory service, such as cold meals. Another sent out dollars-off coupons for its clinic (Sorkin, 1986). "Frills" have been added to attract patients, such as cozy birth centers that provide champagne toasts for the new parents. To the extent that some hospitals are successful in attracting the "cream" of patients, others are worse off, especially if DRG payment rates are involved, because their patient mix no longer includes the less expensive to treat "cream."

A related form of "cream skimming" is the investment in specialty hospitals. By 1987 more than one-third of the 1,375 for-profit hospitals in the United States were devoted exclusively to specialty care, such as psychiatric care, treatment for substance abuse, and physical rehabilitation. This emphasis was prompted partly by the fact that specialized care is not subject to much federal cost-containment pressure; nearly all patients are privately insured, are younger than Medicare recipients, and tend to stay about three times as long as patients in acute care hospitals. Another feature that yields higher profits is that little expensive technology is required. Although the long-term profitability of specialty hospitals may be greatly reduced by government or insurer cost-containment measures, the immediate impact has been to siphon desirable patients away from general hospitals (Freudenheim, 1987b).

By contrast, the nursing home industry—75 percent of which is controlled by for-profit companies—has become somewhat less profitable than it once was because it relies very heavily (over 50 percent) upon government subsidies through Medicare and Medicaid. When government reimbursements were liberal, nursing home chains made huge profits and expanded rapidly. In California the average nursing home made a profit of 41 percent on net equity in 1978–79. In those boom years, for-profit chains grew as much as 900 percent in just four years (see Harrington, 1984). When government funding became more restrictive, however, the chains did not fare so well. For example, Beverly Enterprises, which owned 1,003 nursing homes, lost $30.5 million in 1987, despite revenues of over $2 billion (Feder, 1988).

The profit motive in specialty hospitals (especially those such as nursing homes and psychiatric hospitals, where patients are relatively isolated and powerless) raises serious questions about the quality of care. For example, there were numerous reports of patient neglect and abuse at several Beverly Enterprises nursing homes, and inspections resulted in fifty citations of life-threatening violations over a fifteen-month period. Such institutions had a very high ratio of unskilled workers, often undocumented immigrants, barely earning the minimum wage, with a turnover rate of 78 percent, which led to frequent understaffing (Feder, 1988). Since the nursing home industry has well-organized, powerful political influence and lobbying, it has been successful in persuading legislatures to adopt weak regulations and favorable rates of reimbursement. Nursing home residents and their families, even when represented by consumer interest groups, cannot muster the financial resources or organization to be as powerful in the political arena (Harrington, 1984).

The trends toward proprietarization and corporatization have generally been promoted—directly and indirectly—by government policies, especially under the Reagan administration. At the same time, the federal government and other insurers have increased efforts to control the spiraling cost increases that enhance the profitability of such corporations. These trends are not inevitable, however; the government could, for example, decide to redirect funds into public health care programs. Such policy directions are not likely, however, in the face of the massive political and economic force that these growing corporations wield.

MEDICAL INDUSTRIES

Vast and profitable industries have developed to supply products and processes for medical care. They manufacture, distribute, and market known products, while continuously researching and developing new ones. The most obvious example is the pharmaceutical industry, which markets large numbers of both prescription and over-the-counter drugs. Other industries supply everything from the mundane to the exotic, from the simplest devices to the most complex, including monitors for various organ functions, radiological equipment, laboratory equipment, prosthetic devices, surgical equipment, medical office and hospital supplies and equipment, and intravenous solutions.

Costs

Changing medical technologies involve not only innovations in material objects (e.g., drugs, equipment, and devices), but also the development of new procedures and scientific and technical knowledge bases. Rapidly changing medical technology has been a major source of the increases in hospital and physician-related costs to pay for new technological equipment, to build and adapt spaces to use it, and to hire and supervise the specialized workers to operate it. Estimates from the U.S. Office of Technology Assessment attribute between one-third and three-quarters of increased expenditures for hospital care to the costs of medical technology (Banta et al., 1981).

Similarly, new drugs are often extremely costly, because they involve expensive research and development processes, including the costs of the clinical trials required for federal approval, marketing, product liability insurance, and sizable corporate profit. For example, a year's supply of Factor VIII, used by hemophiliacs for blood clotting, costs $25,000, and a year's supply of growth hormones for children whose bodies do not produce them naturally ranges from $8,000 to $30,000. Drug prices have risen very fast proportionate to other prices in the U.S. economy; while cost-cutting measures by government and private insurers have put some pressure on hospitals and providers to reduce their prices, pharmaceutical prices have not been controlled.

One important component of the cost of drugs in the United States is advertising expenses, which account for an estimated 25 percent of the wholesale price paid by the pharmacist (Roemer, 1986: 17). Marketing is a particularly important factor in profits from prescription drugs; because doctors—not consumers—decide which drug to order, competitive pricing has little impact. Advertising aimed at the physician-prescriber attempts to achieve brand loyalty especially when there is little real difference among the competing products. In 1988, drug companies spent $2.5 billion (or more than $5,000 per doctor) promoting their products (Wilkes and Shuchman, 1989). The pharmaceutical industry has noted that the before-marketing costs of researching, developing, and testing a new drug have about doubled due in part to the difficulties of studying the effectiveness of drugs for chronic (rather than acute) conditions as well as to added measures to assure drug safety. Nevertheless, the industry's return on equity in 1986 was 22.9 percent, compared to 9.6 percent for all manufacturers (Pollack, 1988).

One reason that many medical technologies are so expensive is that they are not *resolutions* of a problem but merely partial *responses* to it. For example, the iron lung was a response to some needs of polio victims, but did not resolve the problem of the disease itself; a resolution came with the development of the polio vaccine. Modern medicine is struggling to respond to many chronic illnesses that are not so amenable to a "technological fix" as were the acute infectious diseases prominent a few decades ago. For example, in 1988 four drugs generated sales of a billion dollars or more each. Two (Tagamet and Zantac) were for ulcers, and two (Vasotec and Capoten) were for high blood pressure and congestive heart failure (Kolata, 1988). The most frequently dispensed drugs are predominantly for chronic illnesses or conditions for which drugs are palliative, not curative: ulcers, hypertension, anxiety, heart disease, arthritis, angina, and menopause. Since the drugs do not actually cure the illnesses, patients must typically take such medication for many years, often for the rest of their lives (Kolata, 1988).

Thus while they may prolong some people's lives, improve some people's functioning, or hold some people's dangerous symptoms in abeyance, even impressive technological developments often do not fully resolve the medical problem. For example, end-stage renal disease is fatal, but there are some very expensive technologies that can keep many patients alive (e.g., in 1987 the cost of in-center dialysis was about $24,000 per year). Nevertheless, these technologies do not actually cure the diseases causing kidney failure, nor can they restore patients to full health. While some recipients may live for several years, nationally only about 30 percent survive more than five years. While some patients are able to function nearly normally, the majority are sufficiently disabled by their illness that they are unable to work outside their home (Plough, 1986: 20, 21). Such medical costs are thus not one-time expenses for a single illness episode, but rather continue to mount so long as recipients live.

Some new technologies do, however, save money. For example, new vaccines can prevent outbreaks of serious diseases. New drugs, for conditions such as ulcers, can make costly surgery unnecessary; however, whether this substitution is money saving depends upon whether the course of drugs is less expensive than an operation.

Another major reason for the increased costs of medical technologies has been the medicalization of problems not previously treated as medical issues (as described in Chapters 9 and 10). The medicalization of menopause, childbirth, old age, hyperactivity, alcoholism and other substance abuse, emotional troubles, and the like has resulted in the prescription of a number of technological medical responses—drugs, devices, and procedures—that have all contributed to the greatly increased cost of treating these "conditions."

Regulation

Many interest groups are involved in the creation and utilization of new medical technologies. Three obvious parties are the manufacturers who profit from their sales, the physicians and hospitals who may choose to employ them, and the regulatory agencies that have varying degrees of power and responsibility over them. Other groups, including research scientists, political figures, media representatives, consumer groups, insurers, and patients, are also involved, sometimes in complex ways. Because of the rapid pace of technological development in medicine and because of the enormous economic, social, and health stakes involved, ongoing critical analysis of medical products and technologies is important. The complexity and sheer quantity of new developments, however, make it difficult for even well-endowed and powerful nations to monitor them adequately. Developing countries are far less able to evaluate and control the use of new products and technologies, so the regulation of medical products marketed by transnational corporations has become a worldwide problem.

In the United States, the Food and Drug Administration (FDA) regulates pharmaceuticals, and has the power to allow or ban their sale and control their labeling; the Federal Trade Commission (FTC) has some additional regulatory authority over the content of advertising claims made for health-related products. In 1938 Congress authorized the FDA controls, but a "grandfather" clause exempted preexisting drugs from scrutiny. Drug regulations required evidence of safety and truth in labelling and, since 1962, proof of efficacy (for a fascinating account of the politics of

FDA regulation, see Silverman and Lee, 1974). Initially, only pharmaceuticals and cosmetics were regulated; in 1976 (after tragedies such as the Dalkan Shield deaths), the FDA was given authority to regulate medical devices. To date, however, medical procedures (such as new forms of surgery) are not regulated or even systematically evaluated.

Medical technologies often have harmful or undesirable side effects. They may even cause illness (iatrogenesis) and death. The evaluation of their safety is difficult, however, partly because it may take years for the bad effects to become evident. For example, in the 1940s and 1950s, unaware of the dangers of radiation, many physicians and dentists used x-rays and other radiological imaging frequently and indiscriminately, thus delivering relatively large doses of radiation to their patients. Since the effects of such radiation are cumulative and may take many years to culminate in disease (which even then may be attributable to multiple causes), the safety of early radioactive technologies was not readily questioned.

Safety is also always relative. The risks of dangerous side effects of a drug or procedure must be weighed against the probabilities and risks of the condition itself as well as of alternative therapies (Banta et al., 1981). For example, oral contraceptives carry the risk of unpleasant, dangerous, and even fatal side effects, but pregnancy and childbirth create serious health risks too. Regulators have not yet resolved issues arising from the fact that safety is also relative to certain characteristics of the patient population. Regulations often restrict drugs that are unsafe for children, for example, but fail to limit those that are unsafe for the elderly. Risks must also be weighed against the potential health benefits. Dangerous side effects might be more acceptable in a drug for potentially fatal AIDS than in one for baldness, weight loss, or acne.

The importance of the powerful regulation of these new products and technologies is amply illustrated by the tragedies created by several dangerous products. Between 1943 and 1970, a synthetic estrogen, diethylstilbestrol (DES), was widely prescribed for women in the United States, despite early and growing evidence of its carcinogenic (cancer-causing) properties and its ineffectiveness for many purposes for which it was prescribed (e.g., preventing miscarriage). By 1971 there was evidence that DES caused iatrogenic disease (such as vaginal cancer) in some daughters born to pregnant recipients; an estimated 2.1 to 3.5 million females may have been thus affected (Weiss, 1983). This case illustrates the effects of poor scientific analysis and shoddy clinical trials, lack of control over physician experimentation with unapproved drugs, and the readiness of a portion of the medical community to prescribe a potent substance that was not fully understood or proven safe and effective (Dutton et al., 1988; see also Apfel and Fisher, 1984; Bell, 1986; Direcks and Hoen, 1986).

A similar tragedy occurred between 1958 and 1962, when some 10,000 children were born with severe birth defects as a result of thalidomide, a sedative prescribed for their mothers to reduce nausea in pregnancy. The drug was not approved in the United States due to the tenacious efforts of a single medical officer with the FDA. The thalidomide disaster spurred the passage of the U.S. Drug Act of 1962 and changed the criteria for testing drug safety (Silverman and Lee, 1974).

The tragedies caused by the Dalkon Shield, an intrauterine device (IUD) for contraception, illustrate the need for greater regulation of medical devices. In 1968 the shield was introduced and entrepreneurially promoted by a respected gynecologist, who later sold the invention to a large pharmaceutical company. The government then had no effective regulation for medical devices. No agency checked the doctor's claims of safety and effectiveness, and the manufacturer had no legal accountability for using those inaccurate claims in its advertising. Several million women in the United States and overseas had the device inserted. Despite numerous reports of serious side effects, massive infections, and dangerous pregnancies due to the IUD, the company did not issue physicians any warnings about its dangers until after the first documented death (Perry and Dawson, 1985; see also Dowie and Johnston, 1987; LaCheen, 1986).

While some evidence pertaining to safety (and effectiveness) can be deduced from the chemical properties of substances and devices, and further data can be gained from experiments on animals, medical industries and the FDA need to test innovations on human subjects. Early procedures for drug approval allowed clinical trials done under uncontrolled circumstances to be used as evidence of safety and effectiveness. Any licensed physician was permitted to experiment on patients with drugs before FDA approval, and pharmaceutical companies provided large quantities of free samples for so-called "clinical trials." There are numerous professional incentives for doctors to experiment to find new applications for approved drugs; such results were publishable sources of professional prestige. Only in the 1970s, however, were experimenters required to obtain the informed consent of patients; previously many subjects did not even know that they were taking experimental drugs.[1] Because of the great medical and commercial interest in the many aspects of women's reproductive lives, women—especially poor women—have been disproportionately used as guinea pigs in medical research (Ford, 1986; Oakley, 1984; Marcelis and Shiva, 1986; Ward, 1986).

The contrast between medical device and drug abuses in the First and

[1]The requirement of informed consent has not been totally effective in eliminating abuses, however, since many patients cannot evaluate information they are given and may not understand the risks. While most universities and hospitals have procedures for monitoring consent, clinical experiments done by individual practitioners or in small clinics are not adequately monitored, and serious abuses are still occurring. For example, in 1987 two anesthesiologists administered—without consent—the drug Dilantin to about 250 women in labor as part of an experiment to determine whether the drug (an approved treatment for epilepsy) could reduce fetal stress in Caesarian births (*New York Times*, June 1, 1988b).

Third World also shows the importance of strong regulation in counteracting the market interests of these industries. Whereas in the United States and other First World countries, regulatory agencies and knowledgeable physicians can prevent the misuse or abuse of pharmaceuticals and other medical products, Third World countries lack the money and expertise necessary to control them. In developing countries, medical industries continue to sell unsafe products that were banned or highly controlled in Western markets.[2]

Profits and Products

The free enterprise model of technological development and marketing in the United States means that the profit motive is a particularly important influence in shaping the creation and marketing of new drugs and technologies. One critic argued that the proliferation of technological inno-

---

[2]Transnational drug corporations have been attracted to the global marketplace, but have frequently exploited developing countries' lack of expertise and inability to control the sale of pharmaceuticals, infant formulas, contraceptives, and the like. Dangerous drugs are sold over the counter in many countries, while the labeling, package inserts, and desk reference information provided by manufacturers fail to mention many dangers and claim many unproven uses. For example, anabolic steroids can cause birth defects, liver tumors, and irreversible masculinization of females, but are readily sold over the counter in Malaysia, Brazil, and several African nations as an appetite stimulant (often specifically for children) to relieve exhaustion, fatigue, and malnutrition (Muller, 1982).

A related exploitation of ther global marketplace was the aggressive and often misleading marketing of infant formulas to Third World families, who could not afford to sustain their babies on purchased formula and lacked the sanitary conditions necessary to prepare and store it. Once they had abandoned nursing their infants, however, mothers were trapped into buying formula, which cost an estimated 85 percent of the family's entire income. Babies became malnourished, dehydrated, and died. In 1981 *Newsweek* estimated that some 1 million children were dying each year from malnutrition and infection due to substitution of commercial formulas for breast milk (cited in Bodenheimer, 1984). Few developing nations had the power, knowledge, or resources to prevent the aggressive marketing of formula, however. In 1977, an international grass-roots boycott was organized against Nestlé (which controlled half of the entire Third World infant formula market) and its many subsidiaries; while never achieving enough leverage to attain a victory, the boycott did pressure Nestlé into a compromise. In 1981, the World Health Organization adopted a clear but voluntary code on the marketing of infant formula; the vote was 118 to 1, with the Reagan administration casting the sole dissenting vote (Norris, 1982; see also Ledogar, 1975).

Commercial misrepresentation is particularly unfortunate for developing nations, which have small health care budgets but massive health care needs. If pharmaceutical companies persuade poor people or poor nations to spend a large proportion of their budgets on expensive commercial preparations for which there are inexpensive, perhaps even homemade substitutes, they are depriving people of the other benefits that money could have bought. Worse yet is when the expensive commercial preparation is ineffective or dangerous. For example, many pharmaceutical companies actively market profitable drugs for diarrhea in developing countries, where conditions make it a common and dangerous problem. Some, such as clioquinol, are ineffective for most causes of diarrhea and have serious side effects (such as neurological damage and blindness); others, such as Lomotil, can stop the flow of diarrhea but exacerbate the more serious problem of dehydration. The best treatment (oral rehydration therapy) is, however, of no commercial value, since the materials used are inexpensive, readily available sugar and salts. The aggressive marketing of the dangerous but profitable drugs thus diverts funds from therapies that could do vastly more good (Muller, 1982).

vation is inevitable, because "expansion is an absolute necessity for capitalist enterprises" (Waitzkin, 1979: 1263). While the profit motive is not the only determining force, it is certainly influential.

On the one hand, the quest for profits has motivated some impressive research; many of the technological advances of bioscientific medicine might not have occurred were it not for the investment of much research time and money. Private enterprise is not the only way a society could organize its research incentive, however; indeed, we gain much—perhaps most—of our medical advances from government-supported research in universities and government research centers. Nevertheless, in the United States many medical changes have come out of the private sector.

On the other hand, the profit orientation has greatly limited the scope of research and development; the medical industries are understandably interested only in new developments that will produce marketable commodities. In the United States, the decision to develop and market a drug depends primarily upon economic considerations; drugs to meet people's actual health needs are often of limited commercial interest (known as "orphan drugs"). The industry is not likely to fund research on a cheap, readily available remedy, even if it may be the best treatment for a condition. For a drug to be profitable, it must be patentable; natural substances and shelf chemicals are not, so they are not researched, even if they may be highly effective. The search for patentable commodities also means that much research is directed to substitute drugs and/or technologies. Many "new" drugs are in fact existing drugs that are only marginally changed to justify a new patent, obtain and hold a market share, or create a new market (e.g., for home use and not just hospital use).

Marketability increasingly depends upon whether the cost of the drug or technology will be reimbursed by third-party payment. For example, if Medicare is not likely to pay for a new treatment for the elderly, then companies are not likely to invest in its development (Pear, 1988a). Drugs for developing nations are likewise of little commercial interest; although large numbers of people need some of these medications, researching and producing them would not be profitable.[3] Pharmaceutical companies are not attracted to developing drugs for small markets; government research institutes do most of what research is done. Many known cures for relatively rare conditions would not be commercially produced if it were not for special government incentives (Asbury, 1981).

[3]This general profit orientation does not mean that individual companies always gauge all policies to maximize profits. For example, when a drug developed by Merck for parasitic worms in livestock and dogs turned out to be a safe and effective treatment for a human parasitic infection causing river blindness among more than 18 million people in Africa, Merck offered to make the drug available without charge through the World Health Organization (*New York Times*, October 22, 1987). Likewise Searle, a leading producer of heart drugs, offered free supplies of certain drugs to needy patients not covered by private or government insurance programs (Altman, 1988a).

Interestingly, recent government incentives have themselves led to high drug prices by eliminating possible competition. The 1983 Orphan Drug Act granted seven-year market monopolies to companies developing treatment for relatively rare diseases. For example, Genentech was granted "orphan drug status" for its version of the human growth hormone, for which it charged some $10,000 to $20,000 for a year's supply—at a hefty gross margin of 90 to 95 percent—for annual sales in 1987 of $86 million (Pollack, 1988).

In the United States, much medical research and new medical technological developments have been directed toward maximizing profits. Sometimes the interests of these corporations coincide with the needs of the sick, but there is no structural reason for this occur. A market-oriented, profit-maximizing industry does not give first priority to the actual needs of the citizenry.

ECONOMIC INTERESTS AND THIRD-PARTY PAYMENT

The system of payment for health care in the United States is extremely complex; indeed, its very complexity makes it more costly. Ultimately, the American people pay all health care costs, but there are three main patterns by which the health care dollars are directed from the people to the providers: by direct payment by the consumer; from government taxation at various levels; and through private insurance companies, both for-profit and not-for-profit. Several large scale agencies in government and the insurance industry have become extremely powerful factors in the health care system, and the interests they represent are influential in dealing with the providers as well as the recipients of health care. Their reimbursement policies and regulations become in effect nationally significant health policies. In many instances, these agencies overlap, such as when the government makes private health insurance companies the fiscal intermediaries for public funds; private companies thus profit by charging for administrative overhead. In addition, the foremost purchasers of private insurance are not the health care recipients but their employers, so the interests of business and other employers figure into this complex system.

Despite our national rhetoric regarding private enterprise, public funding is the single largest source of payments for health care, and reliance upon public funding is steadily increasing. In 1966, Americans paid 49.5 percent of all health care expenditures themselves, with public (federal, state, and local) funding covering only 25.5 percent. Just twenty years later, in 1986, government payments accounted for 41.4 percent of all health care expenditures, compared to the 30.7 percent covered by private insurance and the 25.3 percent coming directly from the patients (Anderson, 1986; see also Schieber and Poullier, 1986; Lohr, 1988).

The existence of insurance for some citizens encouraged the inflation of costs for all, thus increasing the disparity in the affordability of health care for those with ample coverage and those with insufficient or no coverage. In the health care marketplace, demand is not a function of need. Many people need health care but cannot demand it, because they lack the means to pay.

Insurance functions to create the demand for goods and services among persons not wealthy enough to afford them easily otherwise. If a service or health care product is covered by insurance for enough people to create a sufficient market demand, prices spiral upward. For example, the expansion of Medicare and some private insurance coverage to home health care products and services created a profitable market. In 1988, for example, Wall Street analysts were predicting a phenomenal annual growth rate (as much as 20 to 25 percent) for companies producing drugs tailored to home health care delivery (Freudenheim, 1988a). Because both private and public insurance provide piecemeal coverage and relatively weak regulation of the many industries involved, there are few incentives for providers and manufacturers to reduce the costs of needed, insurance-covered services or products.

Private Insurance

The very idea of and need for health insurance is historically relatively recent. Before the turn of the century, medical services consumed a small proportion of a family's budget. Doctors and other healers charged comparatively modest fees, which often were adjusted according to a person's ability to pay or were payable in kind (e.g., with a chicken or sack of potatoes). Pharmaceuticals were simple and inexpensive. The family itself provided most of the nursing care. Even then, however, lost income due to sickness could be devastating to a family.

With the rapid expansion of technologically sophisticated, hospital-centered medicine beginning in the early part of the twentieth century, costs quickly began to climb. Thus citizens encountered a greatly increased risk that the expenses incurred for treatment would exceed the family's ability to pay. The Depression of the 1930s created another major impetus for insurance, as voluntary hospitals experienced massive reductions in income due to patients' inability to pay. They supported (and financially underwrote) health insurance as a way to stabilize their incomes (Feigenbaum, 1987; Fein, 1986; Starr, 1982). In this climate, the idea of using health insurance to spread the financial risks over time and across a population of insured came to fruition.

In industrialized countries of Europe such as Sweden, Denmark, and Switzerland, national programs of compulsory health insurance were developed as early as 1883. These state-subsidized programs were not instituted mainly for medical costs (which were as yet small proportions of people's expenses) but rather for income maintenance—"sick pay." Nevertheless, their existence later enabled European nations to expand national coverage to include medical costs not just for workers but for all citizens (Starr, 1982: 237–240).

Blue Cross, created in the 1930s, was the foremost early form of health insurance in the United States. Actively encouraged by the American Hospital Association, Blue Cross was a not-for-profit hospital insurance plan based upon noncompeting territorial divisions in which participants paid premiums according to communitywide ratings. Although organized labor favored a national health insurance program instead, it accepted the Blue Cross alternative indirectly by including such insurance in bargaining agendas for labor contracts. When commercial insurers discovered that health insurance was an economically viable enterprise, several began to compete by offering coverage for expenses, such as doctors' fees, not insured by Blue Cross. In response Blue Cross developed its companion plan, Blue Shield, for nonhospital services.

Initially, the AMA opposed Blue Cross and other forms of third-party payment on the ideological grounds that they came between the doctor and patients, and restricted doctors' decisions about treatment. The AMA also committed considerable energies and funds to fighting various legislative attempts to create a national compulsory health insurance. Eventually, the medical profession agreed to accept Blue Shield, because it was given some control over the program and believed that such insurance would defuse the momentum toward a national program. By keeping health insurance out of the public sector, the medical profession gained a large measure of control and greatly increased its income (Starr, 1982: 290–334; see also Law, 1974).

Although Blue Cross had the benefit of preferred corporate status and tax treatment, as well as a much lower ratio of administrative costs to profit than commercial insurers, it began to lose its competitive edge in the 1950s. Blue Cross had been conceived as a plan for an entire community, and premium rates were based upon local experience with participants' hospital utilization and costs; risks were thus widely spread. The initial institutional goal was to stabilize hospital use and income; income from insurance itself was not important. The commercial insurers, however, explicitly sought income from insurance; their competitive strategy was to approach employers of low-risk groups and offer them much lower premiums than possible by the community-rating method of Blue Cross. Eventually, Blue Cross had to abandon its communitywide risk pool in order not to lose all the contracts for coverage of lower-risk employees (Feigenbaum, 1987; Starr, 1982: 327–331). The enduring effect of this development has been that certain groups (such as employees of very large corporations and those in occupations with fewer health problems) obtain insurance coverage at comparatively reasonable rates. Others (such as workers in companies with disproportionately large numbers of older and minority employees) are likely to receive little or no employment-related health insurance, because their experience-rated premiums are too expensive for employers to absorb.

Commercial insurance companies make money primarily in two ways: by paying out less in benefits than they receive in premiums, and by investing premium funds before disbursing them as benefits. Commercial insurers generally pay out a much smaller percent of their income in benefits than do Blue Cross and Blue Shield (McCarthy, 1981). Control over such large sums for investment is a significant source of economic and political power for major insurance companies (Bodenheimer et al., 1975; Navarro, 1975). Furthermore, insurance companies' portfolios frequently include investments in other for-profit health care ventures. For example, Connecticut General Insurance (also the holding company for Aetna) merged with the Insurance Company of North America and diversified its holdings; the new corporation, CIGNA, invested in a physician group in California, bought numerous for-profit hospitals in this country and elsewhere, and operates several HMOs. In addition, a subsidiary company acquired substantial investments in several for-profit health care chains, including Humana, HCA, and Beverly Enterprises. Thus CIGNA became the third-largest diversified financial company, ranked by assets, in the U.S. (Wohl, 1984). One growing problem is the lack of regulation of the insurance industry; like the savings and loan industry in the 1980s, some insurance companies in the 1990s are severely undercapitalized, and, when they become insolvent, persons who thought they were insured are left unprotected.

Forms of Private Insurance.   To make benefit expenditures predictable and thereby assuring a desirable profit margin, many commercial insurers offered indemnity plans, in contrast to Blue Shield's earlier service coverage. Indemnity plans specify limits to the costs borne by the insurer by imposing deductibles, co-payments, limits on per-service payments, and annual and/or lifetime ceilings on payments for various types of service (Feigenbaum, 1987). Unlike the service plans offered by Blue Cross, Blue Shield, and some commercial insurers, indemnity plans involve no incentive for the insurer to pressure providers to keep costs down, because the excess is borne by the insured. Since individual health care recipients often have little choice among or leverage over hospitals and other providers, many persons covered by limited indemnity plans find themselves underinsured.

Two other forms of private insurance severely limit the choice of physician and hospital. Preferred provider organizations (PPOs) involve an employer or insurance underwriter's contract with a limited number of doctors, hospitals, and other providers to provide services for the insured at a discounted rate. Insured employees who choose other providers must bear the full difference in cost. While employers and insurance companies are not blind to issues of provider quality, their overriding concern is cost control; under such plans, dissatisfied patients have severely restricted options.

HMOs are prepaid health plans utilizing preferred providers who are either independently contracted or employed by an HMO group practice. Some HMOs, such as Kaiser in California and HIP in New York, are not-for-profit organizations; most, however, such as Maxicare, United Health-care, and various insurance company HMOs (e.g., PruCare) are profit seeking. As the name implies, health maintenance organizations are supposed to be particularly interested in prevention and health maintenance, with the expectation that this emphasis would reduce subsequent costs for acute care and illness treatments. Such long-term savings are difficult to achieve, however, because, as a form of insurance, HMOs are rarely involved in a person's entire illness-causing or preventive experience. An employee may be covered for a few years and then have a different insurer; HMOs also go out of business. Also important factors such as nutrition are outside the control of the HMO.

Cost and Access.   In the 1970s the federal government hoped that HMOs would contain health care costs better than other forms of insurance. It encouraged recipients of government insurance (e.g., Medicare) to use prepaid, preferred provider plans, but the anticipated efficiency gains and cost containment have not resulted, and premiums have risen rapidly (Freudenheim, 1988c). The financial collapse of several HMOs, including the giant Maxicare (which once covered over 2 million persons and paid substantial dividends to investors), left many enrollees uninsured and providers unpaid, highlighting the inadequate regulation of the industry (Freudenheim, 1989c; Holden, 1989).

Both PPOs and HMOs are increasingly involved in the widespread vertical integration of the health care industry. Large investor-owned multihospital systems are linked with PPOs, HMOs, and health insurance companies. For example, HCA bought three HMOs, acquired an insurance company, and planned the expansion of its subsidiary PPO in which insured patients would be encouraged to use HCA facilities (Anderson and Mullner, 1989).

One of the biggest problems for persons counting on private health insurance is that as health costs have escalated rapidly, insurance companies and employers have passed on a significant part of that burden to the insured.[4] Between 1985 and 1987, as health care costs soared, the costs

[4]A growing problem has been that cost-cutting practices by insurers (especially private companies) and providers have made sick people themselves responsible for most of the paperwork for insurance claims. As a result, debilitating illness often results in an inability to collect insurance benefits while bills mount. An entire new business has arisen to process a claimant's paperwork in exchange for a percentage of the resulting benefits, thus further reducing the insured person's actual health care coverage.

borne by employers rose by 35 percent, while those borne by employees increased by 58 percent. Some companies have dramatically raised the deductibles and out-of-pocket expenses to be paid by the employee, while others have dropped family coverage. Yet others have initiated "flexible benefits plans," a euphemism for contributing a fixed amount toward premiums for *all* employee benefits, regardless of costs, and expecting employees to pay the rest (Kramon, 1988a). One study found that in the 1980s the real increase (i.e., adjusted for general inflation) in out-of-pocket medical expenses for recipients averages about 5 percent a year, compared to 0.3 percent a year in the 1970s (Short, 1988).

Exact figures are not available on the number of persons who are *under*insured due to seriously limited health plans; often employees do not discover how poorly they are insured until they are denied benefits during an actual health crisis. Employer cost-cutting measures are likely to lead to an increase in the proportion of Americans who are under- or uninsured (Farley, 1985). Some policy analyst advocates of passing on a greater share of the costs (e.g., through high rates of co-insurance or high deductibles) to the individual argue that people will be more selective and cost conscious if they have to bear a substantial part of the burden. The Rand Health Experiment of 1974–82 found that while cost-sharing did reduce the demands for health services, it did *not* result in good decisions about those demands; in fact, financial barriers reduced the use of health services even when those services were needed and appropriate (Lohr et al., 1986). Greater cost-sharing likewise does not lead to more competitive pricing and consumer "shopping" (Marquis, 1984). In the United States, lack of adequate insurance essentially means severely limited access to health care.

Public Programs

The number, type, and quality of health care programs financed by various levels of government demonstrate the complexity and inadequacy of the U.S. health care system. The federal government, for example, directly provides care for large numbers of persons in the military and their dependents, veterans' hospitals, and federal prisons. The largest federal health insurance programs subsidize some care for the poor (Medicaid) and elderly (Medicare). The federal government also finances much health-related research, and has at times supported medical education and other training programs. State, county, and municipal governments also fund health care, by maintaining, for example, public hospitals, nursing homes, community health services, and health programs. State governments are also co-sponsors of Medicaid and other health services for the indigent. The quality of and access to medical care provided by these many programs vary widely across the nation, but there is no national organization or central planning to coordinate or regulate even the public efforts, much less to connect public and private programs.

Medicare.   Medicare was enacted in 1965 to finance acute medical care mainly for elderly Americans. Coverage was expanded in 1972 to include people with chronic kidney disease or disabilities. By 1985, Medicare covered 30 million Americans. The program has two parts: Part A is hospital insurance, funded by a portion of the Social Security payroll tax. Part B is supplementary medical insurance (SMI) for physicians' services, outpatient care, laboratory fees, and home health care; because it is funded through general federal revenues, its growth as a budget item contributes to the federal deficit and pits health care financing against other expenses, such as defense. Partly in response to the influence of hospitals, doctors, and other interest groups, from the outset Medicare was aimed at the *acute* medical care of the elderly. Chronic illness and long-term care, which are of limited relevance to acute care hospitals and to many doctors, were not part of the plan, even though they affect the health status and economic well-being of the elderly as much or even more than acute illness. Thus Medicare does not cover many needed health services and products.

Before Medicare, only about one-third of the elderly had health insurance; private insurance rates were outside the means of most older Americans. The enactment of Medicare immediately increased the average health care utilization rate among the elderly by more than 30 percent (Sorkin, 1986). Although it dramatically increased access to health care, Medicare failed to protect beneficiaries from destitution in the face of health care costs, because its cost-sharing provisions did not limit liabilities in the event of catastrophic illness and did not cover most long-term or nursing home care.

The financing of Medicare has been problematic from the outset. To overcome the objections to the programs by doctors, insurance companies, hospitals, and various other interest groups, Medicare legislation created less of a public health care program and more of an infusion of public money into private channels (Fein, 1986: 69–92). Initially, there were few cost-control regulations in the program. Partly because of the increased utilization of health care services but largely because of rapidly increasing charges by various providers, the expenditures were far more than anticipated. A limited cost-control measure was introduced in 1972, but it was largely ineffective. Between 1979 and 1982, expenditures under Medicare grew much faster than general inflation: hospital care by a rate of 17.2 percent per year, physician services by a 19.2 percent rate (Gibson et al., 1982; Sorkin, 1986; see also Pear, 1987a). Part of the costliness was due to the fact that high tech medicine and labor-intensive medical care are not as responsive to efficiency and other cost-savings measures as other industries; and part was due simply to overexpansion, greed, and in some case outright fraud on the part of providers, hospitals, and insurance administrators.

While the AMA initially fought against the creation of Medicare, the medical profession has been among its prime beneficiaries, and now generally supports the program and its expansion. To secure the cooperation of physicians, the initial Medicare legislation allowed reimbursement of doctors' "usual and customary fees," so long as those fees were "reasonable." Such vague language, especially in the context of a seldom competitive fee-setting process, led to rapid inflation. Fees increased disproportionate to other rates of inflation; the number of elderly treated increased, and the number of medical services ordered by doctors for their Medicare patients rose markedly. Under Medicare, doctors who had previously treated the needy elderly for a fraction of their normal charges could receive their "customary" full payments. Physicians who had previously been frustrated by their inability to treat their pensioner-patients with the best available methods could, under Medicare, prescribe therapies without prejudice of ability to pay. The influx of Medicare funding provided stability for both physician and hospital income, much as private health insurance had done three decades earlier (Fein, 1986: 80–92). The very complexity of Medicare regulations and reimbursement paperwork, however, adds enormously to the cost of the program. The waste of resources on administrative costs in the United States is particularly highlighted by contrasts with Canada and Great Britain, where insurance company intermediaries are eliminated and providers deal directly with the government rather than struggle with billing and collections (Himmelstein and Woolhandler, 1986; see also Fein, 1986: 157; Lee, 1982).

A major ongoing problem has been that some providers do not accept Medicare rates of reimbursement, so patients must bear the cost of the difference (Fein, 1986: 88–92). Because reimbursement is still based upon fee-for-service rates, there is no incentive for physicians to reduce the number of services or recommend less costly services. New Medicare regulations are regularly being proposed to try to contain costs, to ascertain greater physician cooperation, and to get better care for the moneys spent. The process is essentially a political one in which providers and insurers have disproportionately powerful voices (cf. Marmor et al., 1983b). Whether successful regulations will be enacted or have their desired effect remains to be seen. While Medicare has been an important contribution to the health of covered citizens, it is less and less sufficient for their needs, and less able than ever to cover the increasing proportion of the eligible population. Without major restructuring and massive new sources of funding, Medicare is not a program upon which citizens may rely for the future.

Medicaid.   Medicaid was created at the same time as Medicare, but was organized very differently. Because Medicaid is funded through general revenues rather than a trust fund, and because it is perceived as charity rather than deserved aid, the program is particularly vulnerable to cutbacks at every funding level. Each state operates its own program, with federal contributions varying according to the scope of the state's program, relative level of income, and certain features of providers and recipients. Thus several states that have instituted highly restrictive Medicaid programs do not receive as large a proportion of federal funds as they could with a broader program. The federal program includes health care for persons covered by federal Supplemental Security Income (SSI), which assists blind, disabled, and elderly persons; members of families eligible for Aid to Families with Dependent Children (AFDC); and pregnant women in certain income brackets. Many states have defined the criteria for Medicaid so stringently that they exclude more than half the people who could be covered under federal guidelines (Fein, 1986: 108–112; for a critical history of Medicaid, see Stevens and Stevens, 1974).

Due to deficiencies in Medicare coverage, Medicaid has become a significant source of funding for health care for the elderly. Some states use Medicaid to pay Medicare premiums, deductibles, and co-payments that poor elderly persons cannot afford. Medicaid also covers services, such as long-term care, not provided by Medicare (after recipients have exhausted their resources and become poor enough to meet Medicaid guidelines). In 1983, 37 percent of Medicaid payments were on behalf of Medicare-eligible elderly persons, and 35 percent were on behalf of Medicare-eligible disabled persons. Thus, Medicaid has not functioned primarily as a source of health care for lower-class persons, especially poor children, who accounted for only 12 percent of expenditures. Rather, its main recipients appear to be those who were made poor by the costs of health care in disability and old age (Fein, 1986: 112).

The House Select Committee on Aging reported that 90 percent of single elderly patients "spend down" to the poverty level after one year in a nursing home by paying nursing home charges that average $22,000 per year; half of the couples with one spouse in a nursing home reach poverty level within six months, and the well spouse is left destitute, often with many years of life ahead. Thus Medicaid has become the de facto long-term care supplement to Medicare, paying about half of all expenditures for nursing home care (Crickmer, 1988).

The administrative costs of Medicaid are particularly high. Many states parcel out portions of the program to various local agencies or institutional providers; the several layers multiply administrative costs. Furthermore, unlike Medicare, Medicaid eligibility must be determined by complex formulas and continually reviewed, since agencies have an state-directed imperative to trim rolls and discourage coverage. Medicaid is governed by federal, state, and often local regulations (for patient eligibility, services covered, and the like), the sheer volume and complexity of which create enormous administrative costs. A substantial portion of the funds that Americans believe are used for health care is actually going to the mere administration of public insurance programs (Fein, 1986).

Ironically, the greatest documented abuses of Medicaid funding have been on the part of unscrupulous providers, often abetted by the politically motivated purchasing policies of state and local agencies. For example, in 1971 the California legislature passed the Medical Reform Act, facilitating the assignment of Medicaid recipients to HMOs contracting with the state. The legislature had reasoned that these large health care contractors would be more efficient, reduce utilization (which had become "excessive" under fee-for-service payment plans), and thus be more cost-effective than previous arrangements with independent providers. In fact, however, the welfare HMOs charged more. Compared to other HMOs, which spent about 10 percent of the premium dollar on administration and profits, welfare HMOs used 52 percent of state payments for administration and profits (Lewis, 1976). Subsequent investigations also showed that the utilization of services had been cut by using foreign physicians who spoke limited English, by contracting with proprietary hospitals thirty to fifty miles from the client population, by offering only brief office hours, and by denying emergency services and referrals to specialists (Gabel and Redisch, 1979).

The structure of Medicaid has thus encouraged a two-tiered system of medical care, with the service to those covered by Medicaid being distinctly inferior. Medicaid has, however, increased the access of the poor to *some* medical assistance; after the implementation of the program, poor families used significantly more physician services and hospitalization. It has not given the poor access to mainstream medical care, however; for example, poor children are particularly likely to be treated in hospital outpatient services rather than by private physicians. Nor has the program enabled the poor to obtain sufficient medical attention relative to their generally greater health needs (Marmor, 1983).

The two tiers of the American health care delivery system appear to be further and further apart, as cost-cutting measures make even the middle classes vulnerable to restrictions on the freedom of choice of providers, limitations on covered services, and prohibitively high co-payment levels. While the poor are the first to be limited, more restricted, and less well served, all but the wealthiest in American society are experiencing severe economic limits in their health care. For example, the state of Oregon and Alameda County in California became the first U.S. government units to plan the explicit rationing of health care for the poor by attempting to give priority to medical procedures that save the most lives and give a better quality of life to more people. For example, prenatal care, children's immunizations and certain other preventive measures, and treatment of acute and chronic illnesses are given high priority; organ transplants, plastic surgery, speech therapy, and dental care receive low priority. While for now explicit rationing applies mainly to Medicaid recipients, it is likely to be adopted by insurers of the middle class as well (Gross, 1989).

The Uninsured and Underinsured

Since most private insurance is linked with the fringe benefits of certain kinds of employment, large numbers of Americans have no health insurance whatsoever; others are insured only occasionally or have extremely limited benefits. Premium costs for adequate amounts of insurance are much lower for large group coverage, such as that purchased by businesses, and they are virtually prohibitively expensive for individual purchasers. Table 12.1 shows the percent of the U.S. population in 1984 with various types of health care coverage, by poverty status, race, and age.

In 1987, an estimated 37 million Americans—15.5 percent of all civilian, noninstitutionalized persons—had *no private or public coverage* for their medical expenses. Certain segments of the population were particularly hurt; one-third of all young adults (nineteen to twenty-four years old), one-third of all Hispanics, and more than one-quarter of all blacks were uninsured. Because health insurance is chiefly a benefit of only certain kinds of employment, economic downturns (such as those experienced in the 1970s and 1980s) result in greatly increased numbers of uninsured persons. Many of the manufacturing jobs lost have been re-

TABLE 12.1   Percent of the U.S. Population with Health Care Coverage by Poverty Status, Race, and Age, 1984

| | PERCENT COVERED BY | | | ANY COVERAGE? | | PERCENT OF POPULATION |
	PRIVATE INSURANCE	MEDICARE	PUBLIC ASSISTANCE	YES	NO	
Poverty Status						
In poverty	32	12	32	68	32	15
Under 65	31	2	32	64	36	13
65 and over	42	93	28	97	3	2
Not in poverty	85	11	2	90	10	85
Under 65	86	1	2	89	11	75
65 and over	80	96	3	99	1	10
Race						
White	80	13	4	88	12	85
Under 65	80	1	4	86	14	75
65 and over	77	96	5	99	1	10
Black	57	9	19	80	20	12
Under 65	58	2	18	79	21	11
65 and over	42	92	24	98	2	1
All persons[a]	76	12	6	86	14	100

[a]Includes other race.

Source: Ronald Anderson, Meei-shia Chen, Lu Anne Aday, and Llewellyn Cornelius, "Health status and medical care utilization," *Health Affairs* 6(1), 1987: 139. Reprinted by permission of Project HOPE, Milwood, Virginia.

placed by jobs in the service sector of the economy, few of which carry adequate health insurance benefits. Thus the overall proportion of Americans with sufficient employment-related insurance has decreased substantially in recent years. A 1987 national survey found that 78 percent of the uninsured under the age of sixty-five were workers and their families. Uninsured workers were also disproportionately among the working poor, earning less than $10,000 a year, but were not eligible for Medicaid or other public assistance (Short et al., 1989). Since the lack of insurance severely restricts access to care, the high proportion of uninsured Americans is a national problem (Davis and Rowland, 1983; Freeman et al., 1987).

The number of uninsured children grew 13 percent between 1982 and 1987; about 12 million children have no health insurance. A major reason is cutbacks in Medicaid assistance. While there was more than a 30 percent increase in child poverty compared to the preceding decade, in 1987 Medicaid actually served 400,000 fewer children (Johnson, 1989). Many states have highly restrictive eligibility requirements for Medicaid and other forms of public health care. In 1986, nearly nine million Americans, or 65.9 percent of those with family incomes less than $5,000 and 77.4 percent of those with family incomes between $5,000 and $9,999, were *not* insured by public coverage (Ries, 1987). Furthermore, public programs rarely cover all needed expenses; for example, in 1986, Medicare covered only about 40 percent of elderly persons' actual health care expenses (Dowd, 1987).

Even seemingly small medical expenditures become financially catastrophic for families with low incomes and poor health insurance. One study found that in 1977 two-thirds of all families spending 20 percent or more of their income on medical care and one-half of those spending 10 percent or more were below the poverty level. The growing numbers of persons living in poverty, together with cutbacks in Medicaid funding, make it likely that many Americans will experience financially catastrophic medical bills (Berki, 1986).

Problems of access to and the underutilization of health care services also appear to have grown during the 1980s. One study found that between 1982 and 1986 Americans' overall rate of hospitalization declined from 9 to 7 percent, while per capita physician visits declined from 4.8 to 4.3 percent. Some of this decline may be due to reductions in *over*utilization in response to cost-cutting by providers, insurers, government agencies, and employers. There are indications, however, that the decline is also due to decreased access to physician care for certain segments of the population that are particularly likely to be in poor health: Those who are poor, black, and/or uninsured. Table 12.2 shows indicators of potential underuse of medical care in 1986. It suggests that the lack of insurance, minority status, and low income are all related to the insufficient use of medical services for identifi-

TABLE 12.2   Indicators of Potential Underuse of Medical Care, 1986

PROBLEM	U.S.	LOW INCOME	BLACK	HISPANIC	UNINSURED
Percent with chronic illness without physician visit in a year	17	18	25	22	20
Among persons with one or more physician visits in year, percent with serious symptoms who did not see or contact a physician	41	42	39	53	67
Percent pregnant women without first trimester prenatal care	15	30	17	27	20
Percent of persons with hypertension without blood pressure check in a year	20	15	30	30	22
Percent without a dentist visit in a year	38	57	50	47	—

Source: Howard E. Freeman, Robert J. Blendon, Linda H. Aiken, Seymour Sudman, Connie F. Mullinix, and Christopher R. Corey, "Americans report on their access to health care," Health Affairs 6(1), 1987: 14. Reprinted by permission of Project HOPE, Millwood, Virginia.

able chronic and serious illness (e.g., cancer, heart disease, and stroke), for serious symptoms (e.g., loss of consciousness, unexplained bleeding, and chest pain when exercising), and for prenatal care.

National Health Insurance: The Canadian Model

National health insurance is a perennial issue in the United States. As early as 1914 and with increasing fervor in the 1930s and 1940s, some American health reformers were urging social insurance legislation comparable to that in Europe. These proposals were vigorously fought, especially by insurance companies and the AMA (Starr, 1982: 240–289). The idea of a national health insurance has been raised in Congress many times since (Jonas, 1981), but America has not yet enacted *any* comprehensive health care program for its citizens.

In light of the large numbers of uninsured and underinsured Americans and the rapidly escalating burden of health care expenditures, many U.S. policymakers are debating the merits of the Canadian national health insurance. Since 1972, a national program has covered all Canadian citizens for hospitalization, physician care, and some ancillary services. Private insurers are legally excluded from the health care arena. Health care providers are mostly in the private sector, but the government controls expenses through its monopoly on payment (for example, with a binding fee schedule). Many incentives for excessive surgery and other procedures have been eliminated. Because all citizens are covered by the same level and kind of insurance, administrative costs equal only about 3 percent of health budgets, compared to approximately 12 percent in the United States (Freuden-heim, 1989a).

Control over the hospital sector also keeps costs down. Diagnostic tests are centralized, which provides no profits to physicians or labs. Hospitals are run by each province on an annual budget basis, with no incentives to overbuild or invest in duplicates of expensive technological devices. These controls have enabled the Canadian system to keep its health care expenditures to a much smaller portion of the country's GNP, while providing very high rates of access to health care for all citizens (Coburn et al., 1981; Lee, 1982; Marmor, 1982; Marmor et al., 1983a).

The Canadian system does have several drawbacks, however, compared to health care services afforded by upper-class Americans. There are often long waits, especially for nonemergency hospital procedures. Provincial facilities for some high tech procedures and testing may not be located conveniently. The system also has an operative form of rationing, especially of very expensive services such as organ transplants.

Had the United States enacted a national health program such as Canada's several decades ago, it might have realized similar cost controls and universal health care access. Now, however, vested interests profiting from the laissez-faire American system have become so entrenched, eco-nomically centralized, and powerful that it would be extremely difficult if not impossible to establish any economical national health plan, even one as limited as national health insurance. A few decades ago, U.S. hospitals could have been organized as public facilities, but now many are organized as for-profit businesses with major investments to protect. Expensive high tech medical equipment has already been purchased; excessive hospital rooms have already been built. Likewise, health insurance is big business; without eliminating the profit and paperwork of third-party payments, a national health plan could not realize the kinds of savings of the Canadian system. Stringent government controls would be necessary to prevent na-tional health insurance from creating yet another inflationary spiral of health costs, but is there sufficient political will to take such a strong stand (Marmor et al., 1983a)?

A national insurance program would probably resolve one major as-pect of the current crisis in the U.S. health care system: the access of poor and middle-class people to adequate physician and hospital care. National health insurance also has the potential, if implemented with certain regula-tory safeguards, of improving the quality of care received by nonwealthy citizens. Absent major structural changes to eliminate or greatly restrict profit-taking, however, a national health insurance program would proba-bly not be able to reduce or even control costs.

The American people could decide that affordable health care for all is a sufficiently important value to warrant such structural changes. The enormous political and economic power of the vested interests of hospital corporations, insurance companies, medical industries, and health care providers would almost certainly be utilized to fight those changes. Our society needs to consider whether health care is a basic human right that a government should provide for its citizens. Does a country have obligations to provide universal health care, comparable to universal education? To how much and what kind of health care or medical care do people have a right? What priority should health care expenditures have, relative to other national spending in such cases as the military, education, highways, and the environment? Our society's health policy reflects the larger values of the nation: What kind of a people do we want to be? Perhaps the current crisis in the American health system will encourage public discourse on these broader moral and political issues.

SUMMARY

Continuing our sketch of the U.S. medical system, in this chapter we focused on large-scale organizations such as hospitals, insurance companies, health maintenance organizations, and medical industries. As American medicine has become increasingly specialized and reliant on high technology, these organizations have consolidated their power and economic interests. The corporatization of hospitals has changed the economic situation for patients, and affected the autonomy of physicians and other health care professionals. Insurance companies have become powerful agents in the health care system, creating regulations and controlling access to health services. In an array of poorly articulated programs, government agencies are also significant third-party payers and direct providers of health services. Medical industries, especially those researching and developing new pharmaceuticals and technologies, have substantial economic interests in health-related markets. Always a loosely regulated, relatively unplanned, laissez-faire arrangement, the American health system is now powerfully dominated by large, for-profit industries.

This system has resulted in major problems of access and cost. The quality of care available under the system is mixed; much is outstanding, but much is terrible. While the poor receive generally lower-quality medical care, spending lots of money on medical services does not guarantee good quality. Structural incentives, which are related to profitability, are responsible for both the achievements and failures of the American medical system. The problems of the American system clearly illustrate a key theme emphasized throughout this volume: Health and illness are socially produced, especially by structural features of power and stratification.

CONCLUSION

Throughout this book, we have outlined numerous ideas about how society affects the body, health, and illness. These ideas, however, are not mere abstractions, removed from people's actual lives. Real people get sick, experience afflictions, and try to find help; real people also enjoy health, and successfully use their bodies to enrich themselves and to fulfill their goals. Even seemingly abstract social factors, such as social control, economic organization and cultural practices, are—for individuals—very real in their consequences.

The issues we raise in this text suggest the diverse points at which social arrangements might be changed to help reach the goal of a healthier society. We hope we have stimulated readers to consider many ways to promote health in this society and globally. It is necessary to have a genuinely holistic understanding of the connections between the mind, body, and society to envision the far-ranging possibilities for enhancing health. We need to go way beyond narrow medical conceptions of health and to appreciate the entire web of socioenvironmental contexts that promote health. From such a holistic perspective, we might not only imagine changes in obvious problem areas, such as nutrition, water pollution, occupational health, and health-care financing, but also consider possible health-promoting alterations in areas such as urban landscapes, automobile design, dependent care programs, media messages, and uses of leisure. A broad, holistic perspective to health transforms our ways of thinking about what is relevant to health and illness prevention.

Similarly, we have suggested points of influence for improvements in the prevention and treatment of illness. Since power is such a pivotal factor in both illness causation and treatment, when we envision healthier alternative social arrangements, we should give special attention to considering changes in the exercise of power and to social arrangements that encourage the empowerment of individuals. Likewise, we have noted the importance of access to resources to stay healthy or to get well. Alternative scenarios for a healthier society need to pay close attention to social inequalities and the way we choose to distribute the resources necessary to be well or to be alive.

While the social arrangements that influence our health may seem remote and objectlike, they are human products and as such can be humanly changed. It is necessary, however, for us to move beyond the boundaries of our individual lives to effect many measures that potentially have a wide-ranging ability to prevent illness and death. Our purpose in examining the institutional sources of illness and problems in health care is not to blame but rather to suggest some of the points at which social structure and social policy can be changed. Understanding the complex interrelationships of these arrangements prevents naïve notions that an isolated new program, policy change, or medical innovation will alone produce dramatic changes in people's health. While most envisioned changes are matters of policy and social organization, some needed changes are embedded in cultural values and stubbornly change-resistant social structures; while still human products, they often change more slowly. Nevertheless, becoming aware of the human sources of the social arrangements that shape our lives is a first step in making effective efforts to change those forces.

RECOMMENDED READINGS

Articles

Karen Davis and Diane Rowland, "Uninsured and underserved: Inequities in health care in the United States," *Milbank Memorial Fund Quarterly* 61(2), 1983: 149–176.

Carol McCarthy, "Financing for health care," pp. 272–312 in S. Jonas, ed., *Health Care Delivery in the United States*. New York: Springer, 1981.

J. Warren Salmon, "Profit and health care: Trends in corporatization and proprietization," *International Journal of Health Services* 15(3), 1985: 395–418.

Roberta G. Simmons and Susan Klein Marine, "The regulation of high cost technology medicine: The case of dialysis and transplantation in the U.K.," *Journal of Health and Social Behavior* 25, 1984: 320–334.

Howard Waitzkin, "Health policy in the United States: Problems and alternatives," pp. 475–491 in H. Freeman and S. Levine, eds., *Handbook of Medical Sociology*. Englewood Cliffs, NJ: Prentice-Hall, 1989.

Books

Bradford Gray, ed., *The New Health Care for Profit: Doctors and Hospitals in a Competitive Environment*. Washington, DC: National Academy Press, 1983. This is a useful collection of essays about various ways the pursuit of profit affects the contemporary health care system.

John B. McKinlay, ed., *Issues in the Political Economy of Health Care*. New York: Tavistock, 1984. This volume contains excellent articles on the social production of health and illness, capital interests and the role of the state, for-profit medical care, the pharmaceutical industry, and political-economic relationships between physicians and their sponsors.

Charles E. Rosenberg, *The Care of Strangers: The Rise of America's Hospital System*. New York: Basic, 1987. This book is a fascinating social history of hospitals and the place of various medical professions within them; it offers an excellent background for understanding contemporary policy issues.

Victor W. Sidel and Ruth Sidel, *A Healthy State: An International Perspective on the Crisis in United States Medical Care*. New York: Pantheon, 1983. The authors present a highly readable description of problems with the U.S. health care system; comparisons with the systems of Sweden, Great Britain, the U.S.S.R., and China; and proposals premised on the fundamental human right to health care.

Appendix A

Literature in the Sociology of Health and Illness

I. Social science journals in health and illness

Culture, Medicine, and Psychiatry (D. Reidel), quarterly
International Journal of Health Services (Baywood), quarterly
Journal of Health and Social Behavior (American Sociological Association), quarterly
Medical Anthropology Quarterly (American Anthropological Association and Society
    for Medical Anthropology), quarterly
Social Science & Medicine (Pergamon Press [U.K.]), 24 issues per year
Sociology of Health and Illness: A Journal of Medical Sociology (Basil Blackwell [U.K.]),
    quarterly
Women and Health (Haworth Press), quarterly

II. Sources on current issues, social policy, and health ethics

Disability Studies Quarterly (Brandeis University, Department of Sociology), quarterly
Hastings Center Reports (The Hastings Center), bimonthly
Health/PAC Bulletin (Health Policy Advisory Committee), bimonthly
Health Affairs (Project HOPE), bimonthly
Journal of Health Politics, Policy, and Law (Duke University, Department of Health
    Administration), quarterly
Journal of Public Health Policy (National Association for Public Health Policy), quarterly
Milbank Quarterly (Milbank Memorial Fund), quarterly
The Network News (National Women's Health Network), bimonthly

III. Medical and public health journals

American Journal of Public Health (American Public Health Association), monthly
The Lancet (Lancet [U.K.]), weekly
Medical Care (American Public Health Association, Medical Care Section), monthly
New England Journal of Medicine (Massachusetts Medical Society), weekly

IV. Periodicals with good coverage of health and health policy issues

The Economist (U.K.), monthly
The New York Times, daily
The Wall Street Journal, daily

V. Newsletters and magazines

The Disability Rag (Avacado Press), bi-monthly
Health Facts (Center for Medical Consumers), monthly
Health Letter (Public Citizen's Health Research Group), monthly
Rehab Brief (U.S. Department of Education, National Institute on Disability and Rehabilitation Research), monthly
The Swedish Information Service, occasional factsheets
University of California, Berkeley Wellness Letter (School of Public Health), monthly

VI. Indexes and abstracts

Abstracts in Anthropology
American Statistics Index
Cumulative Index to Nursing and Allied Health Literature
Hospital Literature Index
Index to International Statistics
Index Medicus
Psychological Abstracts
Public Affairs Information Service
Social Sciences Index (most important source for social science journals)
Sociological Abstracts
Statistical Reference Index
Women's Studies Abstracts

VII. Useful bibliographies and dictionaries

Dorland's Illustrated Medical Dictionary
International Bibliography of Social and Cultural Anthropology
Medical Sociology: An Annotated Bibliography, 1972–1982
The Oxford Companion to Medicine

VIII. Sources of current statistical data

U.S. Department of Health and Human Services, Public Health Service, Centers for Disease Control, National Center for Health Statistics:

Advance Data, regular reports of data from *Vital and Health Statistics*, with analysis
Health, United States, annual compendium of data on health and health care.
Monthly Vital Statistics Report
Morbidity and Mortality Weekly Report (publication of the Center for Disease Control in Atlanta, Ga.)
Vital Statistics of the United States, annual report
Vital and Health Statistics, occasional reports

U.S. Dept. of Commerce, Bureau of the Census:

Statistical Abstract of the United States, annual
U.S. Census of Population, every ten years
Current Population Reports, occasional reports between decennial censuses

United Nations Educational, Scientific and Cultural Organization:

Statistical Yearbook, annual

IX. Unpublished Papers

Serious students in the field should attend meetings of professional associations and obtain copies of unpublished papers presented there; these papers are frequently preliminary versions of work that is later published in journals or books, so the unpublished version (while less polished) makes information accessible at least a year earlier. The papers for a conference are often abstracted in a booklet available to registrants. Professional associations have reduced student rates for membership and conference registration. Especially recommended are the meetings of:

American Sociological Association (meets usually in August)
Society for Medical Anthropology (meets as a division of the annual meetings of the American Anthropological Association, usually in November or December)
Society for the Study of Social Problems (meets jointly, usually in August, with the American Sociological Association)

Appendix B

Visual Resources

We have found visual resources, such as films and videos, to be invaluable in teaching the sociology of health and illness. Many of these resources are available in multiple formats (film, VHS, ¾" video). Listed below are the formats we have used, but distributors or film libraries may offer others.

Asbestos: The Way to Dusty Death. ABC News Production, 1978, 16 mm., 52 minutes, color. Depicts effects of asbestos, environmental and occupational health issues, and the politics of regulation.

Barefoot Doctors of Rural China. Diane Li Productions, 1975, 16 mm., 50 minutes, color. Illustrates the use of paramedical workers for massive public health efforts, family planning, and combination of Western and traditional Chinese medical knowledge.

Bottle Babies. Tricontinental Films, 1976, 16 mm., 30 minutes, color. Documents the effects of bottle feeding on the health of Third World babies and examines the role of multinational corporations' marketing of formula.

The Brain. WNET, 1984, VHS, each episode 60 minutes, color. The fourth episode "Stress and Emotion," describes the physiology of stress and how one's sense of control affects capacity to deal with stresses.

The British Way of Health. London Television, 1976, 16 mm., 28 minutes. Illustrates some aspects of the National Health System, with glimpses of three levels of physicians and their work.

The Business of Hunger. Maryknoll World Films, 1979, 16 mm., 28 minutes. Examines the impact of multinational food production for export on the health of people in Third World nations.

Captives of Care. Australian Film Commission, 1973, 16 mm., 50 minutes, color. Docudrama that dramatizes the struggles for autonomy and independence of residents of an institution for persons with disabilities, many of whom were involved in making the film.

Catfish: Man of the Woods. Appalachian Films, 1974, 16 mm., 27 minutes, color. Portrays a traditional herb doctor in the Appalachian Mountains of West Virginia.

China's Only Child. WGBH-BBC co-production, 1983, VHS, 58 minutes, color. Examines China's population problems and policy of having only one child.

Clockwork. California Newsreel, 1982, VHS, 25 minutes, color. Demonstrates the impact of factory production management techniques, from early Taylorism to contemporary computer-assisted regulation.

Crisis at General Hospital. PBS Video, 1984, VHS, color. Examines the impact of inadequate funding for health care, especially for hospitals serving the urban, under-insured poor populations.

D.E.S.: An Uncertain Legacy. National Film Board of Canada and University of California, 16 mm., ¾" video and VHS, 58 minutes, color. Examines the development, use, and subsequent iatrogenic problems of the artificial hormone diethylstilbestrol.

Ending Hunger in the Garden State: Recommendations and Reform. New Jersey Commission on Hunger, 1987, VHS, 35 minutes, color. Probes the extent of the problem of hunger and various responses in one of the wealthiest states.

For Export Only: Pesticides (Part I) *and Pills* (Part II). Icarus, 16mm, ¾" video and VHS, 56 minutes each, color. Discusses the pesticides and pharmaceuticals that have been banned or highly restricted in the United States, but are still produced here for export to Third World countries, which have little effective means to control or ban these substances that harm public health and the environment.

Healing. National Film Board of Canada, 1978, 16 mm., 56 minutes, color. Documentary that examines Christian faith-healing in a modern society.

Health Care on the Critical List. Public Policy Production, 1985, VHS, 55 minutes (30-minute edition also available), color. Analyzes rising U.S. health care costs and the problems of equity in the health care system; illustrates HMO, PPO, and DRG concepts as approaches to controlling costs, but raises concerns about the long-range quality of health care.

Holistic Health: The New Medicine. Hartley, 1978, 16 mm., 34 minutes, color. Shows twelve leading practitioners of contemporary approaches to medicine that attempt to treat the whole person—body, mind, and spirit.

Hospice: An Alternative Way to Care for the Dying. Billy Budd Films, 1979, 16 mm., 25 minutes, color. Documents the hospice movement, which emphasizes holistic caring for the dying patient and family, typically in the home.

Hospital. Zipporah Films, 1969, 16 mm., 84 minutes, black and white. Frederick Wiseman's *cinéma verité* documentary (no narration) that records everyday occurrences in a metropolitan hospital.

Hungry for Profit. Robert Richter Productions, 1984, 16 mm., 86 minutes, color. Explores the role of multinational agribusiness in worsening problems of hunger in the Third World by encouraging the use of inappropriate technologies and the growth of export crops in the quest for profits.

The Killing Ground. ABC News Production, 1979, 16 mm., 52 minutes, color. Examines the environmental and public health effects of toxic waste dumping, and critically looks at the politics of regulation and cleanup.

Madness and Medicine. ABC, 1977, 16 mm., 51 minutes, color. Critically examines mental institutions, their treatment programs (in particular drug therapies, electroshock, and psychosurgery), and postrelease care.

Medicine in China. Felix Greene, 1973, ¾" video, 25 minutes, color. Describes early postrevolutionary changes in health care and health in China.

The Mind. WNET, 1988, VHS, each episode 60 minutes, color. The episodes "Aging" and "Pain and Healing" are particularly useful.

Modern Times. United Artists, 1936, VHS and 16 mm., 87 minutes, black and white. This classic Charlie Chaplin film satirizes the assembly line and other modern conditions of industrial labor.

No Heroic Measures. Carle Medical Communications, 1984, ¾" video or VHS, 23 minutes, color. Explores the ethical, legal, and emotional issues involved in the withdrawal of technological life supports.

Nurse, Where Are You? CBS, 1980, ¾" video, 49 minutes, color. Depicts the nursing shortage and its effects, nurses' roles and status, and unionization.

The Politics of Food. Yorkshire Television, 1988, VHS, 2 hours, color. Covers political sources of hunger and famine, problems with food aid, politics and agricultural policies, and alternative political approaches.

Rational Suicide. CBS (from the "Sixty Minutes" series), 16 mm., 16 minutes, color. Explores various aspects of "death with dignity"; includes interviews with terminally ill patients, their families, and advocates for various approaches to dealing with dying.

The Reckoning. California Newsreel, 1979, 16 mm., 27 minutes, color. Describes research about the health impacts of unemployment in two British cities; disproportionate footage of researchers looking at computer print-outs.

Rich Man's Medicine, Poor Man's Medicine. Icarus, 1976, 16 mm., 45 minutes, color. Compares traditional native healing with high-priced, highly technological medicine in Gabon, Senegal, and Kenya.

The Skin Horse. Central Independent Television PIC, 1983, VHS, 1 hour, color. Evocative documentary that deals with sexuality and disability.

Song of the Canary. New Day Films, 1978, 16 mm., 57 minutes, color. Provocatively examines occupational health problems, using case studies of chemical and textile workers.

Strange Sleep. PBS ("Nova" series), 1980, VHS, 45 minutes, color. Docudrama that covers the invention of anesthesia and the social factors surrounding its acceptance.

Taking Our Bodies Back: The Women's Health Movement. Cambridge Documentary Films, 1974, 16 mm., 33 minutes, color. Examines the development and issues of the women's health movement; contains graphic material about self-help techniques and abortion.

The Therapeutic Touch: Healing in the New Age. Hartley, 1978, 16 mm., 35 minutes, color. Depicts the work of Dr. Delores Krieger, professor of nursing at New York University, who trains health professionals in the use of therapeutic touch, a form of paranormal healing.

Tibetan Medicine: A Buddhist Approach to Healing. Hartley, 1976, 16 mm., 29 minutes, color. Discusses Tibetan medicine, an interesting contrast to Western biomedicine, that heals both the physical and psychic being.

Titticut Follies. Zipporah Films, 1967, 16 mm., 89 minutes, black and white. Frederick Wiseman's controversial *cinéma verité* documentary (no narration) about a hospital for the criminally insane that illustrates a total institution, with different worlds of staff and inmates.

Who Lives, Who Dies. Public Policy Productions, 1987, VHS, 60 minutes, color. Explores the crisis in the U.S. health care system, and raises issues of health care spending, equity, rationing, and priorities in national spending.

Bibliography

Albrecht, Gary L., and Judith A. Levy
    1982   "The professionalization of osteopathy: Adaptation in the medical marketplace," *Research in the Sociology of Health Care* 2: 161–202.

Alexander, Jacqui
    1988   "The ideological construction of risk: An analysis of corporate health programs in the 1980s," *Social Science and Medicine* 26(5): 559–567.

Alexander, Linda
    1982   "Illness maintenance and the new American sick role," pp. 351–367 in N. J. Chrisman and T. W. Maretzki, eds., *Clinically Applied Anthropology*. Dordrecht, Netherlands: D. Reidel.

Alexander, Ralph W., and Joseph Fedoruk
    1986   "Epidemic psychogenic illness in a telephone operators' building," *Journal of Occupations and Medicine* 28(1): 42–45.

Altman, Charles F.
    1985   *Social Policies in Western Industrialized Societies*. Berkeley: Institute of International Studies, University of California.

Altman, Lawrence
    1988a   "Maker gives free heart medicine to needy," *New York Times,* April 6.
    1988b   "U.S. moves to improve death certificate." *New York Times,* October 18.

Altman, Lawrence, and Elisabeth Rosenthal
    1990   "Changes in medicine bring pain to healing profession," *New York Times,* Februaury 18.

American Psychiatric Association
    1980   *Diagnostic and Statistical Manual of Mental Disorders*. Washington, DC: American Psychiatric Association.

American Public Health Association Chartbook
    1975   *Health Work in America*. Washington, DC: American Public Health Association.

Anderson, Gerard F.
    1986   "National medical care spending," *Health Affairs* 5(3): 123–130.

Anderson, Robert A.
    1978   *Stress Power.* New York: Human Sciences Press.

Anderson, Ronald, Meei-shia Chen, Lu Anne Aday, and Llewellyn Cornelius
    1987   "Health status and medical care utilization," *Health Affairs* 6(1):
                136–156.

Anderson, Ronald, and Ross M. Mullner
    1989   "Trends in the organization of health services," pp. 144–165 in
                H. E. Freeman and S. Levine, eds., *Handbook of Medical Sociology.*
                Englewood Cliffs, NJ: Prentice-Hall.

Andreoni, Diego
    1986   *The Costs of Occupational Accidents and Diseases.* Occupational
                Safety and Health Series, No. 54. Geneva: International Labour
                Organization.

Aneshensel, Carol S., and Leonard I. Pearlin
    1987   "Structural contexts of sex differences in stress," pp. 75–95 in R.
                Barnett, L. Biener, and G. K. Baruch, eds., *Gender and Stress.* New
                York: The Free Press.

Angel, Ronald
    1989   "The health of the Mexican origin population," pp. 82–94 in
                P. Brown, ed., *Perspectives in Medical Sociology.* Belmont, CA:
                Wadsworth.

Angel, Ronald, and Peggy Thoits
    1987   "The impact of culture on the cognitive structure of illness," *Cul-
                ture, Medicine, and Psychiatry* 11(4): 465–494.

Anspach, Renee
    1977   "From stigma to identity politics: Political activism among physi-
                cally disabled and former mental patients," *Social Science and Medi-
                cine* 13A: 765–773.
    1988   "Notes on the sociology of medical discourse: The language
                of case presentation," *Journal of Health and Social Behavior* 29:
                357–375.

Antonovsky, Aaron
    1979   *Health, Stress and Coping.* San Francisco: Jossey Bass.
    1984   "The sense of coherence as a determinant of health," *Advances*
                1(3): 37–50.
    1987   *Unraveling the Mystery of Health: How People Manage Stress and Stay
                Well.* San Francisco: Jossey Bass.

Apfel, Roberta, and Susan M. Fisher
    1984   *To Do No Harm: DES and the Dilemmas of Modern Medicine.* New
                Haven: Yale University Press.

Aries, Nancy, and Louanne Kennedy
    1986   "The health labor force: The effects of change," pp. 196–207 in
                P. Conrad and R. Kern, eds., *The Sociology of Health and Illness.*
                New York: St. Martin's Press.

Ariès, Philippe
    1974   *Western Attitudes Toward Death: From the Middle Ages to the Present.*
                Baltimore: Johns Hopkins University Press.

Armstrong, David
    1983   *Political Anatomy of the Body: Medical Knowledge in Britain in the Twentieth Century.* Cambridge: Cambridge University Press.

Asbury, Carolyn H.
    1981   "Medical drugs of limited commercial interest: Profit alone is a bitter pill," *International Journal of Health Services* 11(3): 451–462.

Atkinson, Paul
    1978   "From honey to vinegar: Lévi-Strauss in Vermont," pp. 168–188 in P. Morley and R. Wallis, eds., *Culture and Curing.* Pittsburgh: University of Pittsburgh Press.

Atkinson, Thomas, Ramsay Liem, and Joan Liem
    1986   "The social costs of unemployment: Implications for social support," *Journal of Health and Social Behavior* 27: 317–331.

Attie, Ilana, and J. Brooks-Gunn
    1987   "Weight concerns as chronic stressors in women," pp. 218–254 in R. Barnett, L. Biener, and G. K. Baruch, eds., *Gender and Stress.* New York: The Free Press.

Back, Aaron
    1981   *Occupational Stress: The Inside Story.* Oakland, CA: Institute for Labor and Mental Health.

Baer, Hans A.
    1984   "A comparative view of a heterodox health system: Chiropractic in America and Britain," *Medical Anthropology* 8: 151–168.
    1987   "Divergence and convergence in two systems of manual medicine: Osteopathy and chiropractic in the United States," *Medical Anthropology Quarterly* n.s. 1(2): 176–193.

Bakal, Donald A.
    1979   *Psychology and Medicine.* New York: Springer.

Baker, Dean
    1981   "The use and health consequences of shift work," pp. 107–122 in V. Navarro and D. M. Berman, eds., *Health and Work Under Capitalism: An International Perspective.* Farmingdale, NY: Baywood.

Baker, Susan B., Stephen Teret, and Erich M. Daub
    1987   "Injuries," pp. 177–206 in S. R. Levine and A. Lilienfeld, eds., *Epidemiology and Health Policy.* New York: Tavistock.

Banta, H. David
    1986   "Medical technology and developing countries: The case of Brazil," *International Journal of Health Services* 16(3): 363–373.

Banta, H. David, Clyde J. Behney, and Jane Sisk Willems
    1981   *Toward Rational Technology in Medicine: Considerations for Health Policy.* New York: Springer.

Banta, H. David, and Kerry Britten Kemp
    1982   *The Management of Health Care Technology in Nine Countries.* New York: Springer.

Barchas, Patricia, and Sally P. Mendoza, eds.
    1984a   *Social Cohesion: Essays Toward a Sociophysiological perspective.* Westport, CT: Greenwood.

1984b   *Social Hierarchies: Essays Toward a Sociophysiological Perspective.* Westport, CT: Greenwood.

Barker-Benfield, Ben
1975   "Sexual surgery in late nineteenth-century America," *International Journal of Health Services* 5(2): 279–298.

Barnet, Richard J., and Ronald E. Mueller
1974   *Global Reach.* New York: Simon and Schuster.

Barnett, Rosalind, Lois Biener, and Grace K. Baruch, eds.
1987   *Gender and Stress.* New York: The Free Press.

Barnouw, Erik
1978   *The Sponsor: Notes on a Modern Potentate.* New York: Oxford University Press.

Barron, James
1989   "Unnecessary Surgery," *New York Times Magazine,* April 16, pp. 25–26, 43–46.

Bartrop, R. W., L. Lazarus, L. Luckhurst, L. Kiloh, and R. Penny
1977   "Depressed lymphocyte function after bereavement," *Lancet* 1(8,016): 834–836.

Bates, Maryann
1987   "Ethnicity and pain: A biocultural model," *Social Science and Medicine* 24(1): 47–50.

Becker, E. Lovell
1986   *International Dictionary of Medicine and Biology.* New York: Wiley.

Becker, Howard
1963   *Outsiders: Studies in the Sociology of Deviance.* New York: The Free Press.
1967   "History, culture, and subjective experience: An exploration of the social bases of drug-induced experiences," *Journal of Health and Social Behavior* 8(3): 163–176.

Becker, Howard, Blanche Geer, Everett Hughes, and Anselm Strauss
1961   *Boys in White.* Chicago: University of Chicago Press.

Beckman, Howard and R. M. Frankl
1984   "The effects of physician's behavior on the collection of data," *Annals of Internal Medicine* 101(5): 692–696.

Beecher, Henry K.
1956   "Relationship of the significance of wound to the pain experience," *Journal of the American Medical Association* 161: 1604–1613.
1959   *Measurement of Subjective Responses: Quantitative Effects of Drugs.* New York: Oxford University Press.

Belkin, Lisa
1988   "Town revives a hospital and itself," *New York Times,* December 1.
1990   "Many in medicine are calling rules a professional malaise," *New York Times,* February 19.

Bell, Susan
1986   "A new model of medical technology development: A case study of DES," *Research in the Sociology of Health Care* 4: 1–32.
1987   "Changing ideas: The medicalization of menopause," *Social Science and Medicine* 24(6): 535–542.

Bennett, Jon, and Susan George
1987   *The Hunger Machine: The Politics of Food.* Cambridge: Polity Press.

Ben-Sira, Zeev
1985   "Potency: A stress-buffering link in the coping-stress-disease relationship," *Social Science and Medicine* 21(4): 397–406.

Benson, Herbert
1979   "The relaxation response: Techniques and clinical applications," pp. 331–351 in D. Sobel, ed., *Ways of Health.* New York: Harcourt, Brace, Jovanovich.

Berger, Peter
1967   *The Sacred Canopy: Elements of a Sociological Theory of Religion.* Garden City, NY: Doubleday.

Berger, Peter, and Thomas Luckmann
1967   *The Social Construction of Reality.* Garden City, NY: Doubleday.

Bergsma, Jurrit
1981   *Health Care: Its Psychosocial Dimensions.* Pittsburgh: Duquesne University Press.

Berki, Sylvester E.
1986   "A look at catastrophic medical expenses and the poor," *Health Affairs* 5(4): 138–145.

Berkman, Lisa F., and S. Leonard Syme
1979   "Social networks, host resistance, and mortality: A nine-year follow-up study of Alameda County residents," *American Journal of Epidemiology* 109:186–204.

Berlant, Jeffrey L.
1975   *Profession and Monopoly: A Study of Medicine in Great Britain and the United States.* Berkeley: University of California Press.

Berliner, Howard S.
1975   "A larger perspective on the Flexner Report," *International Journal of Health Services* 5(4): 573–592.
1976   "Starr wars," *International Journal of Health Services* 13(4): 671–675.

Berliner, Howard S., and Robb K. Burlage
1987   "Proprietary hospital chains and academic medical centers," *International Journal of Health Services* 17(1): 27–45.

Berman, Daniel M.
1978   *Death on the Job: Occupational Health and Safety Struggles in the United States.* New York: Monthly Review Press.

Bieliauskas, Linas
1982   *Stress and Its Relationship to Health and Illness.* Boulder, CO: Westview.

Birke, Lynda
1986   *Women, Feminism and Biology: The Feminist Challenge.* New York: Methuen.

Black, Douglas
1980   *Inequalities in Health: Report of a Research Working Group.* London: Department of Health and Social Services.

Blair, Gwenda
    1979   "Why Dick can't stop smoking: The politics of our national addiction," *Mother Jones* 4(1): 31–42.

Blaxter, Mildred
    1983   "The causes of disease: Women talking," *Social Science and Medicine* 17: 59–69.

Blaxter, Mildred, and Elizabeth Paterson
    1982   *Mothers and Daughters: A Three Generational Study of Health Attitudes and Behavior.* London: Heinemann.

Bloom, Samuel W.
    1979   "Socialization for the physician's role: A review of some contributions of research to theory," pp. 3–52 in E. C. Shapiro and L. M. Loenstein, eds., *Becoming a Physician: Development of Values and Attitudes in Medicine.* Cambridge, MA: Ballinger.

Bloor, Michael
    1976   "Bishop Berkeley and the adenotonsillectomy enigma: An exploration of variation in the social construction of medical disposals," *Sociology: The Journal of the British Sociological Association* 10(1): 43–61.

Bloor, Michael, M. Samphier, and L. Prior
    1987   "Artefact explanations of inequalities in health: An assessment of the evidence," *Sociology of Health and Illness* 9(3): 231–263.

Blyton, Paul
    1985   *Changes in Working Time: An International Review.* New York: St. Martin's Press.

Bodenheimer, Thomas S.
    1984   "The transnational pharmaceutical industry and the health of the world's people," pp. 187–216 in J. B. McKinlay, ed., *Issues in the Political Economy of Health Care.* New York: Tavistock.

Bodenheimer, Thomas S., Steven Cummings, and Elizabeth Harding
    1975   "Capitalizing on illness: The health insurance industry," pp. 69–84 in V. Navarro, ed., *Health and Medical Care in the U.S.: A Critical Analysis.* Farmingdale, NY: Baywood.

Bogin, Meg
    1982   *The Path to Pain Control.* Boston: Houghton Mifflin.

Bologh, Roslyn
    1981   "Grounding the alienation of self and body: A critical, phenomenological analysis of the patient in western medicine," *Sociology of Health and Illness* 3(2): 188–206.

Bolton, Ralph
    1989   "Introduction: The AIDS pandemic, a global emergency," *Medical Anthropology* 10: 93–104.

Bookchin, Murray
    1962   *Our Synthetic Environment.* New York: Harper and Row.

Bordo, Susan
    1989   "The body and the reproduction of femininity: A feminist appropriation of Foucault," pp. 13–33 in A. Jaggar and S. Bordo,, eds., *Gender/Body/Knowledge: Feminist Reconstructions of Being and Knowing.* New Brunswick, NJ: Rutgers University Press.

Botkin, Daniel B., and Edward A. Keller
    1982   *Environmental Studies.* Columbus, OH: Charles E. Merrill.
Boudreau, Thomas J.
    1978   "Physical activity, health, and social policies," pp. 239–250 in F.
                Landry and W.A.R. Orban, eds., *Physical Activity and Human Well-
                Being.* Miami: Symposia Specialists.
Braden, Charles S.
    1963   *Spirits in Rebellion: The Rise and Development of New Thought.* Dallas:
                Southern Methodist University Press.
Braudel, Fernand
    1973   *Capitalism and Material Life: 1400–1800.* New York: Harper and
                Row.
Braverman, Harry
    1974   *Labor and Monopoly Capital.* New York: Monthly Review Press.
Brenner, M. Harvey
    1976   *Estimating the Social Costs of Economic Policy: Implications for Mental
                and Physical Health, and Criminal Aggression.* Report to the Congres-
                sional Research Service of the Library of Congress and Joint Eco-
                nomic Committee of Congress. Washington, DC: Government
                Printing Office.
    1979   "Mortality and the national economy," *Lancet* 2(8,142): 568–573.
Brodeur, Paul
    1974   *Expendable Americans.* New York: Viking.
Brody, Jane E.
    1975   "Physicians' views unchanged on use of estrogen therapy," *New
                York Times,* December 5.
    1983   "Research lifts blame from many of the obese," *New York Times,*
                March 24.
Brown, Carol A.
    1978   "The division of laborers: Allied health professions," pp. 73–82
                in S. Wolfe, ed., *Organization of Health Workers and Labor Conflict.*
                Farmingdale, NY: Baywood.
    1983   "Women workers in the health service industry," pp. 105–116 in
                E. Fee, ed., *Women and Health: The Politics of Sex in Medicine.* Far-
                mingdale, NY: Baywood.
Brown, E. Richard
    1979   *Rockefeller Medicine Men: Medicine and Capitalism in America.* Berke-
                ley: University of California Press.
Brown, George W.
    1976   "Social causes of disease," pp. 291–333 in D. Tuckett, ed., *An
                Introduction to Medical Sociology.* London: Tavistock.
Brown, Leigh Patricia
    1988   "Designs take heed of human frailty," *New York Times,* April 14.
Brown, Lester, William U. Chandler, Christopher Flavin, Jodi Jacobson, Cynthia
Pollock, Sandra Postel, Linda Starke, Edward C. Wolf.
    1987   *State of the World, 1987.* New York: W. W. Norton.
Brown, Phil, and Steven C. Funk
    1986   "Tardive dyskinesia: Barriers to the professional recognition of
                an iatrogenic disease," *Journal of Health and Social Behavior* 27:
                116–132.

Burkholder, John R.
1974   "The law knows no heresy: Marginal religious movements and the courts," pp. 27–52 in I. Zaretsky and M. Leone, eds., *Religious Movements in Contemporary America*. Princeton: Princeton University Press.

Burkitt, Denis P.
1973   "Some disease characteristics of modern Western civilisation," *British Medical Journal* 1: 274–278.

Burns, Robert B.
1979   *The Self Concept*. New York: Longman.

Burrell, Craig D., and Cecil G. Sheps, eds.
1978   *Primary Health Care in Industrialized Nations*. New York: New York Academy of Sciences.

Bury, Michael
1982   "Chronic illness as biographical disruption," *Sociology of Health and Illness* 4(2): 167–182.

Buss, Terry F., and Stevens F. Redburn
1983   *Mass Unemployment: Plant Closings and Community Mental Health*. Beverly Hills: Sage.

Butler, Samuel
[1901] 1960 *Erewhon*. New York: New American Library.

Buytendijk, Jacobus
1974   *Prolegomena to an Anthropological Physiology*. Pittsburgh: Duquesne University Press.

Byrne, Patrick S., and Barrie E. Long
1976   *Doctors Talking to Patients*. London: Her Majesty's Stationery Office.

Cahnman, Werner J.
1968   "The stigma of obesity," *Sociological Quarterly* 9(3): 283–299.

Califano, Joseph A.
1989   "Billions blown on health," *New York Times*, April 12.

Callahan, Daniel
1987   *Setting Limits: Medical Goals in an Aging Society*. New York: Simon and Schuster.
1989   *What Kind of Life: The Limits of Medical Progress*. New York: Simon and Schuster.

Calnan, Michael
1984   "Clinical uncertainty: Is it a problem in the doctor-patient relationship?" *Sociology of Health and Illness* 6(1): 74–85.
1987   *Health and Illness: The Lay Perspective*. New York: Tavistock.

Cameron, H. M., and E. McGoogan
1981   "Prospective study of 1152 hospital autopsies: Inaccuracies in death certification," *Journal of Pathology* 133: 273–283.

Cannon, Walter B.
1929   *Bodily Changes in Pain, Hunger, Fear, and Rage*. New York: Harper and Row.
1942   " 'Voodoo' death," *American Anthropologist* 44: 169–181.

Caplan, Gerald, and Marie Killilea
    1976   *Support Systems and Mutual Help: Multidisciplinary Explorations.* New
                York: Grune and Stratton.

Caplan, Robert D.
    1972   "Organizational stress and individual strain: A sociopsychological
                study of risk factors in coronary heart disease among administra-
                tors, engineers, and scientists." Unpublished Ph.D. dissertation,
                The University of Michigan.

Carpenter, Eugenia S.
    1980   "Children's health care and the changing role of women," *Medical
                Care* 18(12): 1208–1218.

Cartwright, Anne
    1967   *Patients and Their Doctors.* New York: Atherton.

Cartwright, Samuel A.
    1851   "Report on the diseases and physical pecularities of the Negro
                race," *New Orleans Medical and Surgical Journal* 7: 691–715.

Cash, Thomas F., Barbara Winstead, and Louis Janda
    1986   "The great American shape-up," *Psychology Today* 20(4): 30–37.

Cassedy, James H.
    1977   "Why self-help? Americans alone with their diseases, 1800–
                1850," pp. 31–48 in G. Risse, R. L. Numbers, and J. W. Leavitt,
                eds., *Medicine Without Doctors: Home Health Care in American History.*
                New York: Science History.

Cassell, Eric J.
    1976   "Disease as an 'it': Concepts of disease revealed by patients' presen-
                tation of symptoms," *Social Science and Medicine* 10: 143–146.
    1982   "The nature of suffering and the goals of medicine," *New England
                Journal of Medicine* 306: 639–645.
    1986   "Ideas in conflict: The rise and fall (and rise and fall) of new views
                of disease," *Daedalus: Journal of the American Academy of Arts and
                Sciences* 115(2): 19–41.

Cassidy, Claire M., Hans Baer, and Barbara Becker
    1985   "Selected references on professionalized heterodox health sys-
                tems in English-speaking countries," *Medical Anthropology Quar-
                terly* 17(1): 10–18.

Castelman, Barry J., and Manuel Vera-Vera
    1981   "Impending proliferation of asbestos," pp. 271–308 in V. Navarro
                and D. M. Berman, eds., *Health and Work Under Capitalism: An
                International Perspective.* Farmingdale, NY: Baywood.

Center for Philosophy and Public Policy
    1985   "Air pollution: The role and limits of consent," *Report from the
                Center for Philosophy and Public Policy,* volume 5, number 5. Hy-
                attsville, Md.: University of Maryland.

Center for Study of Responsive Law
    1982   *Eating Clean: Food Safety and the Chemical Harvest.* Washington, DC:
                Center for Study of Responsive Law.

Chapkis, Wendy
    1986   *Beauty Secrets.* Boston: South End Press.

Charles, Nicke, and Marion Kerr
1987   "Food for feminist thought," *Sociological Review* 34(3): 537–572.

Charmaz, Kathy
1983   "Loss of self: A fundamental form of suffering of the chronically ill," *Sociology of Health and Illness* 4: 167–182.
1987   "Struggling for a self: Identity levels of the chronically ill," *Research in the Sociology of Health Care* 6: 283–321.

Chase, Laurie
1980   "Mass psychogenic illness," *Science for the People* 12(2): 18–19.

Chassin, Mark R., Jacqueline Kosecoff, R. E. Park, Constance Winslow, Katherine Kahn, Nancy Merrick, Joan Keesey, Arlene Fink, David Solomon, and Robert Brook
1987   "Does inappropriate use explain geographic variations in the use of health care services? A study of three procedures," *Journal of the American Medical Association* 258(18): 2533–2537.

Chavkin, Wendy, ed.
1984   *Double Exposure: Women's Health Hazards on the Job and at Home.* New York: Monthly Review Press.

Cherfas, Jeremy, and Roger Lewin, eds.
1980   *Not Work Alone: A Cross-Cultural View of Activities Superfluous to Survival.* Beverly Hills: Sage.

Chernin, Kim
1981   *The Obsession: Reflections on the Tyranny of Slenderness.* New York: Harper and Row.

Chesler, Phyllis
1972   *Women and Madness.* Garden City, NY: Doubleday.

Chrisman, Noel J.
1977   "The health-seeking process: An approach to the natural history of illness," *Culture, Medicine, and Psychiatry* 1: 351–377.

Chronic Pain Letter
1988   *Chronic Pain Letter: An Information Source for the Sufferer* 5(1).

Cicourel, Aaron V.
1983   "Hearing is not believing: Language and the structure of belief in medical communication," pp. 221–239 in S. Fisher and A. Todd, eds., *The Social Organization of Doctor-Patient Communication.* Norwood, NJ: Ablex.

Claybrook, Joan, and staff of *Public Citizen*
1984   *Retreat from Safety.* New York: Pantheon.

Cleary, Paul D.
1987   "Gender differences in stress-related disorders," pp. 39–72 in R. Barnett, L. Biener, and G. K. Baruch, eds., *Gender and Stress.* New York: The Free Press.

Clines, Francis X.
1987   "Britain's health service: Is it curing or hurting?" *New York Times,* June 3.

Cobb, Leonard A., George Thomas, David H. Dillard, K. Alvin Merendino, and
Robert A. Bruce
    1959   "An evaluation of internal mammary artery ligation by a double-
                blind technic," *New England Journal of Medicine* 260: 1115–1118.

Cobb, Sydney, and Stanislav Kasl
    1977   *Termination: The Consequence of Job Loss.* Publication No. 77-224.
                Cincinnati: National Institute for Occupational Safety and
                Health.

Coburn, David, and C. Lesley Biggs
    1986   "Limits to medical dominance: The case of chiropractic," *Social
                Science and Medicine* 22: 1035–1046.

Coburn, David, Carl D'Arcy, Peter Ness, and George M. Torrance, eds.
    1981   *Health and Canadian Society: Sociological Perspective.* Pickering,
                Ont.: Fitzhenry and Whiteside.

Coburn, David, George M. Torrance, and Joseph M. Kaufert
    1983   "Medical dominance in Canada in historical perspective: The rise
                and fall of medicine?" *International Journal of Health Services* 13 (3):
                407–432.

Cockburn, Alexander
    1988   "Live souls," *Zeta Magazine* 1(2): 5–15.

Cockerham, William C.
    1978   *Medical Sociology.* Englewood Cliffs, NJ: Prentice-Hall.

Cohen, Stanley, and Laurie Taylor
    1976   *Escape Attempts: The Theory and Practise of Resistance to Everyday Life.*
                London: Allen Lane.

Comaroff, Jean
    1976   "Communicating information about non-fatal illnesses: The strate-
                gies of a group of general practitioners," *Sociological Review* 24(2):
                269–290.
    1978   "Medicine and culture: Some anthropological perspectives," *So-
                cial Science and Medicine* 12B: 247–254.
    1982   "Medicine: Symbol and ideology," pp. 49–68 in P. Wright and A.
                Treacher, eds., *The Problem of Medical Knowledge: Examining the
                Social Construction of Medicine.* Edinburgh: Edinburgh University
                Press.
    1984   "Medicine, time, and the perception of death," *Listening* 19(2):
                155–169.
    1985   *Body of Power, Spirit of Resistance: The Culture and History of a South
                African People.* Chicago: University of Chicago Press.

Comaroff, Jean, and Peter Maguire
    1981   "Ambiguity and the search for meaning: Childhood leukaemia in
                the modern clinical context," *Social Science and Medicine* 15B(2):
                115–123.

Conrad, Peter
    1975   "The discovery of hyperkinesis: Notes on the medicalization of
                deviant behavior," *Social Problems* 23(1): 12–21.
    1985   "The meaning of medications: Another look at compliance," *So-
                cial Science and Medicine* 20: 29–37.
    1986   "The social meaning of AIDS," *Social Policy* 17(1): 51–56.

1987   "The experience of illness: Recent and new directions," *Research in the Sociology of Health Care* 6: 1–31.

1988   "Worksite health promotion: The social context," *Social Science and Medicine* 26(5): 485–489.

Conrad, Peter, and Joseph W. Schneider

1980   *Deviance and Medicalization: From Badness to Sickness.* St. Louis: C. V. Mosby.

Coombs, Robert H.

1978   *Mastering Medicine: Professional Socialization in Medical School.* New York: The Free Press.

Cooper, Richard S.

1987   "Has the period of rising mortality in the Soviet Union come to an end?" *International Journal of Health Services* 17(3): 515–519.

Cooper, Richard S., and Arthur Schatzkin

1982   "The pattern of mass disease in the U.S.S.R.: A product of socialist or capitalist development," *International Journal of Health Services* 12(3): 459–480.

Corea, Gena

1977   *The Hidden Malpractice: How American Medicine Mistreats Women.* New York: Jove/Harcourt, Brace, Jovanovich.

Coulter, Harris L.

1984   "Homoeopathy," pp. 57–79 in J. W. Salmon, ed., *Alternative Medicines: Popular and Policy Perspectives.* New York: Tavistock.

Cowie, Bill

1976   "The cardiac patient's perception of his heart attack," *Social Science and Medicine* 10: 87–96.

Coyne, James, and Kenneth Holroyd

1982   "Stress, coping and illness: A transactional perspective," pp. 103–127 in T. Millon, C. Green, and R. Meagher, eds., *Handbook of Clinical Health Psychology.* New York: Plenum.

Crane, Diana

1975   "Decision to treat critically ill patients: A comparison of social versus medical considerations," pp. 301–333 in J. B. McKinlay, ed., *Health Care Consumers, Professionals, and Organizations.* Milbank Reader, No. 2. Cambridge, MA: MIT Press.

Crawford, Robert

1977   "You are dangerous to your health: The ideology and politics of victim blaming," *International Journal of Health Services* 7(4): 663–680.

1984   "A cultural account of 'health': Control, release, and the social body," pp. 60–103 in J. B. McKinlay, ed., *Issues in the Political Economy of Health Care.* New York: Tavistock.

Crewe, Nancy M., and Irving K. Zola, eds.

1983   *Independent Living in America.* San Francisco: Jossey-Bass.

Crichton, Anne

1981   *Health Policy Making: Fundamental Issues in the U.S.A., Canada, Great Britain, and Australia.* Ann Arbor, MI: Health Administration Press.

Crickmer, Barry T.
    1988   "How to handle long-term health care," *New York Times*, January 18.

Crittenden, Ann
    1981   "Bangladesh hunger linked to feudal system," *New York Times*, December 11.

Csikszentmihalyi, Mihaly
    1978   "Body and behavior: A new look at the mind-body problem," pp. 283–302 in F. Landry and W.A.R. Orban, eds., *Physical Activity and Human Well-Being*. Miami: Symposia Specialists.

Csordas, Thomas
    1983   "The rhetoric of transformation in ritual healing," *Culture, Medicine, and Psychiatry* 7(4): 333–375.

Csordas, Thomas, and Steven Cross
    1976   "Healing of memories: Psychotherapeutic ritual among Catholic Pentecostals," *Journal of Pastoral Care* 30: 245–257.

Culyer, A. J., and Bengt Jonsson, eds.
    1986   *Public and Private Health Services: Complementaries and Conflicts*. Oxford: Basil Blackwell.

Cummings, Judith
    1984   "Restrictions on smoking spreading Across U.S.," *New York Times*, February 1.

Dahlgren, Goeran, and Finn Diderichsen
    1986   "Strategies for equity in health: Report from Sweden," *International Journal of Health Services* 16(4): 517–537.

Danaher, Kevin
    1985a   "How the U.S. and Europe caused Africa's famine," *Utne Reader* 11: 101–103.
    1985b   "Myths of African hunger," *Science for the People* 17(5): 15–18, 30.

Daniels, Arlene K.
    1969   "The captive professional: Bureaucratic limitations in the practice of military psychiatry," *Journal of Health and Social Behavior* 10(4): 255–265.
    1972   "Military psychiatry: The emergence of a subspecialty," pp. 145–162 in E. Freidson and J. Lorber, eds., *Medical Men and Their Work*. Chicago: Aldine Atherton.

Davies, Celia
    1982   "The regulation of nursing work: An historical comparison of Britain and the U. S. A.," *Research in the Sociology of Health Care* 2: 121–160.

Davis, Joel
    1984   *Endorphins: New Waves in Brain Chemistry*. Garden City, NY: Doubleday.

Davis, Karen, and Diane Rowland
    1983   "Uninsured and underserved: Inequities in health care in the United States," *Milbank Memorial Fund Quarterly* 61(2): 149–176.

Davis-Floyd, Robbie
    1987   "Obstetric training as a rite of passage," *Medical Anthropology Quarterly* 1(3): 288–318.

Derber, Charles
　　1983　　　"Sponsorship and the control of physicians," *Theory and Society* 12: 561–601.
　　1984　　　"Physicians and their sponsorship: The new medical relations of production," pp. 217–254 in J. B. McKinlay, ed., *Issues in the Political Economy of Health Care*. New York: Tavistock.

Devisch, Renaat
　　1987　　　"Interweaving the vital flow and the symbolic function in healing," paper presented to American Anthropological Association.

Devisch, Renaat, and Antoine Gailly
　　1985　　　"A therapeutic self-help group among Turkish women, Dertleşmek: 'The sharing of sorrow,' " *Psichiatria e Psicoterapie Analitica* 4(2): 133–152.

Diamond, Marian Cleeves
　　1988　　　*Enriching Heredity: The Impact of the Environment on the Anatomy of the Brain*. New York: The Free Press.

DiMatteo, M. Robin, and Howard S. Friedman
　　1982　　　*Social Psychology and Medicine*. Cambridge, Mass.: Oelgeschlager, Gunn, and Hain, Publishers.

Dingwall, Robert
　　1976　　　*Aspects of Illness*. New York: St. Martin's Press.

Direcks, Anita, and Ellen't Hoen
　　1986　　　"DES: The crime continues," pp. 41–49 in K. McDonnell, ed., *Adverse Effects: Women and the Pharmaceutical Industry*. Toronto: Women's Educational Press.

Doherty, William J., and Thomas L. Campbell
　　1988　　　*Families and Health*. Beverly Hills: Sage.

Dohrenwend, Barbara, and Leonard Pearlin
　　1982　　　"Report on stress and life events," pp. 55–88 in G. R. Elliott and C. Eisdorfer, eds., *Stress and Human Health*. New York: Springer.

Dolan, Andrew K.
　　1980　　　"Antitrust law and physician dominance of other practitioners," *Journal of Health, Politics, and Law* 4: 675–689.

Donahue, John M.
　　1986　　　*The Nicaraguan Revolution in Health*. South Hadley, MA: Bergin and Garvey.
　　1989　　　"International organizations, health services, and nation building in Nicaragua," *Medical Anthropology Quarterly* 3(3): 258–269.

Donnelly, Patrick G.
　　1982　　　"The origins of the Occupational Safety and Health Act of 1970," *Social Problems* 30(1): 13–25.

Donovan, Rebecca
　　1987　　　"Poorly paid home health care workers subsidize an industry" [letter to the editor], *New York Times*, May 16.

Douglas, Mary
　　1966　　　*Purity and Danger: An Analysis of Concepts of Pollution and Taboo*. London: Routledge and Kegan Paul.
　　1970　　　*Natural Symbols: Explorations in Cosmology*. London: Barrie and Jenkins.

Dow, James
  1986   "Universal aspects of symbolic healing: A theoretical synthesis,"
              American Anthropologist 88(1): 56–69.
Dowd, Maureen
  1987   "U.S. health care faulted in Senate," *New York Times*, January 13.
Dowie, Mark, and Tracy Johnston
  1987   "A case of corporate malpractice and the Dalkon Shield," pp.
              629–637 in H. D. Schwartz, ed., *Dominant Issues in Medical Sociol-
              ogy.* New York: Random House.
Doyal, Lesley, and Imogen Pennell
  1981   *The Political Economy of Health.* Boston: South End Press.
  1983   "Women, health and the sexual division of labour: A case study of
              the women's health movement in Britain," *Critical Social Policy* 7:
              1–33.
Drinka, George Frederick
  1984   *The Birth of Neurosis: Myth, Malady, and the Victorians.* New York:
              Simon and Schuster.
Droge, David, Paul Arntson, and Robert Norton
  1986   "The social support function in epilepsy self-help groups," *Small
              Group Behavior* 17(2): 139–163.
Drummond, Hugh
  1980   *Doctor Drummond's Spirited Guide to Health Care in a Dying Empire.*
              New York: Grove.
Dubos, René
  1959   *The Mirage of Health.* Garden City, NY: Doubleday.
  1968   *Man, Medicine and Environment.* Baltimore: Penguin.
Dunn, Frederick L., and Craig Janes
  1986   "Introduction: Medical anthropology and epidemiology," pp. 3–
              34 in C. Janes, R. Stall, and S. Gifford, eds., *Anthropology and
              Epidemiology: Interdisciplinary Approaches to the Study of Health and
              Disease.* Boston: D. Reidel.
Dunnell, Karen, and Ann Cartwright
  1972   *Medicine Takers, Prescribers, and Hoarders.* London: Routledge and
              Kegan Paul.
Durkheim, Emile
  [1893] 1964 *The Division of Labor in Society.* New York: The Free Press.
  [1895] 1938 *Rules of the Sociological Method.* New York: The Free Press.
  [1897] 1951 *Suicide: A Study in Sociology.* New York: The Free Press.
  [1915] 1965 *The Elementary Forms of the Religious Life.* New York: Collier/
              Macmillan.
Dutton, Diana
  1986   "Social class, health and illness," pp. 31–62 in L. Aiken and D.
              Mechanic, eds., *Applications of Social Science to Clinical Medicine and
              Health Policy.* New Brunswick, NJ: Rutgers University Press.
Dutton, Diana, Thomas A. Preston, and Nancy E. Pfund
  1988   *Worse Than the Disease: Pitfalls of Medical Progress.* New York: Cam-
              bridge University Press.
Dye, James W.
  1981   "Man a machine: A philosophical critique," *Journal of Biological
              Experience: Studies in the Life of the Body* 3(2): 44–60.

Eastwell, Harry D.
1982   "Voodoo death and the mechanism for dispatch of the dying in East Arnheim, Australia," *American Anthropologist* 84(1): 5–18.

Eckholm, Erik
1977   *The Picture of Health: Environmental Sources of Disease.* New York: W. W. Norton.
1989   "River blindness: Conquering an ancient scourge," *New York Times Magazine,* January 8.

Economist, The
1985   "The western way to die," 296 (7,409): 75–78.

Ehrenreich, Barbara, and John Ehrenreich
1978   "Hospital workers: Class conflicts in the making," pp. 41–49 in S. Wolfe, ed., *Organization of Health Workers and Labor Conflict.* Farmingdale, NY: Baywood.

Ehrenreich, Barbara, and Deirdre English
1973   *Witches, Midwives, and Nurses: A History of Women Healers.* Old Westbury, NY: The Feminist Press.
1978   *For Her Own Good: 150 Years of the Experts' Advice to Women.* Garden City, NY: Doubleday.

Elias, Norbert
1978   *The Civilizing Process,* Vol. 1. New York: Urizen.
1982   *Power and Civility.* New York: Pantheon.
1985   *The Loneliness of Dying.* Oxford: Basil Blackwell.

Elling, Ray H.
1981   "Political economy, cultural hegemony, and mixes of traditional and modern medicine," *Social Science and Medicine* 15A: 89–99.
1986   *The Struggle for Workers' Health: A Study of Six Industrialized Countries.* Farmingdale, NY: Baywood.

Emerson, Joan P.
1970   "Behavior in private places: Sustaining definitions of reality in gynecological examinations," pp. 74–97 in H. P. Dreitzel, ed., *Recent Sociology #2: Patterns of Communicative Behavior.* New York: Macmillan.

Engel, George L.
1971   "Sudden and rapid death during psychological stress: Folklore or folk wisdom?" *Annals of Internal Medicine* 74: 771–782.
1976   "Psychologic factors in instantaneous cardiac death," *New England Journal of Medicine* 294: 664–665.
1977   "The need for a new medical model: A challenge for biomedicine," *Science* 196: 129–136.

Englehardt, H. Tristam
1978   "The disease of masturbation: Values and the concept of disease," pp. 15–24 in J. W. Leavitt and R. L. Numbers, eds., *Sickness and Health in America.* Madison: University of Wisconsin Press.

Engels, Friedrich
[1845] 1973 *The Conditions of the Working Class in England in 1844.* Moscow: Universal.

Engler, Rick
1986   "Political power aids health and safety," *In These Times,* January 15–21: 16–17.

Epstein, Paul, and Randall Packard
   1987   "Ecology and immunity," *Science for the People* 19(1): 10–20.

Epstein, Samuel S.
   1978   *The Politics of Cancer.* San Francisco: Sierra Club Books.

Evans, Robert G.
   1974   "Supplier-induced demand: Some empirical evidence and implica-
               tions," pp. 162–173 in M. Perlman, ed., *The Economics of Health
               and Medical Care.* London: Macmillan.
   1983   "Health care in Canada: Patterns of funding and regulation,"
               Journal of Health Politics, Policy, and Law 8(1): 1–43.

Everett, Melissa
   1984   "Coffee: How it gets to your cup," *Whole Life Times,* January–
               February: 20–23.

Eyer, Joseph
   1975   "Hypertension as a disease of modern society," *International Jour-
               nal of Health Services* 5: 539–558.
   1977   "Prosperity as a cause of death," *International Journal of Health
               Services* 7: 125–150.
   1984   "Capitalism, health and illness," pp. 23–58 in J. B. McKinlay, ed.,
               Issues in the Political Economy of Health Care. New York: Tavistock.

Eyer, Joseph, and Peter Sterling
   1977   "Stress-related mortality and social organization," *Review of Radi-
               cal Political Economics* 9(1): 1–44.

Fagerhaugh, Shizuko, and Anselm Strauss
   1977   *Politics of Pain Management: Staff-Patient Interaction.* Reading, MA:
               Addison-Wesley.
   1980   "How to manage your patient's pain . . . and how not to," *Nursing*
               80: 44–47.

Fallon, April E., and Paul Rozin
   1985   "Sex differences in perception of desirable body shape," *Journal of
               Abnormal Psychology* 94(1): 102–105.

Fanon, Franz
   1963   *The Wretched of the Earth.* New York: Grove.

Farb, Peter, and George Armelagos
   1980   *Consuming Passions: The Anthropology of Eating.* Boston: Houghton
               Mifflin.

Farley, Pamela J.
   1985   "Who are the underinsured?" *Milbank Memorial Fund Quarterly* 63:
               476–503.

Fauci, Anthony
   1988   "How far will AIDS spread in the United States," *The Futurist* 22
               (4): 41–42.

Feder, Barnaby
   1988   "What ails a nursing home empire," *New York Times,* December 11.

Feigenbaum, Susan
   1987   "Risk bearing in health care finance," pp. 105–144 in C. J.
               Schramm, ed., *Health Care and Its Costs.* New York: W. W. Norton.

Fein, Rashi
    1986   *Medical Care, Medical Costs: The Search for a Health Insurance Policy.*
                Cambridge: Harvard University Press.

Feller, Barbara
    1983   "Americans needing help to function at home," *Advance Data,*
                Report Number 92.

Fenn, Richard
    1978   *Toward a Theory of Secularization.* SSSR Monograph Series, No. 1.
                Storrs, CT: Society for the Scientific Study of Religion.
    1982   *Liturgies and Trials: The Secularization of Religious Language.* Ox-
                ford: Basil Blackwell.

Feshback, Murray
    1984   "Soviet health problems," *Society* 21(3): 79–89.

Festinger, Leon
    1957   *A Theory of Cognitive Dissonance.* Palo Alto: Stanford University
                Press.

Fettner, Ann Guidici
    1987   "Where there's smoke, there's ire," *Village Voice* 32(5): 25.

Feuerstein, Michael, and Eric Skjei
    1979   *Mastering Pain.* New York: Bantam.

Field, Mark G.
    1973   "The concept of the 'health system' at the macrosociological
                level," *Social Science and Medicine* 7: 763–785.
    1976   "The modern medical system: The Soviet variant," pp. 82–101 in
                C. Leslie, ed., *Asian Medical Systems: A Comparative Study.* Berkeley:
                University of California Press.

Fielding, Jonathan E., and Kenneth J. Phenow
    1988   "Health effects of involuntary smoking," *New England Journal of
                Medicine* 319(22): 1452–1460.

Figlio, Karl
    1982   "How does illness mediate social relations?: Workmen's compensa-
                tion and medico-legal practices, 1890–1940," pp. 174–217 in P.
                Wright and A. Treacher, eds., *The Problem of Medical Knowledge:
                Examining the Social Construction of Medicine.* Edinburgh: Edin-
                burgh University Press.

Findlay, Steven
    1988   "There's no place like home," *U. S. News and World Report,* January
                25: 68–70.

Fine, Doris R.
    1988   "Women caregivers and home health workers: Prejudice and ineq-
                uity in home health care," *Research in the Sociology of Health Care* 7:
                105–117.

Fine, Michelle, and Adrienne Asch
    1988   "Disability beyond stigma: Social interaction, discrimination and
                activism," *Journal of Social Issues* 44(1): 3–21.

Fischer, Claude
    1983   "The friendship cure-all," *Psychology Today* 17(1): 74–78.

Fisher, Sue
    1983   "Doctor talk/Patient talk: How treatment decisions are negotiated

in doctor-patient communication," pp. 135–157 in S. Fisher and A. Todd, eds., *The Social Organization of Doctor-Patient Communication*. Norwood, NJ: Ablex.

1986   *In the Patient's Best Interest: Women and the Politics of Medical Decisions*. New Brunswick, NJ: Rutgers University Press.

Flexner, Abraham
1910   *Medical Education in the United States and Canada*. Bulletin, Number 4. New York: Carnegie Foundation for the Advancement of Teaching.

Ford, Anne Rochon
1986   "Hormones: Getting out of hands," pp. 27–40 in K. McDonnell, ed., *Adverse Effects: Women and the Pharmaceutical Industry*. Toronto: Women's Educational Press.

Foucault, Michel
1973   *The Birth of the Clinic: An Archaeology of Medical Perception*. New York: Tavistock.
1978   *The History of Sexuality: An Introduction*. New York: Pantheon.

Fougeyrollas, Patricia
1985   "Adaptation and rehabilitation of the functionally disabled: Guidelines for the future." Paper presented to the Canadian Congress of Rehabilitation.

Fox, Renée C.
1957   "Training for uncertainty," pp. 207–241 in R. K. Merton, G. C. Reader, and P. L. Kendall, eds., *The Student Physician*. Cambridge: Harvard University Press.

Frank, Jerome D.
1973   *Persuasion and Healing*. New York: Shocken.

Franke, Richard W.
1987   "The effects of colonialism and neo-colonialism on the gastronomic patterns of the Third World," pp. 455–479 in M. Harris and E. B. Ross, eds., *Food and Evolution: Toward a Theory of Food Habits*. Philadelphia: Temple University Press.

Franke, Richard W., and Barbara H. Chasin
1981   *Seeds of Famine: Ecological Destruction and the Development Dilemma in the West African Sahel*. Montclair, NJ: Allanheld, Osmun.

Frankel, Glenn
1986   "Even the diseases are segregated," *International Herald Tribune*, July 17.

Frankenberg, Ronald
1986   "Sickness as cultural performance: Drama, trajectory, and pilgrimage—Root metaphors and the making social of disease," *International Journal of Health Services* 16(4): 603–626.

Frankenhaeuscr, Marianne
1981   "Coping with stress at work," *International Journal of Health Services* 11(4): 491–510.

Frankenhaeuser, Marianne, and Bertil Gardell
1976   "Underload and overload in working life: Outline of a multidisciplinary approach," *Journal of Human Stress* 2(3): 35–46.

Freeman, Howard E., Robert J. Blendon, Linda H. Aiken, Seymour Sudman, Connie F. Mullinix, and Christopher R. Corey
    1987   "Americans report on their access to health care," *Health Affairs* 6(1): 6–18.

Freidson, Eliot
    1970   *Profession of Medicine: A Study of the Sociology of Applied Knowledge.* New York: Dodd, Mead.

French, Howard
    1988   "Poor overwhelm New York hospitals," *New York Times,* December 4.
    1989   "Tiny miracles become huge public health problems," *New York Times,* February 19.

Freudenheim, Milt
    1987a   "Debate widens over expanding use and growing cost of medical tests," *New York Times,* May 30.
    1987b   "Specialty health care booms," *New York Times,* November 24.
    1988a   "The boom in home health care," *New York Times,* May 2.
    1988b   "Doctors' concern: Fixing prices and price fixing," *New York Times,* December 18.
    1988c   "Prepaid programs for health care encounter snags," *New York Times,* January 31.
    1989a   "Debating Canadian health model," *New York Times,* June 29.
    1989b   "Maxicare Health seeks bankruptcy protection," *New York Times,* March 17.

Freund, Peter E. S.
    1982   *The Civilized Body: Social Domination, Control and Health.* Philadelphia: Temple University Press.

Friedl, John
    1982   "Explanatory models of black lung: Understanding the health-related behavior of Appalachian coal miners," *Culture, Medicine, and Psychiatry* 6(1): 3–10.

Friedman, Gary D.
    1987   *Primer of Epidemiology* (third edition). New York: McGraw Hill.

Friedman, Meyer, and Ray H. Rosenman
    1974   *Type A Behavior and Your Heart.* New York: Fawcett Crest.

Friedmann, Georges
    1961   The Anatomy of Work. Glencoe, IL: The Free Press.

Fromm, Eric
    1965   *Escape from Freedom.* New York: Avon Books.

Funkenstein, Daniel, S. H. King, and M. E. Drolette
    1957   *Mastery of Stress.* Cambridge: Harvard University Press.

Gabel, John R., and Michael A. Redisch
    1979   "Alternative physician payment methods: Incentives, efficiency, and National Health Insurance," *Milbank Memorial Fund Quarterly* 57(1): 38–59.

Garfield, Jon
    1980   "Alienated labor, stress, and coronary disease," *International Journal of Health Services* 10(4): 551–559.

Garrison, Vivian
    1977   "Doctor, espiritista, or psychiatrist: Health-seeking behavior in a Puerto Rican neighborhood of New York City," *Medical Anthropology* 1(2): 67–183.

Garson, Barbara
    1977   *All the Livelong Day.* New York: Penguin.
    1988   *The Electronic Sweatshop.* New York: Simon and Schuster.

Gartner, Alan, and Tom Joe
    1987   "Introduction," pp. 1–6 in A. Gartner and T. Joe, eds., *Images of the Disabled, Disabling Images.* New York: Praeger.

Geertz, Clifford
    1964   "Ideology as a cultural system," pp. 47–76 in D. Apter, ed., *Ideology and Discontent.* New York: The Free Press.

Gelber, Alexis, Larry Rohter, Joseph Harnes, and Eric Schine
    1981   "Pesticides' global fallout," *Newsweek* 98 (August 17): 53.

Gellhorn, Eric
    1969   "The consequences of the suppression of overt movements in emotional stress: A neurophysiological interpretation," *Confinia Neurologica* 32: 289–299.

George, Susan
    1982   *How the Other Half Dies.* Montclair, NJ: Allanheld, Osmun.

Gertman, Paul M.
    1981   "Physicians as guiders of health services use," pp. 258–279 in J. B. McKinlay, ed., *Health Care Consumers, Professionals, and Organizations.* Milbank Reader, No. 2. Cambridge, MA: MIT Press.

Gibson, Robert, Katherine Levit, H. Lazenby, and Daniel Waldo
    1984   "National health expenditures, 1983," *Health Care Financing Review,* 6: 1–30.

Gibson, Robert, Daniel Waldo, and Katherine Levit
    1982   "National health expenditures, 1982," *Health Care Financing Review* 5(1): 13–15.

Gill, Derek
    1980   *The British National Health Service: A Sociologist's Perspective.* Bethesda, MD: U.S. Department of Health and Human Services, Public Health Services, National Institutes of Health.

Gill, Derek, and Stanley R. Ingman
    1986   "Geriatric care and distributive justice: Problems and prospects," *Social Science and Medicine* 23(12): 1205–1215.

Gill, Sam D.
    1981   *Sacred Words: A Study of Navajo Religion and Prayer.* Westport, CT: Greenwood.

Glaberson, William
    1987   "Misery on the meatpacking line," *New York Times,* June 14.

Glaser, Barney, and Anselm Strauss
    1965   *Awareness of Dying.* Chicago: Aldine.
    1968   *Time for Dying.* Chicago: Aldine.

Glass, David
    1977   "Stress behavior patterns and coronary disease," *American Scientist* 65: 177–187.

Glassman, Marjorie
    1980   "Misdiagnosis of senile dementia: Denial of care to the elderly,"
                Social Work 25(4): 288–292.

Glassner, Barry
    1989   "Fitness and the postmodern self," *Journal of Health and Social
                Behavior* 30: 180–191.

Glenn, Evelyn Nakano, and Roslyn L. Feldberg
    1977   "Degraded and deskilled: The proletarianization of clerical work,"
                Social Problems 25(1): 52–64.

Gliedman, John
    1979   "The wheelchair rebellion," *Psychology Today* 13(3): 59–64, 99–
                101.

Gliedman, John, and William Roth
    1980   "The unexpected minority: Why society is so mystified by handi-
                cap," *New Republic* 182(5): 26–30.

Goffman, Erving
    1959   *The Presentation of Self in Everyday Life.* Garden City, NY: Double-
                day.
    1961   *Asylums.* Garden City, NY: Doubleday.
    1963   *Stigma: Notes on the Management of Spoiled Identity.* Englewood
                Cliffs, NJ: Spectrum/Prentice-Hall.

Gold, Allan R.
    1988   "Competition squeeze seen in leading to more medical antitrust
                cases," *New York Times*, December 8.

Goldblatt, Philip, Mary Moore, and Albert Stunkard
    1965   "Social factors in obesity," *Journal of the American Medical Association*
                192: 97–102.

Goldsmith, Frank, and Lorin E. Kerr
    1982   *Occupational Safety and Health.* New York: Human Sciences Press.

Goldstein, Michael S., Dennis Jaffe, Carol Sutherland, and Josie Wilson
    1987   "Holistic physicians: Implications for the study of the medical
                profession," *Journal of Health and Social Behavior* 28(2): 103–119.

Good, Byron
    1977   "The heart of what's the matter: The semantics of illness in Iran,"
                Culture, Medicine, and Psychiatry 1: 25–58.

Good, Byron, and Mary-Jo Delvecchio Good
    1981   "The meaning of symptoms: A cultural hermeneutic model for
                clinical practice," pp. 165–196 in A. Kleinman and L. Eisenberg,
                eds., *The Relevance of Social Science for Medicine.* Dordrecht, Nether-
                lands: D. Reidel.

Good, Charles M.
    1987   *Ethnomedical Systems in Africa: Patterns of Traditional Medicine in Ru-
                ral and Urban Kenya.* New York: Guilford.

Good, Mary-Jo Delvecchio and Byron Good
    1982   "Patient requests in primary care clinics," pp. 275–295 in N. J.
                Chrisman and T. W. Maretzki, eds., *Clinically Applied Anthropology.*
                Dordrecht, Netherlands: D. Reidel.

Gordon, Deborah
1988   "Tenacious assumptions in Western medicine," pp. 19–56 in M.
            Lock and D. R. Gordon, eds., *Biomedicine Examined*. Dordrecht,
            Netherlands: Kluwer.

Gore, Susan
1978   "The effect of social support in moderating the health conse-
            quences of unemployment," *Journal of Health and Social Behavior*
            19: 157–165.

Gould, Jeffrey, Becky Davey, and Randall Stoffard
1989   "Socioeconomic differences in rates of Cesarean section," *New
            England Journal of Medicine*, 321(4): 233–239.

Gould-Martin, Katherine, and Chorswang Ngin
1981   "Chinese Americans," pp. 130–171 in A. Harwood, ed., *Ethnicity
            and Medical Care*. Cambridge: Harvard University Press.

Graham, Hilary
1985   "Providers, negotiators, and mediators: Women as the hidden
            carers," pp. 25–52 in E. Lewin and V. Oleson, eds., *Women, Health,
            and Healing: Toward a New Perspective*. New York: Tavistock.

Gray, Alastair McIntosh
1982   "Inequalities in health, The Black Report: A summary and com-
            ment," *International Journal of Health Services* 12(3): 349–380.

Gray, Bradford, ed.
1983   *The New Health Care for Profit: Doctors and Hospitals in a Competitive
            Environment*. Washington, DC: National Academy Press.

Green, Jeremy
1983   "Detecting the hypersusceptible worker: Genetics and politics in
            industrial medicine," *International Journal of Health Services* 13(2):
            247–264.

Green, Linda Buckley
1989   "Consensus and coercion: Primary health care and the Guatema-
            lan state," *Medical Anthropology Quarterly* 3(3): 246–257.

Gritzer, Glenn
1981   "Occupational specialization in medicine: Knowledge and market
            explanations," *Research in the Sociology of Health Care* 2: 251–283.

Groopman, Leonard C.
1987   "Medical internship as moral education: An essay on the system
            of training physicians," *Culture, Medicine, and Psychiatry* 11: 207–
            227.

Gross, Jane
1989   "What medical care the poor can have: Lists are drawn up," *New
            York Times*, March 27.

Grossinger, Richard
1980   *Planet Medicine*. Garden City, NY: Doubleday.

Gruchow, William
1979   "Catecholamine activity and infectious disease episodes," *Journal
            of Human Stress* 5(3): 11–17.

Guarasci, Richard
1987   "Death by cotton dust," pp. 76–92 in S. L. Hills, ed., *Corporate
            Violence*. Totowa, NJ: Rowman and Littlefield.

Guarnaccia, Peter, and Pablo Farias
　　1988　　"The social meaning of *nervios:* A case study of a Central American woman," *Social Science and Medicine* 26(12): 1223–1231.

Gubrium, Jabor F.
　　1975　　*Living and Dying at Murray Manor.* New York: St. Martin's Press.

Guillemin, Jeanne H., and L. L. Holmstrom
　　1986　　*Mixed Blessings: Intensive Care for Newborns.* New York: Oxford University Press.

Gusfield, Joseph R.
　　1981　　*The Culture of Public Problems: Drinking-Driving and the Symbolic Order.* Chicago: University of Chicago Press.

Gussow, Joan Dye, ed.
　　1978　　*The Feeding Web: Issues in Nutritional Ecology.* Palo Alto: Bull.

Guttmacher, Sally, and Lourdes Garcia
　　1975　　"Social science and health in Cuba: Ideology, planning and health," pp. 507–522 in S. R. Ingman and A. E. Thomas, eds., *Topias and Utopias in Health.* The Hague: Mouton.

Haber, Suzanne N., and Patricia Barchas
　　1984　　"The regulatory effect of social rank on behavior after amphetamine administration," pp. 119–132 in P. Barchas and S. P. Mendoza, eds., *Social Hierarchies: Essays Toward a Sociophysiological Perspective.* Westport, CT: Greenwood.

Hacker, Andrew, ed.
　　1983　　*U/S: A Statistical Portrait of the American People.* New York: Viking.

Haehn, Klaus-Dieter
　　1980　　"Heilpraktikerbesuche chronisch Kranker: Frequenz und Motivation," *Diagnostik* 13: 145–146.

Hahn, Harlan
　　1988　　"The politics of physical differences: Disability and discrimination," *Journal of Social Issues* 44(1): 39–47.

Hahn, Robert A.
　　1985a　　"Between two worlds: Physicians as patients," *Medical Anthropology Quarterly* 16(4): 87–98.
　　1985b　　"A world of internal medicine: Portrait of an internist," pp. 51–111 in R. A. Hahn and A. D. Gaines, eds., *Physicians of Western Medicine.* Dordrecht, Netherlands: D. Reidel.
　　1987　　"Divisions of labor: Obstetrician, woman, and society in *Williams Obstetrics,* 1903–1985," *Medical Anthropology Quarterly* 1(3): 256–282.

Hahn, Robert A., and Arthur Kleinman
　　1983　　"Biomedical practice and anthropological theory: Frameworks and directions," *American Review of Anthropology* 12: 305–333.

Ham, Christopher
　　1982　　*Health Policy in Britain.* New York: Macmillan.

Hammond, Phillip E.
　　1974　　"Religion, pluralism, and Durkheim's integration thesis," pp. 115–142 in A. Eister, ed., *Changing Perspectives in the Scientific Study of Religion.* New York: Wiley.

Haraszti, Miklos
    1978   *A Worker in a Worker's State.* New York: Universe.

Harburg, Ernest, Edwin H. Blakelock, and Peter J. Roeper
    1979   "Resentful and reflective coping with arbitrary authority and
                blood pressure," *Psychosomatic Medicine* 41(3): 189–202.

Harburg, Ernest, John C. Erfurt, Louise Haunstein, Catherine Chape, William
Schull, and M. A. Schork
    1973   "Socio-ecological stress, suppressed hostility, skin color, and black-
                white male blood pressure, Detroit," *Psychosomatic Medicine* 35:
                276–296.

Harding, Jim
    1981   "The pharmaceutical industry as a public-health hazard and as an
                institution of social control," pp. 274–291 in D. Coburn, C.
                D'Arcy, P. Ness, and G. M. Torrance, *Health and Canadian Society:
                Sociological Perspective.* Pickering, Ont.: Fitzhenry and Whiteside.
    1986   "Mood-modifiers and elderly women in Canada: The medicali-
                zation of poverty," pp. 51–86 in K. McDonnell, ed., *Adverse Ef-
                fects: Women and the Pharmaceutical Industry.* Toronto: Women's
                Educational Press.

Harrington, Charlene
    1984   "The nursing home industry," pp. 144–154 in M. Minkler and C.
                L. Estes, eds., *Readings in the Political Economy of Aging.* Farming-
                dale, NY: Baywood.

Harris, Marvin
    1985   *The Sacred Cow and the Abominable Pig: Riddles of Food and Culture.*
                New York: Simon and Schuster.

Harwood, Alan
    1977   *Rx: Spiritist as Needed: A Study of a Puerto Rican Community Mental
                Health Resource.* New York: Wiley.
    1981a   "Mainland Puerto Ricans," pp. 397–481 in A. Harwood, ed., *Eth-
                nicity and Medical Care.* Cambridge: Harvard University Press.

Harwood, Alan, ed.,
    1981b   *Ethnicity and Medical Care.* Cambridge: Harvard University Press.

Hatfield, Elaine, and Susan Sprecher
    1986   *Mirror, Mirror . . . : The Importance of Looks in Everyday Life.* Albany:
                State University of New York Press.

Hayes, Dennis
    1989   *Behind the Silicon Curtain: The Seductions of Work in a Lonely Era.*
                Boston: South End Press.

Hayes-Bautista, David E.
    1976   "Modifying the treatment: Patient compliance, patient control,
                and medical care," *Social Science and Medicine* 10: 233–238.

Haynes, S. G., M. Feinleib, and W. B. Kannel
    1980   "The relationship of psychosocial factors to coronary heart dis-
                ease in the Framingham Study, III: Eight-year incidence of coro-
                nary heart disease," *American Journal of Epidemiology* 3: 37–58.

Health Letter
    1987   "Tranquilizing air traffic controllers," 3(12): 11–12.

Heggenhougen, Kris, Patrick Vaughan, Eustace Muhondwa, and J. Rutabanzibwa-Ngaiza
1987   *Community Health Workers: The Tanzanian Experience.* Oxford: Oxford Medical Publications, Oxford University Press.

Heidenheimer, Arnold J., and Nils Elvander, eds.
1980   *The Shaping of the Swedish Health System.* New York: St. Martin's Press.

Helman, Cecil
1978   " 'Feed a cold, starve a fever'—Folk models of infection in an English suburban community and their relation to medical treatment," *Culture, Medicine, and Psychiatry* 2: 107–137.
1985   "Communication in primary care: The role of patient and practitioner explanatory models," *Social Science and Medicine* 20(9): 923–931.

Henifin, Mary Sue, and Joan Bertin
1984   "Making healthy babies: It's not just women's work," *Science for the People,* March–April: 18–22.

Henley, Nancy M.
1977   *Body Politics.* Englewood Cliffs, NJ: Prentice-Hall.

Hentoff, Nat
1986a   "No wonder God punishes her by making her blind," *Village Voice,* 31(46) November 18: 27.
1986b   "Separate and unequal," *Village Voice,* 31(12) March 25: 24.

Herzlich, Claudine
1973   "Health and illness: A social-psychological analysis," *European Monographs in Social Psychology,* vol. 5. London: Academic Press.

Herzlich, Claudine, and Janine Pierret
1987   *Illness and Self in Society.* Baltimore: Johns Hopkins University Press.

Hess, John L.
1987   "Malthus then and now," *Nation,* 244(15): 496–500.

Hessler, Richard M., and Andrew C. Twaddle
1982   "Sweden's crisis in medical care: Political and legal changes," *Journal of Health Politics, Policy, and Law* 7(2): 440–459.

Hevesi, Dennis
1989   "Polls show discontent with health care," *New York Times,* February 15.

Heyward, William L., and James W. Curran
1988   "The epidemiology of A.I.D.S. in the U.S.," *Scientific American* 259(4): 72–81.

Hilbert, Richard A.
1984   "The acultural dimensions of chronic pain: Flawed reality construction and the problem of meaning," *Social Problems* 31(4): 365–378.

Hilfiker, David
1983   "Allowing the debilitated to die: Facing our ethical choices," *New England Journal of Medicine* 308: 718.
1984   "Making medical mistakes," *Harper's Magazine* 268(1606): 59–65.
1986   "A doctor's view of modern medicine," *New York Times Magazine,* February 23.

Hill, Carole E.
1973   "Black healing practices in the rural South," *Journal of Popular Culture* 6(4): 849–853.

Hill, Rolla B., and Robert Anderson
1988   *The Autopsy: Medical Practice and Public Policy*. Boston: Butterworth.

Hills, Stuart L., ed.
1987   *Corporate Violence*. Totowa, NJ: Rowman and Littlefield.

Himmelstein, David, Steffie Woolhandler, Martha Harnly, Michael Bader, Ralph Silber, Howard Backer and Alice Jones
1984   "Patient transfers: Medical practice as social triage," *American Journal of Public Health* 74: 494–496.

Himmelstein, David, and Steffie Woolhandler
1986   "Cost without benefit: Administrative waste in U.S. health care," *New England Journal of Medicine* 134(7): 441–445.

Hinds, Michael de Courcy
1987   "Consumer Groups' Dishonor Roll of '87," *New York Times*, December 5.

Hochschild, Arlie
1983   *The Managed Heart: Commercialization of Human Feeling*. Berkeley: University of California Press.

Hoffman, Lily M.
1989   *The Politics of Knowledge: Activist Movements in Medicine and Planning*. Ithaca: State University of New York Press.

Hokanson, J. E., and M. Burgess
1962   "The effects of three types of aggression on vascular processes," *Journal of Abnormal and Social Psychology* 648: 446–449.

Holden, John M.
1989   "Maxicare posts $17.2 million loss; regulators contest Chapter 11 status," *American Medical News*, April 21.

Holmes, Thomas H., and Richard H. Rahe
1967   "The social readjustment rating scale," *Journal of Psychosomatic Research* 11: 213–218.

Homola, Samuel
1968   *Backache: Home Treatment and Prevention*. West Nyack, NY: Parker.

Horn, James J.
1985   "Brazil: The health care model of the military modernizers and technocrats," *International Journal of Health Services* 15(1): 47–68.

Horn, Joshua S.
1969   *Away with All Pests: An English Surgeon in People's China, 1954–1969*. New York: Monthly Review Press.

Horobin, Gordon, and Jim McIntosh
1983   "Time, risk, and routine in general practice," *Sociology of Health and Illness* 5(3): 312–331.

Horton, Elizabeth
1985a   "Unfriendly persuasion," *Science Digest* 93(12): 214.
1985b   "Why don't we buckle up?" *Science Digest* 93(2): 22.

House, James S.
    1974   "Occupational stress and coronary heart disease: A review and theoretical integration," *Journal of Health and Social Behavior* 15: 17–27.
    1981   *Work Stress and Social Support.* Reading, MA: Addison-Wesley.

House, James S., Anthony J. McMichael, James A. Wells, Berton H. Kaplan, and Lawrence R. Landerman
    1979   "Occupational stress and health among factory workers," *Journal of Health and Social Behavior* 20(2): 139–160.

Howard, Robert
    1985   *Brave New Workplace.* New York: Penguin.

Hughes, David
    1988   "When nurse knows best: Some aspects of nurse/doctor interaction in a casualty department," *Sociology of Health and Illness* 10(1): 1–22.

Hunger, U.S.A.: A Report by the Citizens' Board of Inquiry into Hunger and Malnutrition in the United States.
    1968   Boston: Beacon.

Illich, Ivan
    1975   *Medical Nemesis: The Expropriation of Health.* London: Calder and Boyars.

Ingleby, David
    1982   "The social construction of mental illness," pp. 123–143 in P. Wright and A. Treacher, eds., *The Problem of Medical Knowledge: Examining the Social Construction of Medicine.* Edinburgh: Edinburgh University Press.

Institute of Medicine
    1986   *For-Profit Enterprise in Health Care.* Washington, DC: National Academy Press.

In These Times
    1986   "Swedish road to better conditions," January 18: 17.

Irwin, Susan, and Brigitte Jordan
    1987   "Knowledge, practice, and power: Court-ordered Cesarean section," *Medical Anthropology Quarterly* 1(3): 319–334.

Ivancevich, John M., and Michael T. Matteson
    1988   "Type A behavior and the healthy individual," *British Journal of Medical Psychology* 61: 37–56.

Iverem, Esther
    1988   "New York's home health-care system facing a labor crisis," *New York Times*, January 28.

Jackall, Robert
    1977   "The control of public faces in a commercial work situation," *Urban Life* 6(3): 277–302.

Jackson, Michael
    1983   "Knowledge of the body," *Man* 18: 327–345.

Jacobson, Alan M., and Joan B. Leibovich
    1984   "Psychological issues in diabetes mellitus," *Psychosomatics* 25(1): 7–15.

Jahoda, Marie, Paul Lazarsfeld, and Harry Zeisel
   1971   *Marienthal: The Sociography of an Unemployment Community.* Chicago: Aldine Atherton.

Janes, Craig
   1986   "Migration and hypertension: An ethnography of disease risk in an urban Samoan community," pp. 175–211 in C. Janes, R. Stall, and S. Gifford, eds., *Anthropology and Epidemiology: Interdisciplinary Approaches to the Study of Health and Disease.* Dordrecht, Holland: D. Reidel.

Jeffery, Roger
   1979   "Normal rubbish: Deviant patients in casualty departments," *Sociology of Health and Illness* 1(1): 90–107.

Johnson, Allen
   1978   "In search of the affluent society," *Human Nature* 1: 50–59.

Johnson, Daniel M., J. Sherwood Williams, and David Bromley
   1986   "Religion, health and healing: Findings from a southern city," *Sociological Analysis* 47(1): 66–73.

Johnson, James H., and Irwin G. Sarason
   1978   "Life stress, depression and anxiety: Internal-external control as a moderator variable," *Journal of Psychosomatic Research* 22: 205–208.

Johnson, Julie
   1989   "Children's health seen as declining," *New York Times,* March 2.

Johnson, Thomas M.
   1987   "Premenstrual syndrome as a Western culture-specific disorder," *Culture, Medicine, and Psychiatry,* 11: 337–356.

Jonas, Steven
   1981   "National health insurance," pp. 438–470 in S. Jonas, ed., *Health Care Delivery in the United States.* New York: Springer.

Jones, R. Kenneth
   1985   "The development of medical sects," pp. 1–22 in R. K. Jones, ed., *Sickness and Sectarianism: Exploratory Studies in Medical and Religious Sectarianism.* London: Gower.

Jones, Russell A.
   1982   "Expectations and illness," pp. 145–167 in H. S. Friedman and M. R. DiMatteo, eds., *Interpersonal Issues in Health Care.* New York: Academic.

Jourard, Sidney M.
   1964   *The Transparent Self.* New York: D. Van Nostrand.

Kagan, Aubrey, and Lennart Levi
   1974   "Health and environment: Psychosocial stimuli, a review," *Social Science and Medicine* 8: 225–241.

Kahn, Robert L.
   1981   "Work and health: Some psychosocial effects of advanced technology," pp. 17–37 in B. Gardell and C. Johansson, eds., *Working Life.* New York: Wiley.

Kaplan, Howard, Robert Johnson, Carol Bailey, and William Simon
   1987   "The sociological study of AIDS: A critical review of the literature and suggested research agenda," *Journal of Health and Social Behavior* 28: 140–157.

Kaplan, Jay, Stephen Manuck, Thomas Clarkson, Frances Lusso, David Taub, and
Eric Miller
    1983   "Social stress and atherosclerosis in normocholesterolemic mon-
           keys," *Science* 220(4,598): 733–735.

Karasek, Robert, Dean Baker, Frank Marxer, Anders Ahlbom, and Tores Theorell
    1981   "Job decision latitude, job demands, and cardiovascular disease: A
           prospective study of Swedish men," *American Journal of Public
           Health* 71: 694–705.

Karliner, Joshua N., and Daniel Faber
    1988   "The other revolution: Nicaragua's environmental crisis," *Utne
           Reader,* January–February: 54–65.

Kasl, Stanislav V.
    1975   "Issues in patient adherence to health care regimens," *Journal of
           Human Stress* 1(1,975): 5–17.

Kasl, Stanislav V., and Sidney Cobb
    1966   "Health behavior, illness behavior, and sick role behavior," *Ar-
           chives of Environmental Health* 12: 246–266.

Kasl, Stanislav V., Alfred S. Evans, and James C. Niederman
    1985   "Psychosocial risk factors in the development of infectious mono-
           nucleosis," pp. 341–362 in S. Locke, R. Ader, H. Besedovsky, N.
           Hall, G. Solomon, and T. Strom, eds., *Foundations of Psychoneuroim-
           munology.* New York: Aldine.

Kassirer, J. P., and G. A. Gorry
    1978   "Clinical problem solving: A behavioral analysis," *Annals of Inter-
           nal Medicine* 89: 245–255.

Kastenbaum, Robert
    1971   "Getting there ahead of time," *Psychology Today* 5: 52–54, 83–84.

Katz, Alfred
    1979   "Self-help groups: Some clarifications," *Social Science and Medicine*
           13A: 491–494.

Katz, Alfred, and Eugene I. Bender, eds.
    1976   *The Strength in Us: Self-Help Groups in the Modern World.* New York:
           New Viewpoints.

Katz, Alfred, and Lowell Levin
    1980   "Self-care is not a solipsistic trap: A reply to critics," *International
           Journal of Health Services* 10: 329–336.

Kaufert, Patricia
    1988   "Menopause as process or event: The creation of definitions in
           biomedicine," pp. 331–349 in M. Lock and D. R. Gordon, eds.,
           Biomedicine Examined. Dordrecht, Netherlands: Kluwer.

Kaufert, Patricia, and Sonja M. McKinlay
    1985   "Estrogen-replacement therapy: The production of medical
           knowledge and the emergence of policy," pp. 113–138 in E.
           Lewin and V. Olesen, eds., *Women, Health, and Healing: Toward a
           New Perspective.* London: Tavistock.

Kaufman, Caroline
    1987   "Rights and the provision of health care: A comparison of Can-
           ada, Great Britain, and the United States," pp. 491–510 in H. D.
           Schwartz, ed., *Dominant Issues in Medical Care.* New York: Random
           House.

Kaufman, Martin
    1971   *Homeopathy in America: The Rise and Fall of a Medical Heresy.* Balti-
                more: Johns Hopkins University Press.
Kaufman, Sharon R.
    1988   "Toward a phenomenology of boundaries in medicine: Chronic
                illness experience in the case of stroke," *Medical Anthropology Quar-
                terly* 2(4): 338–354.
Kearl, Michael
    1989   *Endings: A Sociology of Death and Dying.* New York: Oxford.
Kessler, Ronald C., James House, and Blake Turner
    1987   "Unemployment and health in a community sample," *Journal of
                Health and Social Behavior* 28: 51–59.
Kessler, Ronald C., and Camille B. Wortman
    1989   "Social and psychological factors in health and illness," pp. 69–86
                in H. Freeman and S. Levine, *Handbook of Medical Sociology* (fourth
                edition). Englewood Cliffs, NJ: Prentice-Hall.
Kiev, Ari
    1968   *Curanderismo: Mexican-American Folk Psychiatry.* New York: The
                Free Press.
Kingsport Study Group
    1978   "Smells like money," *Southern Exposure* 6(2): 59–65.
Kinley, David, Arnold Levinson, and Frances Moore-Lappé
    1981   "The myth of humanitarian foreign aid," *Nation,* 233(2): 41–43.
Kircher, Tobias, Judith Nelson, and Harold Burdo
    1985   "The autopsy as a measure of accuracy of the death certificate,"
                New England Journal of Medicine 313: 1263–1269.
Kiritz, Stewart, and Rudolf H. Moos
    1974   "Physiological effects of social environments," *Psychosomatic Medi-
                cine* 36(2): 96–114.
Kirmayer, Laurence J.
    1988   "Mind and body as metaphors: Hidden values in biomedicine,"
                pp. 57–94 in M. Lock and D. R. Gordon, eds., *Biomedicine Exam-
                ined.* Dordrecht, Netherlands: Kluwer.
Kleiman, Dena
    1985   "Changing way of death: Some agonizing choices," *New York
                Times,* January 24.
Klein, David, Jackob Najman, Arthur Kohrman, and Clarke Munro
    1982   "Patient characteristics that elicit negative responses from family
                physicians," *Journal of Family Practice* 14(5): 881–888.
Klein, Rudolf
    1983   *The Politics of the National Health Service.* London: Longman.
Kleinfield, N. R.
    1986   "The ever-fatter business of thinness," *New York Times,* Septem-
                ber 7.
Kleinman, Arthur
    1978   "The failure of Western medicine," *Human Nature* 1: 63–68.
    1980   *Patients and Healers in the Context of Culture: An Exploration of the
                Borderland Between Anthropology, Medicine, and Psychiatry.* Berkeley:
                University of California Press.

1984   "Indigenous systems of healing: Questions for professional, popular, and folk care," pp. 138–164 in J. W. Salmon, ed., *Alternative Medicine: Popular and Policy Perspectives.* New York: Tavistock.

1988   *The Illness Narratives: Suffering, Healing, and the Human Condition.* New York: Basic.

Kleinman, Arthur, Peter Kunstadter, E. Russell Alexander, and James L. Gate, eds.

1978   *Culture and Healing in Asian Societies.* Cambridge, MA: Schenkman.

Koenig, Barbara

1988   "The technological imperative in medical practice: The social creation of a 'routine' treatment," pp. 465–496 in M. Lock and D. R. Gordon, eds., *Biomedicine Examined.* Dordrecht, Netherlands: Kluwer.

Kolata, Gina

1988   "Companies search for next $1 billion drug," *New York Times,* November 28.

1989   "Ambivalence over pill grows with risk data," *New York Times,* January 8.

Konner, Melvin

1987   *Becoming a Doctor: A Journey of Initiation in Medical School.* New York: Viking.

Koos, Earl L.

1954   *The Health of Regionville.* New York: Columbia University Press.

Kotarba, Joseph A.

1975   "American acupuncturists: The new entrepreneurs of hope," *Urban Life* 4(2): 149–177.

1977   "The chronic pain experience," pp. 257–272 in J. Douglas, ed., *Existential Sociology.* Cambridge: Cambridge University Press.

Kotzsch, Ronald

1985   "How our food choices affect the world," *East West Journal,* June: 15–19.

Kramon, Glenn

1988a   "Employees paying ever-bigger share of medical costs," *New York Times,* November 22.

1988b   "Good medicine, better business," *New York Times,* May 15.

1988c   "Outpatient strategy fails to cut health costs," *New York Times,* March 8.

Kuhn, Thomas S.

1970   *The Structure of Scientific Revolutions.* International Encyclopedia of Unified Science, Vol. 2, No. 2. Chicago: University of Chicago Press.

Kunitz, Stephen, and Jerrold Levy

1981   "Navajos," pp. 337–396 in A. Harwood, ed., *Ethnicity and Medical Care.* Cambridge, MA: Harvard University Press.

Kunzle, David

1981   *Fashion and Fetishism: A Social History of the Corset, Tight-Lacing and Other Forms of Body Sculpture in the West.* London: Rowan and Littlefield.

Kutner, Nancy
1982   "Cost-benefit issues in U.S. national health legislation: The case of the end-stage renal disease program," *Social Problems* 30(1): 51–63.

LaCheen, Cary
1986   "Population control and the pharmaceutical industry," pp. 89–136 in K. McDonnell, ed., *Adverse Effects: Women and the Pharmaceutical Industry.* Toronto: Women's Educational Press.

Lack, Dorothea Z.
1982   "Women and pain: Another feminist issue," *Women and Therapy* 1(1): 55–63.

Laing, Ronald, and Aaron Esterson
1965   *Sanity, Madness and the Family.* New York: Basic.

Lakoff, Robin T., and Raquel L. Scherr
1984   *Face Value: The Politics of Beauty.* Boston: Routledge and Kegan Paul.

Lardy, Nicholas R.
1983   *Agriculture in China's Modern Economic Development.* Cambridge: Cambridge University Press.

Larned, Deborah
1977   "The epidemic of unnecessary hysterectomy," pp. 195–208 in C. Dreifus, ed., *Seizing Our Bodies: The Politics of Women's Health.* New York: Vintage.

LaRocco, James M., and James S. House
1980   "Social support, occupational stress and health," *Journal of Health and Social Behavior* 21: 202–218.

Larson, Magali Sarfatti
1979   "Professionalism: Rise and fall," *International Journal of Health Services* 9(4): 607–627.

Lasch, Christopher
1979   *The Culture of Narcissism.* New York: W. W. Norton.

Latham, Michael C.
1987   "Strategies for the control of malnutrition and the influence of the nutritional sciences," pp. 330–345 in J. Price, G. Hinger, J. Leslie, and C. Hoisington, eds., *Food Policy: Integrating Supply, Distribution and Consumption.* Baltimore: Johns Hopkins University Press.

Latour, Bruno, and Steve Woolgar
1979   *Laboratory Life: The Social Construction of Scientific Fact.* Beverly Hills: Sage.

Lauer, Robert H.
1973   "The social readjustment scale and anxiety: A cross-cultural study," *Journal of Psychosomatic Research* 17: 171–174.

Laumann, E. O., J. H. Gagnon, S. Michaels, R. T. Michael, and J. S. Coleman
1989   "Monitoring the AIDS epidemic in the United States: A network approach," *Science* 244: 1186–1189.

Law, Sylvia
1974   *Blue Cross—What Went Wrong?* New Haven: Yale University Press.

Lawrence, Linda, and Thomas McLemore
  1983   "1981 National Ambulatory Medical Care Survey," *Advance Data*,
            Report Number 88.

Lawrence, Philip
  1958   "Chronic illness and socioeconomic status," pp. 37–49 in E. G.
            Jaco, ed., *Patients, Physicians and Illness*. New York: The Free Press.

Lazarus, Ellen S.
  1988   "Theoretical considerations for the study of the doctor-patient
            relationship: Implications of a perinatal study," *Medical Anthropol-
            ogy Quarterly* 2(1): 34–58.

Lazarus, Richard, ed.
  1966   *Psychological Stress and the Coping Process*. New York: McGraw Hill.

Leavitt, Judith W.
  1987   "The growth of medical authority: Technology and morals in
            turn-of-the-century obstetrics," *Medical Anthropology Quarterly* 1(3):
            230–255.

Ledogar, Robert J.
  1975   *Hungry for Profits: U.S. Food and Drug Multinationals in Latin Amer-
            ica*. New York: IDOC/North America.

Lee, Sidney
  1982   "Health policy, a social contract: A comparison of the United
            States and Canada," *Journal of Public Health Policy* 3(3): 293–301.

Lefcourt, Harold M.
  1973   "The function of the illusions of control and freedom," *American
            Psychologist* 28: 417–425.

Leichter, Howard M.
  1979   *A Comparative Approach to Policy Analysis: Health Care Policies in Four
            Nations*. Cambridge: Cambridge University Press.

Leiderman, Deborah, and Jean-Anne Grisso
  1985   "The GOMER phenomenon," *Journal of Health and Social Behavior*
            26: 222–231.

Lennerlof, Lennart
  1988   "Learned helplessness at work," *International Journal of Health Ser-
            vices* 18(2): 207–222.

Lerner, Michael
  1979   "Surplus powerlessness," *Social Policy* 9: 1–10.

Leslie, Charles, ed.
  1976   *Asian Medical Systems: A Comparative Study*. Berkeley: University of
            California Press.

Levi, Lennart
  1978   "Quality of the working environment: Protection and promotion
            of occupational mental health," *Working Life in Sweden* 8.
  1981   *Preventing Work Stress*. Reading, MA: Addison-Wesley.

Levin, Lowell S., and Ellen L. Idler
  1981   *The Hidden Health Care System: Mediating Structures and Medicine*.
            Cambridge, MA: Ballinger.

Levin, Lowell S., Alfred H. Katz, and Erik Holst
  1976   *Self-Care: Lay Initiatives in Health*. New York: Prodist.

Levine, Jon D., N. C. Gordon, and H. Fields
1978   "Mechanism of placebo analgesia," *Lancet* 2(23): 654–657.

Levine, Sol R., and Abraham Lilienfeld, eds.
1987   *Epidemiology and Health Policy.* New York: Tavistock.

Levins, Richard, and Richard Lewontin
1985   *The Dialectical Biologist.* Cambridge: Harvard University Press.

Lewin, Tamar
1987a   "Company sues its workers' doctors," *New York Times,* June 9.
1987b   "Sudden nurse shortage threatens hospital care," *New York Times,* July 7.
1989   "Ailing parent: Women's burden grows," *New York Times,* November 24.

Lewis, Charles E.
1969   "Variance in the incidence of surgery," *New England Journal of Medicine* 281: 880–884.
1976   "Health maintenance organizations: Guarantors of access to medical care?" pp. 220–240 in C. Lewis, R. Fein, and D. Mechanic, eds., *A Right to Health: The Problem of Access in Primary Care.* New York: Wiley-Interscience.

Lewis, Ioan M.
1971   *Ecstatic Religion: An Anthropological Study of Spirit Possession and Shamanism.* Harmondsworth, England: Penguin.

Lewis, Paul
1987   "World hunger fund still growing," *New York Times,* June 28.

Liem, Ramsay
1981   "Economic change and unemployment: Context of illness," pp. 54–78 in E. Mishler, L. AmaraSingham, S. Hauser, R. Liem, S. Osherson, and N. Waxler, eds., *Social Contexts of Health, Illness, and Patient Care.* Cambridge: Cambridge University Press.

Light, Donald W.
1980   *Becoming Psychiatrists: The Professional Transformation of Self.* New York: Norton.
1986   "Corporate medicine for profit," *Scientific American* 255(6): 38–45.

Light, Donald W., and Sol Levine
1988   "The changing character of the medical profession: A theoretical overview," *Milbank Quarterly* 66(supplement 2): 10–32.

Light, Donald W., and Alexander Schuller, eds.
1986   *Political Values and Health Care: The German Experience.* Cambridge, MA: MIT Press.

Lilienfeld, Abraham, and David Lilienfeld
1980   *Foundations of Epidemiology* (second edition). New York: Oxford University Press.

Lin, Nan, Mary W. Woelfel, and Steven C. Light
1985   "The buffering effect of social support subsequent to an important life event," *Journal of Health and Social Behavior* 26: 247–263.

Lindheim, Roslyn
1985   "New design parameters for healthy places," *Places* 2(4): 17–27.

Lipowski, Zbigniew J.
1973   "Affluence, information inputs, and health," *Social Science and Medicine* 7: 517–529.

Little, Marilyn
1982   "Conflict and negotiation in a new role: The family nurse practitioner," *Research in the Sociology of Health Care* 2: 31–59.

Lock, Margaret
1982   "Models and practice in medicine: Menopause as syndrome or life transition," *Culture, Medicine, and Psychiatry* 6(3): 261–280.
1986   "Speaking 'truth' to illness: Metaphor, reification, and a pedagogy for patients." Paper presented to the American Anthropological Association.

Locke, Steven, Robert Ader, Hugo Besedovsky, Nicolas Hall, George Solomon, and Terry Strom, eds.
1985   *Foundations of Psychoneuroimmunology.* New York: Aldine.

Locker, David
1981   *Symptoms and Illness: The Cognitive Organization of Disorder.* New York: Tavistock.

Lohr, Kathleen, R. H. Brook, C. J. Kamberg, G. Goldberg, A. Leibowitz, J. Keesey, D. Reboussin, and J. P. Newhouse
1986   *Use of Medical Care in the Rand Health Insurance Experiment: Diagnosis and Service-Specific Analysis in a Randomized Control Trial.* Santa Monica, CA: Rand.

Lohr, Steve
1988   "British health service faces a crisis in funds and delays," *New York Times,* August 7.

Longmore, Paul K.
1987   "Screening stereotypes: Images of disabled people in television and motion pictures," pp. 65–78 in A. Gartner and T. Joe, eds., *Images of the Disabled, Disabling Images.* New York: Prager.

Low, Setha M.
1985   *Culture, Politics, and Medicine in Costa Rica.* Bedford Hills, NY: Redgrave.

Lowe, Marian, and Ruth Hubbard, eds.
1983   *Woman's Nature.* New York: Pergamon.

Lubitz, Jim, and Ronald Priboda
1984   "Uses and costs of Medicare services in the last two years of life," *Health Care Financing Review* 5: 117–131.

Luce, Gay Gaer
1971   *Biological Rhythms in Human and Animal Physiology.* New York: Dover.

Luft, Harold
1983   "Economic incentives and clinical decisions," pp. 103–123 in B. Gray, ed., *The New Health Care for Profit: Doctors and Hospitals in a Competitive Environment.* Washington, DC: National Academy Press.

Lundberg, Ulf
    1976   "Urban commuting: Crowdedness and catecholamine excretion,"
                Journal of Human Stress 2(3): 26–31.

Lurie, Elinore E.
    1981   "Nurse practitioners: Issues in professional socialization," *Journal of Health and Social Behavior* 22: 31–48.

Lynch, James
    1979   *The Broken Heart.* New York: Basic.
    1985   *The Language of the Heart.* New York: Basic.

MacDougall, J. M., T. M. Dembroski, J. E. Dimsdale, and T. Hackett
    1985   "Components of Type A, hostility and anger-in: Further relationships to angiographic findings," *Health Psychology* 4: 137–152.

MacLennan, Carol A.
    1988   "From accident to crash: The auto industry and the politics of injury," *Medical Anthropology Quarterly* 2(3): 233–250.

MacMahon, Bryan, and Thomas F. Pugh
    1970   *Epidemiologic Principles and Methods.* Boston: Little, Brown.

Mairs, Nancy
    1987   "Hers," *New York Times,* July 9.

Malcolm, Andrew H.
    1988   "In health care policy, the latest word is fiscal," *New York Times,* October 23.

Maloney, H. Newton
    1987   "Anti-cultism: The ethics of psychologists' reactions to new religions." Paper presented to the American Psychological Association.

Malthus, Thomas Robert
  [1798] 1965 *Essay on the Principle of Population as It Affects the Future Improvements of Society,* reprinted as *First Essay on Population, 1798.* New York: Kelley.

Mann, Jonathan M., James Chin, Peter Piot, and Thomas Quinn
    1988   "The international epidemiology of A.I.D.S.," *Scientific American* 259(4): 82–89.

Mansour, Jared
    1987   "Eating culture: Food as junk commodity," *Critique* 25: 14–16.

Marcelis, Carla, and Mira Shiva
    1986   "EP drugs: Unsafe by any name," pp. 11–26 in K. McDonnell, ed., *Adverse Effects: Women and the Pharmaceutical Industry.* Toronto: Women's Educational Press.

Maretzki, Thomas, and Eduard Seidler
    1985   "Biomedicine and naturopathic healing in West Germany: A historical and ethnomedical view of a stormy relationship," *Culture, Medicine, and Psychiatry* 9(4): 383–421.

Marmor, Theodore
    1982   "Canada's path, America's choice: Lessons from the Canadian experience with National Health Insurance," pp. 77–96 in R. L. Numbers, ed., *Compulsory Health Insurance: The Continuing American Debate.* Westport, CT: Greenwood Press.

1983   "Rethinking national health insurance," pp. 187–206 in T. Marmor, ed., *Political Analysis and American Medical Care*. Cambridge: Cambridge University Press.

Marmor, Theodore, Wayne L. Hoffman, and Thomas C. Heagy
1983a   "National Health Insurance: Some lessons from the Canadian experience," pp. 165–186 in T. Marmor, ed., *Political Analysis and American Medical Care*. Cambridge: Cambridge University Press.

Marmor, Theodore, Donald Wittman, and Thomas C. Heagy
1983b   "The politics of medical inflation," pp. 61–75 in T. Marmor, ed., *Political Analysis and American Medical Care*. Cambridge: Cambridge University Press.

Marmot, M. G., M. Kogevinas, and M. A. Elston
1987   "Social/economic status and disease," *Annual Review of Public Health* 8: 111–135.

Marquis, M. Susan
1984   *Cost-Sharing and the Patient's Choice of Provider*. Santa Monica, CA: Rand.

Marshall, Carolyn
1987   "Fetal protection policies: An excuse for workplace hazard," *Nation* 244(16): 532–534.

Martin, Catherine Gould, and Chors Wang Ngin
1981   "Chinese-Americans," pp. 130–171 in A. Harwood, ed., *Ethnicity and Medical Care*. Cambridge: Harvard University Press.

Massachusetts Rehabilitation Hospital
1978   "Breaking out of the pain cycle through the Boston Pain Unit," *Dimensions*, Spring: 1–4.

Mausner, Judith S., and Anita Bahn
1985   *Epidemiology: An Introductory Text* (second edition). Philadelphia: W. B. Saunders.

Maxwell, Robert J.
1981   *Health and Wealth: An International Study of Health Care Spending*. Lexington, MA: Lexington Books.

May, Clifford
1985   "Reporter's notebook: Images far from Ethiopia's famine," *New York Times*, April 7.

McCarthy, Carol
1981   "Financing for health care," pp. 272–312 in S. Jonas, ed., *Health Care Delivery in the United States*. New York: Springer.

McCarty, Richard, Karin Horwatt, and Maria Konarska
1988   "Chronic stress and sympathetic-adrenal medullary responsiveness," *Social Science and Medicine* 26(3): 333–341.

McCrea, Frances
1983   "The politics of menopause: The discovery of a deficiency disease," *Social Problems* 13(1): 111–123.

McDonald, Catherine A.
1981   "Political-economic structures—Approaches to traditional and modern medical systems," *Social Science and Medicine* 15A: 101–108.

McElroy, Ann, and Patricia K. Townsend
    1985   *Medical Anthropology in Ecological Perspective.* Boulder, CO: West-view.

McGuire, Meredith B.
    1982   *Pentecostal Catholics: Power, Charisma, and Order in a Religious Movement.* Philadelphia: Temple University Press.
    1983   "Words of power: Personal empowerment and healing," *Culture, Medicine, and Psychiatry* 7: 221–240.
    1985   "Religion and Healing," pp. 268–284 in P. Hammond, ed., *The Sacred in a Secular Age.* Berkeley: University of California Press.
    1987   *Religion: The Social Context.* Belmont, CA: Wadsworth.
    1988   *Ritual Healing in Suburban America,* with the assistance of Debra Kantor. New Brunswick, NJ: Rutgers University Press.

McGuire, Meredith B., and Debra J. Kantor
    1987   "Belief systems and illness experiences: The case of non-medical healing groups," *Research in the Sociology of Health Care* 6: 221–248.

McIntosh, Jim
    1974   "Processes of communication, information-seeking, and control associated with cancer," *Social Science and Medicine* 8A: 157–187.

McKee, Janet
    1988   "Holistic health and the critique of Western medicine," *Social Science and Medicine* 26(8): 775–784.

McKeown, Thomas
    1979   *The Role of Medicine: Dream, Mirage, or Nemesis?* Princeton: Princeton University Press.

McKinlay, John B.
    1972   "The sick role, illness, and pregnancy," *Social Science and Medicine* 6: 561–572.
    1975   "Who is really ignorant—Physician or patient?" *Journal of Health and Social Behavior* 16: 3–11.
    1978   "Social network influences on morbid episodes and the career of help-seeking," pp. 77–101 in L. Eisenberg and A. Kleinman, eds., *The Relevance of Social Science for Medicine.* Dordrecht, Netherlands: D. Reidel.
    1985   "Towards the proletarianization of physicians," *International Journal of Health Services* 15(2): 161–195.
    1986   "A case for refocusing upstream: The political economy of illness," pp. 484–498 in P. Conrad and R. Kern, eds., *The Sociology of Health and Illness: Critical Perspectives.* New York: St. Martin's Press.

McKinlay, John B., ed.
    1984   *Issues in the Political Economy of Health Care.* New York: Tavistock.
    1985   *Milbank Quarterly* 66 (supplement 2).

McKinlay, John B., and Joan Archer
    1985   "Towards the proletarianization of physicians," *International Journal of Health Services* 15(2): 161–195.

McKinlay, John B., and Sonja M. McKinlay
    1977   "The questionable effect of medical measures on the decline of mortality in the United States in the twentieth century," *Milbank Memorial Fund Quarterly* 55: 405–428.

McKinlay, John B., Sonja McKinlay, and Robert Beagle Role
1989   "Trends in death and disease and the contribution of medical measures," pp. 14–45 in H. E. Freeman and S. Levine, eds., *Handbook of Medical Sociology* (fourth edition). Englewood Cliffs, NJ: Prentice-Hall.

McKinlay, John B., and John D. Stoeckle
1988   "Corporatization and the social transformation of doctoring," *International Journal of Health Services* 18(2): 191–205.

McQueen, David, and Johannes Siegrist
1982   "Social factors in the etiology of chronic disease: An overview," *Social Science and Medicine* 16: 353–367.

Mechanic, David
1976   "Illness, illness behavior, and help-seeking," pp. 161–175 in D. Mechanic, ed., *The Growth of Bureaucratic Medicine*. New York: Wiley.
1978   *Medical Sociology*. New York: The Free Press.
1986   *From Advocacy to Allocation: The Evolving American Health Care System*. New York: The Free Press.

Medvedev, Z., and R. Medvedev
1971   *A Question of Madness*. New York: Alfred Knopf.

Melamed, Elissa
1983   *Mirror, Mirror: The Terror of Not Being Young*. New York: Linden.

Melosh, Barbara
1982   *The Physician's Hand: Work, Culture, and Conflict in American Nursing*. Philadelphia: Temple University Press.

Melzack, Ronald, and Peter Wall
1983   *The Challenge of Pain*. New York: Basic.

Members of the Working Party
1975   "Occupational accidents," pp. 65–90 in Members of the Working Party, eds., *Research for a Better Work Environment: A Summary of Reports on Four Central Research Areas*. Stockholm: LiberFörlag.

Merton, Robert K., George C. Reader, and Patricia L. Kendall, eds.
1957   *The Student Physician*. Cambridge: Harvard University Press.

Michaels, David
1988   "Waiting for the body count: Corporate decision-making and bladder cancer in the U.S. dye industry," *Medical Anthropology Quarterly* 2(3): 215–232.

Milio, Nancy
1985   "Health policy and the emerging tobacco reality," *Social Science and Medicine* 21(6): 603–613.

Miller, Frances H.
1983   "Secondary income from recommended treatment: Should fiduciary principles constrain physician behavior?" pp. 153–169 in B. Gray, ed., *The New Health Care for Profit: Doctors and Hospitals in a Competitive Environment*. Washington, DC: National Academy Press.

Millman, Marcia
1976   *The Unkindest Cut: Life in the Backrooms of Medicine*. New York: William Morrow.
1980   *Such a Pretty Face: Being Fat in America*. New York: W. W. Norton.

Millon, Theodore, Catherine Green, and Robert Meagher, eds.
1982   *Handbook of Clinical Health Psychology.* New York: Plenum.

Mills, C. Wright
1956   *White Collar.* New York: Oxford University Press.

Mintz, Sidney
1979   "Time, Sugar, and Sweetness," *Marxist Perspectives* 8: 56–73.

Mishler, Elliott
1984   *The Discourse of Medicine: Dialectics of Medical Interviews.* Norwood, NJ: Ablex.

Mizrahi, Terry
1986   *Getting Rid of Patients: Contradictions in the Socialization of Physicians.* New Brunswick, NJ: Rutgers University Press.

Moerman, Daniel
1979   "Anthropology of symbolic healing," *Current Anthropology* 20(1): 59–66.
1983   "Physiology and symbols: The anthropological implications of the placebo effect," pp. 156–167 in L. Romanucci-Ross, D. Moerman, L. Tancredi, eds., *The Anthropology of Medicine: From Culture to Method.* South Hadley, MA: Bergin and Garvey.

Moody, Edward
1974   "Magical therapy: An anthropological investigation of contemporary satanism," pp. 355–382 in I. Zaretsky and M. Leone, eds., *Religious Movements in Contemporary America.* Princeton: Princeton University Press.

Moore, Wilbert E., and Melvin Tumin
1949   "Some social functions of ignorance," *American Sociological Review* 14: 787–795.

Moore-Lappé, Frances, and Joseph Collins
1977   *Food First: Beyond the Myth of Scarcity.* New York: Houghton Mifflin.
1986   *World Hunger, Twelve Myths.* New York: Grove.

Morantz-Sanchez, Regina M.
1985   *Sympathy and Science: Women Physicians in American Medicine.* New York: Oxford.

Morgan, John H., ed.
1983   *Third World Medicine and Social Change: A Reader in Social Science and Medicine.* Lanham, MD: University Press of America.

Morgan, Lynn
1989   " 'Political will' and community participation in Costa Rican primary health care," *Medical Anthropology Quarterly* 3(3): 232–245.

Morgan, Myfanwy, D. Patrick, and J. Charlton
1984   "Social network and psychological support among disabled people," *Social Science and Medicine* 19: 489–497.

Morone, James A., and Andrew B. Dunham
1984   "The waning of professional dominance: DRGs and the hospitals," *Health Affairs* 3(1): 73–87.

Moroney, Robert M.
1980   *Families, Social Services, and Social Policy: The Issue of Shared Responsibility.* U.S. Department of Health and Human Services (DHHS Publication No. [ADM] 80-846). Washington, DC: Government Printing Office.

Moss, Abigail
1987   "Recent declines in hospitalization: United States, 1983–86," *Advance Data,* Report No. 140.

Moss, Gordon Ervin
1973   *Illness, Immunity, and Social Interaction.* New York: Wiley.

Moss, Ralph W.
1980   *The Cancer Syndrome.* New York: Grove.

Muller, Jessica H., and Barbara A. Koenig
1988   "On the boundary of life and death: The definition of dying by medical residents," pp. 351–374 in M. Lock and D. R. Gordon, eds., *Biomedicine Examined.* Dordrecht, Netherlands: Kluwer.

Muller, Mike
1982   *The Health of Nations.* London: Faber and Faber.

Mumford, Lewis
1963   *Technics and Civilization.* New York: Harcourt, Brace, and World.
1970   *The Conduct of Life.* New York: Harcourt, Brace, Jovanovich.

Murphy, Jane M.
1964   "Psychotherapeutic aspects of shamanism on St. Lawrence Island, Alaska," pp. 53–83 in A. Kiev, ed., *Magic, Faith, and Healing.* New York: The Free Press.

Murphy, Robert F.
1987   *The Body Silent.* New York: Henry Holt.

Myers, Sumner
1972   "Turning transit subsidies into compensatory transportation," *City* 6(3): 20–25.

National Institute on Disability and Rehabilitation Research
1986   "Rehabilitation of nonwhite disabled people," *Rehab Brief,* volume IX number 20.
1987   "Low back pain," *Rehab Brief,* volume IX, number 9.

National Safety Council
1986   *Accident Facts:* 1986 Edition. Chicago: National Safety Council.

Navarro, Vicente
1975   "The political economy of medical care," *International Journal of Health Services* 5(1): 65–94.
1981   "Work, ideology, and science: The case of medicine," pp. 11–38 in V. Navarro and D. M. Berman, eds., *Health and Work Under Capitalism: An International Perspective.* Farmingdale, NY: Baywood.
1988   "Professional dominance or proletarianization?: Neither," *Milbank Quarterly* 66(supplement 2): 57–75.
1989   "Race *or* class, or race *and* class," *International Journal of Health Services* 19(2): 311–314.

Navarro, Vicente, and Daniel M. Berman, eds.
1981   *Health and Work Under Capitalism: An International Perspective.* Farmingdale, NY: Baywood.

Neal, Helen
1978   *The Politics of Pain.* New York: McGraw Hill.

Nelkin, Dorothy, and Michael S. Brown
1984   *Workers at Risk: Voices from the Workplace.* Chicago: University of Chicago Press.

Nelson, Bryce
1983   "Bosses face less risk than the bossed," *New York Times,* April 3.

New York Times
1979   "A.M.A. softens a policy critical of chiropractors," July 25.
1984   "Heart disease deaths are dropping, but why?" November 18.
1986a   "Census study reports 1 in 5 adults suffers from disability," December 23.
1986b   "Your cigarettes or your job, workers are told," January 25.
1987   "Alcohol-related deaths seen under-reported; autopsies find diagnostic errors," July 21.
1987   "Merck offers free distribution of new river blindness drug," October 22.
1988a   "Hospitals' handling of uninsured patients faulted," March 30.
1988b   "Pregnant women received drug, without consent, hospital says," June 1.
1989   "For mothers, elderly present second burden," May 13.

Newman, Sandra J.
1976   *Housing Adjustments of Older People.* Ann Arbor: Institute for Social Research, University of Michigan.

Nichter, Mark
1987   "Kyasanur forest disease: An ethnography of a disease of development," *Medical Anthropology Quarterly* 1(4): 406–423.

Nightingale, Florence
1860   *Notes on Nursing: What It Is, and What It Is Not.* New York: Appleton.

Noble, Kenneth B.
1986   "Certain numbers can kill," *New York Times,* December 28.

Norbeck, Edward, and Margaret Lock, eds.
1987   *Health, Illness, and Medical Care in Japan.* Honolulu: University of Hawaii Press.

Norris, Ruth, ed.
1982   *Pills, Pesticides, and Profits: The International Trade in Toxic Substances.* Croton on Hudson, NY: North River Press.

Novack, Dennis, Robin Plumer, Raymond Smith, Herbert Ochitill, Gary R. Morrow, and John M. Bennett
1979   "Changes in physician attitude toward telling the cancer patient," *Journal of the American Medical Association* 241(9): 897–900.

Nuckolls, Katherine B., John Cassel, and Berton V. Kaplan
1972   "Psychosocial assets, life crisis, and the prognosis of pregnancy," *American Journal of Epidemiology* 95: 431–441.

Nudelman, Arthur E.
1976   "The maintenance of Christian Science in scientific society," pp. 42–60 in R. Wallis and P. Morley, eds., *Marginal Medicine*. New York: The Free Press.

Numbers, Ronald L.
1977   "Do it yourself the sectarian way," pp. 49–72 in G. Risse, R. L. Numbers, and J. W. Leavitt, eds., *Medicine Without Doctors: Home Health Care in American History*. New York: Science History.

Numbers, Ronald L., ed.
1982   *Compulsory Health Insurance: The Continuing American Debate*. Westport, CT: Greenwood.

Oakley, Ann
1984   *The Captured Womb: A History of the Medical Care of Pregnant Women*. Oxford: Basil Blackwell.

O'Donnel, Mary
1978   "Lesbian health care: Issues and literature," *Science for the People*, May–June: 18–19.

Ohrbach, Susie
1981   *Fat Is a Feminist Issue*. New York: Berkeley.

Oken, Donald
1961   "What to tell cancer patients—A study of medical attitudes," *Journal of the American Medical Association* 175: 1120–1128.

Omran, Abdel R.
1971   "The epidemiologic transition: A theory of the epidemiology of population change," *Milbank Memorial Fund Quarterly* 49: 509–538.

O'Neill, Brian, Ronald S. Karpf, and Susan P. Baker
1984   *The Injury Fact Book*. Lexington, MA: D. C. Heath.

Osherson, Samuel, and Lorna AmaraSingham
1981   "The machine metaphor in medicine," pp. 218–249 in E. Mishler et al., *Social Contexts of Health, Illness, and Patient Care*. Cambridge: Cambridge University Press.

Osterweis, Marian, Arthur Kleinman, and David Mechanic, eds.
1987   *Pain and Disability: Clinical, Behavioral, and Public Policy Perspectives*. Washington, DC: Institute of Medicine, National Academy Press.

Overfield, Theresa
1985   *Biologic Variation in Health and Illness*. Menlo Park, CA: Addison-Wesley.

Paget, Marianne A.
1983   "On the work of talk: Studies in misunderstandings," pp. 55–73 in S. Fisher and A. Todd, eds., *The Social Organization of Doctor-Patient Communication*. Norwood, NJ: Ablex.

Panides, Wallace C., and Robert C. Ziller
1981   "The self-perception of children with asthma and asthma enuresis," *Journal of Psychosomatic Research* 25: 51–56.

Parker, Richard
1981   "Lappé take dictators off the dole," *Mother Jones* 6(1) January: 12–13.

Parsons, Talcott
    1951   *The Social System.* Glencoe, IL: The Free Press.
    1966   *Societies: Evolutionary and Comparative Perspectives.* Englewood Cliffs, NJ: Prentice-Hall.
    1972   "Definitions of health and illness in light of American values and social structure," pp. 107–127 in E. G. Jaco, ed., *Patients, Physicians, and Illness.* New York: Macmillan.

Payer, Lynn
    1988   *Medicine and Culture: Varieties of Treatment in the United States, England, West Germany, and France.* New York: Henry Holt.

Pear, Robert
    1984   "Interpreting the results of the yearly U.S. physical," *New York Times,* January 22.
    1987a   "Medicare expansion imperiled by high costs," *New York Times,* September 20.
    1987b   "Physicians contend systems of payment have eroded status," *New York Times,* December 26.
    1988a   "Fate of newest treatments is often determined by Medicare," *New York Times,* January 14.
    1988b   "Hospitals' Medicare profits drop; decline may curb access to care," *New York Times,* January 28.

Pearlin, Leonard I.
    1983   "Role strains and personal stress," pp. 3–32 in H. B. Kaplan, ed., *Psychosocial Stress: Trends in Theory and Research.* New York: Academic.

Pearlin, Leonard I., Morton Lieberman, Elizabeth Menaghan, and Joseph Mullan
    1981   "The stress process," *Journal of Health and Social Behavior* 22: 337–356.

Pearlin, Leonard I., and Carm Schooler
    1978   "The structure of coping," *Journal of Health and Social Behavior* 19: 2–21.

Pellegrino, Edmund D.
    1976   "Prescribing and drug ingestion: Symbols and substances," *Drug Intelligence and Clinical Pharmacy* 10: 624–630.

Pelletier, Kenneth R.
    1977   *Mind as Healer, Mind as Slayer.* New York: Dell.
    1981   *Longevity: Fulfilling Our Biological Potential.* New York: Dell.
    1985   *Healthy People in Unhealthy Places: Stress and Fitness of Work.* New York: Dell.

Pendleton, David, and Stephen Bochner
    1980   "The communication of medical information in general practice consultations as a function of patients' social class," *Social Sccience and Medicine* 14A(6): 669–673.

Perry, Susan, and Jim Dawson
    1985   *Nightmare: Women and the Dalkon Shield.* New York: Macmillan.

Peterson, Iver
    1986   "Surge in Indians' diabetes linked to their history," *New York Times,* February 18.

Pettingale, K. W.
   1985   "Towards a psychobiological model of cancer: Biological consider-
               ations," *Social Science and Medicine* 20(8): 779–787.

Pfeffer, Richard M.
   1979   *Working for Capitalism*. New York: Columbia University Press.

Physicians' Task Force on Hunger in America
   1985   *Hunger in America: The Growing Epidemic*. Middletown, CT: Wes-
               leyan University Press.

Pilisuk, Marc, and Susan H. Parks
   1986   *The Healing Web: Social Networks and Human Survival*. Hanover,
               NH: University Press of New England.

Plough, Alonzo L.
   1986   *Borrowed Time: Artificial Organs and the Politics of Extending Lives*.
               Philadelphia: Temple University Press.

Polefrone, Joanna M., and Stephen B. Manuck
   1987   "Gender differences in cardiovascular and neuroendocrine re-
               sponses to stressors" pp. 13–38 in R. Barnett, L. Biener, and G. K.
               Baruch, eds., *Gender and Stress*. New York: The Free Press.

Pollack, Andrew
   1988   "The troubling cost of drugs that offer hope," *New York Times*,
               February 9.

Pollard, Sidney
   1972   "Factory discipline in the industrial revolution," pp. 76–81 in M.
               Cherniavsky, A. J. Slavin, and S. Ewen, eds., *Social Textures of West-
               ern Civilization: The Lower Depths*, Vol. 11. Waltham, MA: Xerox
               College.

Poloma, Margaret
   1985   "An empirical study of perception of healing among Assemblies
               of God members," *Pneuma* 7(1): 61–82.

Population Reference Bureau
   1982   *Population Bulletin* 37(2): 30–31.

Posner, Tina
   1977   "Magical elements in orthodox medicine," pp. 141–158 in R.
               Dingwall, C. Heath, M. Reid, and M. Stacey, eds., *Health Care and
               Health Knowledge*. London: Croom Helm.

Pratt, Lois
   1976   *Family Structure and Effective Health Behavior*. Boston: Houghton
               Mifflin.

Pratt, Lois, Arthur Seligman, and George Reader
   1957   "Physicians' views on the level of medical information among pa-
               tients," *American Journal of Public Health* 47: 1277–1283.

Prout, Marianne, Theodore Colton, and Robert A. Smith
   1987   "Cancer epidemiology and health policy," pp. 117–156 in S. R.
               Levine and A. Lilienfeld, eds., *Epidemiology and Health Policy*. New
               York: Tavistock.

Raffel, Marshall W.
   1984   *Comparative Health Systems*. University Park: Pennsylvania State
               University Press.

Rahe, Richard, and Arthur J. Ransom
    1968   "Life change patterns surrounding illness experience," *Journal of Psychosomatic Research* 11: 341–345.

Ramsey, Matthew
    1977   "Medical power and popular medicine: Illegal healers in 19th century France," *Journal of Social History* 10(4): 560–587.

Rawls, Rebecca
    1980   "Reproductive hazards in the workplace," *Chemical and Engineering News* 58: 28–30, 41.

Reed, Wornie L.
    1986   "Suffer the children: Some effects of racism on the health of black infants," pp. 272–280 in P. Conrad and R. Kern, eds., *The Sociology of Health and Illness: Critical Perspectives.* New York: St. Martin's Press.

Reinhardt, Uwe E.
    1987   "Resource allocation in health care: The allocation of life styles to providers," *Milbank Quarterly* 65(2): 153–176.

Reinhold, Robert
    1987   "As hospitals close, rural America tries to cope with a void," *New York Times,* July 6.
    1988   "Crisis in emergency rooms: More symptoms than cures," *New York Times,* December 8.

Relman, Arnold S.
    1980   "The new medical-industrial complex," *New England Journal of Medicine* 303: 963–970.

Renner, Michael
    1988   "Rethinking the role of the automobile," *Worldwatch Paper,* No. 84. Washington, DC: Worldwatch Institute.

Reverby, Susan
    1987a   "A caring dilemma: Womanhood and nursing in historical perspective," *Nursing Research* 36(1): 5–11.
    1987b   *Ordered to Care: The Dilemma of American Nursing, 1850–1945.* Cambridge: Cambridge University Press.

Richardson, James T.
    1987   "Battle for legitimacy: Psychiatry and the new religions in America." Paper presented to the Conférence Internationale de Sociologie Religieuse.

Richardson, Stephen A., Norman Goodman, Albert Hastdorf, and Stanford Dornbush
    1963   "Variant reactions to physical disabilities," *American Sociological Review* 28: 429–435.

Ries, Peter
    1987   "Health care coverage by age, sex, race, and family income: United States, 1986," *Advance Data,* Report No. 139.

Riska, Elianne
    1985   *Power Politics and Health: Forces Shaping American Medicine.* Helsinki: The Finnish Society of Letters.

Risse, Guenter, Ronald L. Numbers, and Judith W. Leavitt, eds.
    1977   *Medicine Without Doctors: Home Health Care in American History.* New York: Science History.

Ritenbaugh, Cheryl
    1982   "Obesity as a culture-bound syndrome," *Culture, Medicine, and Psychiatry* 6(4): 347–361.

Robbins, Thomas, and Dick Anthony
    1982   "Deprogramming, brainwashing, and the medicalization of deviant religious groups," *Social Problems* 29(3): 283–297.

Robinson, A. A.
    1988   "The motor vehicle, stress, and circulatory system," *Stress Medicine* 4: 73–176.

Robinson, Elizabeth T.
    1983   "The world's worst social disease—hunger," *Whole Life Times,* September–October: 24–27.

Rodwin, Victor G.
    1984   *The Health Planning Predicament: France, Quebec, England, and the United States.* Berkeley: University of California Press.

Roebuck, Julian, and Robert Bruce Hunter
    1975   "Medical quackery as deviant behavior," pp. 72–82 in F. Scarpitti and P. McFarlane, eds., *Deviance: Action, Reaction, Interaction.* Reading, MA: Addison-Wesley.

Roemer, Milton I.
    1985   *National Strategies for Health Care Organization: A World Overview.* Ann Arbor: Health Administration Press.

    1986   *An Introduction to the U. S. Health Care System.* New York: Springer.

Roemer, Milton I., and Ruth J. Roemer
    1981   *Health Care Systems and Comparative Manpower Policies.* New York: Marcel Dekker.

Romalis, Shelly
    1985   "Struggle between providers and recipients: The case of birth practices," pp. 174–208 in E. Lewin and V. Oleson, eds., *Women, Health, and Healing.* New York: Tavistock.

Rosenberg, Charles E.
    1987   *The Care of Strangers: The Rise of America's Hospital System.* New York: Basic.

Rosenhan, David L.
    1973   "On being sane in insane places," *Science* 179: 250–258.

Rosenman, Ray H., Richard J. Brand, C. David Jenkins, Meyer Friedman, Reuben Strauss, and Moses Wurm
    1975   "Coronary heart disease in the Western Collaborative Group Study: Final follow-up experience of 8½ years," *Journal of the American Medical Association* 233: 872–877.

Rosenthal, Marilynn
    1987   *Health Care in the People's Republic of China: Moving Toward Modernization.* Boulder, CO: Westview.

    1988   *Dealing with Medical Malpractice: The British and Swedish Experience.* Durham, NC: Duke University Press.

Rosett, Richard
    1984   *Doing Well by Doing Good: Investor-Owned Hospitals.* Chicago: Center for Health Administration Studies, University of Chicago.

Rosner, David
 1986   *A Once Charitable Enterprise: Hospitals and Health Care in Brooklyn
             and New York, 1885–1915.* Princeton: Princeton University Press.

Ross, Elizabeth
 1975   *Wheat for the Future: Famine or Feast.* New York: World View.

Ross, H. Laurence, and Graham Hughes
 1986   "Drunk driving: What not to do," *Nation* 243(20): 663–664.

Roth, Julius
 1972   "Some contingencies of the moral evaluation and control of clien-
             tele: The case of the hospital emergency service," *American Journal
             of Sociology* 77: 839–856.
 1976   *Health Purifiers and Their Enemies: A Study of the Natural Health
             Movement in the United States with a Comparison to Its Counterpart in
             Germany.* London: Croom Helm.
 1984   "The application of 'sociological wisdom' to issues of cost escala-
             tion and cost containment," *Research in the Sociology of Health Care*
             3: 257–280.

Rubel, Arthur, Carl O'Nell, and Rolando Collado-Ard'on
 1984   *Susto: A Folk Illness.* Berkeley: University of California Press.

Rushing, William
 1984   "Social factors in the rise of hospital costs," *Research in the Sociology
             of Health Care* 3: 27–114.

Ruzek, Sheryl B.
 1979   *The Women's Health Movement.* New York: Praeger.

Ryan, William
 1971   *Blaming the Victim.* New York: Vintage.

Sacks, Oliver
 1984   *A Leg to Stand On.* New York: Summit.

Sagan, Leonard
 1987   *The Health of Nations.* New York: Basic.

Salmon, J. Warren
 1984   "Organizing Medical Care for Profit," pp. 143–186 in J. B.
             McKinlay, ed., *Issues in the Political Economy of Health Care.* New
             York: Tavistock.
 1985   "Profit and health care: Trends in corporatization and proprietiza-
             tion," *International Journal of Health Services* 15(3): 395–418.

Sandler, Dale, Richard B. Everson, and Allen Wilcox
 1988   "Passive smoking in adulthood and cancer rise," *American Journal
             of Epidemiology* 121(1): 37–48.

Sapolsky, Robert M.
 1982   "The endocrine stress-response and social status in the wild ba-
             boon," *Hormones and Behavior* 16: 279–292.

Schachter, Stanley
 1968   "Obesity and Eating," *Science* 16: 751–756.

Scheder, Jo C.
 1988   "A sickly-sweet harvest: Farmworker diabetes and social equality,"
             Medical Anthropology Quarterly 2(3): 251–277.

Scheer, Jessica, and Nora Croce
    1988   "Impairment as a human constant: Cross-cultural and historical
                perspectives on variation," *Journal of Social Issues* 44(1): 23–37.

Schensul, Stephen L., and Jean J. Schensul
    1982   "Healing resource use in a Puerto Rican community," *Urban An-
                thropology* 11(1): 59–79.

Scheper-Hughes, Nancy, and Margaret M. Lock
    1986   "Speaking 'truth' to illness: Metaphor, reification, and a pedagogy
                for patients," *Medical Anthropology Quarterly* 17: 137–140.
    1987   "The mindful body: A prolegomenon to future work in medical
                anthropology," *Medical Anthropology* 1: 6–41.

Schepers, Rita
    1985   "The legal and institutional development of the Belgian medical
                profession in the nineteenth century," *Sociology of Health and Illness*
                7(3): 314–341.

Schieber, George, and Jean-Pierre Poullier
    1986   "International health-care spending," *Health Affairs* 5(3): 111–
                122.

Schiff, Robert L., Daiv Ansell, James Schlosser, Ahamed Idris, Ann Morrison, and
Steven Whitman
    1986   "Transfers to a public hospital," *New England Journal of Medicine*
                314(9): 552–559.

Schmale, Arthur H.
    1972   "Giving up as a final common pathway to changes in health," pp.
                20–40 in Z. Lipowski, ed., *Advances in Psychosomatic Medicine,* Vol.
                8. Basel: S. Karger.

Schmeck, Harold M.
    1985   "73% of Americans suffer headaches," *New York Times,* October
                22.

Schnall, Peter L., and Rochelle Kern
    1981   "Hypertension in American society: An introduction to historical
                materialist epidemiology," pp. 73–89 in P. Conrad and R. Kern,
                eds., *The Sociology of Health and Illness* (second edition). New York:
                St. Martin's Press.

Schneider, Joseph W., and Peter Conrad
    1980   "In the closet with illness: Epilepsy, stigma potential, and informa-
                tion control," *Social Problems* 28(1): 32–45.
    1983   *Having Epilepsy: The Experience and Control of Illness.* Philadelphia:
                Temple University Press.

Schneider, Keith
    1987   "New product on farms in Midwest: Hunger," *New York Times,*
                September 29.

Schneider, Michael
    1975   *Neurosis and Civilization: A Marxist-Freudian Synthesis.* New York:
                Seabury.

Schrank, Jeffrey
    1977   *Snap, Crackle, and Popular Taste.* New York: Dell.

Schreiber, Janet M., and John Homiak
    1981   "Mexican Americans," pp. 264–336 in A. Harwood, ed., *Ethnicity and Medical Care*. Cambridge: Harvard University Press.

Schur, Edwin M.
    1984   *Labeling Women Deviant: Gender, Stigma, and Social Control*. New York: Random.

Schwartz, Barry
    1973   "Waiting, exchange, and power: The distribution of time in social systems," *American Journal of Sociology* 79: 841–870.

Schwartz, Hillel
    1986   *Never Satisfied: A Cultural History of Diets, Fantasies, and Fat*. New York: Macmillan.

Schwartz, Howard D., Peggy L. de Wolf, and James K. Skipper, Jr.
    1987   "Gender, professionalization, and occupation anomie: The case of nursing," pp. 559–569 in H. D. Schwartz, ed., *Dominant Issues in Medical Sociology*. New York: Random House.

Schwartz, Miriam
    1984   "A sociological reinterpretation of the controversy over 'unnecessary surgery,' " *Research in the Sociology of Health Care* 3: 159–200.

Science for the People
    1985   "Medicine's new discovery: Workers," 17(4): 8.

Science News
    1978   "Doctors' strike lowered death rate," October 28: 293.

Scitovsky, Anne, and Alexander M. Capron
    1986   "Medical care at the end of life: The interaction of economics and ethics," *Annual Review of Public Health* 7: 59–75.

Scotch, Richard K.
    1988   "Disability as the basis for a social movement: Advocacy and the politics of definition," *Journal of Social Issues* 44(1): 159–172.

Scott, Clarissa S.
    1974   "Health and healing practices among five ethnic groups in Miami, Florida," *Public Health Reports* 89(6): 524–532.

Scully, Diana
    1980   *Men Who Control Women's Health: The Miseducation of Obstetrician-Gynecologists*. Boston: Houghton Mifflin.

Segall, Alexander, and Lance W. Roberts
    1980   "A comparative analysis of physician estimates and levels of knowledge among patients," *Sociology of Health and Illness* 2(3): 317–334.

Seligman, Martin
    1975   *Helplessness: On Depression, Development, and Death*. San Francisco: W. H. Freeman.

Selik, Richard M., Kenneth G. Castro, Marguerite Pappaivanou, and James W. Buehler
    1989   "Birthplace and the risk of AIDS among Hispanics in the United States," *American Journal of Public Health* 79(7): 836–839.

Selye, Hans
    1956   *The Stress of Life*. New York: McGraw Hill.
    1975   *Stress Without Distress*. New York: New American Library.

Sennett, Richard, and Jonathan Cobb
    1972   *The Hidden Injuries of Class.* New York: Vintage.

Serrin, William
    1989   "Playing down unemployment," *Nation* 248(3): 84–88.

Severo, Richard
    1980   "Dispute arises over Dow studies on genetic damage to workers,"
                New York Times, February 5.

Shabecoff, Philip
    1987a   "Panel says caesarians are used too often," *New York Times,* Novem-
                ber 3.
    1987b   "Vast changes in environment seen," *New York Times,* November 4.

Sheehan, John
    1982   "Cost-benefit analysis: A technique gone awry," pp. 51–74 in J. S.
                Lee and W. N. Rom, eds., *Legal and Ethical Dilemmas in Occupa-
                tional Health.* Ann Arbor, MI: Ann Arbor Science.

Sheehan, Susan
    1984   *Kate Quinton's Days.* New York: New American Library.

Shekelle, Richard B., S. B. Hulley, J. Neaton, J. Billings, N. Borhani, T. Gerace, D.
Jacobs, N. Lasser, M. Mittlemark, J. Stamler for the MRFIT Research Group.
    1985   "The MRFIT behavior pattern study, II: Type A behavior pattern
                and incidence of coronary heart disease," *American Journal of
                Epidemiology* 122: 559–570.

Sherrill, Robert
    1977   "Raising hell on the highways," *New York Times Magazine,* Novem-
                ber 27.

Shilts, Randy
    1987   *And the Band Played On: Politics, People, and the AIDS Epidemic.* New
                York: St. Martin's Press.

Short, Pamela F.
    1988   "Trends in employee health benefits," *Health Affairs* 7(3): 186–
                196.

Short, Pamela F., Alan C. Monheit, and Karen Beauregard
    1989   *Uninsured Americans: A 1987 Profile.* Rockville, MD: National Cen-
                ter for Health Services Research and Health Care Technology
                Assessment.

Shorter, Edward
    1982   *A History of Women's Bodies.* New York: Basic.

Shulman, Lawrence C., and Joanne E. Mantell
    1988   "The AIDS crisis: A United States health care perspective," *Social
                Science and Medicine* 26(10): 979–988.

Sicherman, Barbara
    1978   "The uses of a diagnosis: Doctors, patients, and neurasthenia,"
                pp. 25–38 in J. Leavitt and R. L. Numbers, eds., *Sickness and
                Health in America.* Madison: University of Wisconsin Press.

Sidel, Ruth, and Victor Sidel
    1982   *The Health of China: Current Conflicts in Medical and Human Services
                for 1 Billion People.* Boston: Beacon.

Sidel, Victor W., and Ruth Sidel
    1983   *A Healthy State: An International Perspective on the Crisis in United States Medical Care.* New York: Pantheon.

Siegrist, Richard B., Jr.
    1983   "Wall Street and the for-profit hospital management companies," pp. 35–50 in B. Gray, ed., *The New Health Care for Profit: Doctors and Hospitals in a Competitive Environment.* Washington, DC: National Academy Press.

Sigerist, Henry B.
    1960   *On the History of Medicine.* New York: M. D. Publications.

Silverman, Milton, and Philip R. Lee
    1974   *Pills, Profits, and Politics.* Berkeley: University of California Press.

Silverstein, Bret
    1984   *Fed Up.* Boston: South End.

Simmons, Roberta G., and Susan Klein Marine
    1984   "The regulation of high cost technology medicine: The case of dialysis and transplantation in the U.K.," *Journal of Health and Social Behavior* 25: 320–334.

Simon, Philip J.
    1983   *Reagan in the Workplace: Unraveling the Health and Safety Net.* Washington, DC: Center for Study of Responsive Law.

Simonelli, Jeanne M.
    1987   "Defective modernization and health in Mexico," *Social Science and Medicine* 24(1): 23–36.

Sivard, Ruth
    1987   *World Military and Social Expenditures, 1987–88.* Washington, DC: World Priorities.

Skultans, Vieda
    1974   *Intimacy and Ritual: A Study of Spiritualism, Mediums, and Groups.* London: Routledge and Kegan Paul.

Small, Gary W., and Jonathan F. Borus
    1983   "Outbreak of illness in a school chorus," *New England Journal of Medicine* 308(1): 632–635.

Smith, Barbara Ellen
    1981   "Black lung: The social production of disease," *International Journal of Health Services* 11(3): 343–359.
    1987   *Digging Our Own Graves: Coal Miners and the Struggle over Black Lung Disease.* Chicago: University of Chicago Press.

Smith, Robert C., and George Zimny
    1988   "Physicians' emotional reactions to patients," *Psychosomatics* 29(4): 392–397.

Snell, Bradford
    1982   "American ground transport," pp. 316–338 in J. H. Skolnick and E. Currie, eds., *Crisis in American Institutions.* Boston: Little, Brown.

Snow, John
    [1855] 1936 *On the Mode of Communication of Cholera,* reprinted as *Snow on Cholera.* New York: Hafner.

Snow, Loudell F.
1974   "Folk medical beliefs and their implications for care of patients,"
            Annals of Internal Medicine 81: 82–96.

Snyder, Patricia
1983   "The use of nonprescribed treatments by hemodialysis patients,"
            Culture, Medicine, and Psychiatry 7: 57–76.

Society of Actuaries and Association of Life Insurance Medical Directors of
America
1983   *1979 Build Study.* New York: Metropolitan Life Insurance Company.

Soderstrom, Lee
1980   "The Canadian experience," pp. 224–238 in A. Levin, ed., *Regulating Health Care: The Struggle for Control.* New York: Academy of Political Science.

Soldo, Beth J.
1985   "In-home services for the dependent elderly," *Research on Aging* 7: 281–304.

Solomon, George F.
1985   "The emerging field of psychoneuroimmunology," *Advances: Journal of the Institute for the Advancement of Health* 2(1): 6–19.

Sontag, Susan
1972   "The double standard of aging," *Saturday Review,* September 23: 29–38.
1978   *Illness as Metaphor.* New York: Farrar, Straus, and Giroux.

Sorkin, Alan L.
1986   *Health Care and the Changing Economic Environment.* Lexington, MA: D. C. Heath.

Spillane, Robert
1984   "Stress at work: A review of Australian research," *International Journal of Health Services* 14(4): 589–604.

Spruit, Ingeborg P., and Daan Kromhout
1987   "Medical sociology and epidemiology: Convergences, divergences, and legitimate boundaries," *Social Science and Medicine* 25(6): 579–587.

Stannard, Charles
1973   "Old folks and dirty work: The social conditions for patient abuse in a nursing home," *Social Problems* 20(3): 329–342.

Stark, Elizabeth
1985   "Break the pain habit," *Psychology Today* 19(5): 31–34.

Starr, Paul
1982   *The Social Transformation of American Medicine.* New York: Basic.

Stearns, Carol Zisowitz, and Peter N. Stearns
1986   *Anger: The Struggle for Emotional Control in America's History.* Chicago: University of Chicago Press.

Stebbins, Kenyon Rainier
1986   "Curative medicine, preventive medicine, and health status: The influence of politics on health status in a rural Mexican village," *Social Science and Medicine* 23(2): 139–148.

Stein, Howard F.
1986   " 'Sick people' and 'trolls': A contribution to the understanding of the dynamics of physician explanatory models," *Culture, Medicine, and Psychiatry* 10: 221–229.

Stein, Leonard I.
1967   "The doctor-nurse game," *Archives of General Psychiatry* 16: 699–703.

Steinmetz, Suzanne K.
1978   "Battered parents," *Society* 15: 54–55.

Stellman, Jeanne
1977   *Women's Work, Women's Health.* New York: Pantheon.

Stellman, Jeanne, and Susan M. Daum
1971   *Work is Dangerous to Your Health.* New York: Pantheon.

Stellman, Jeanne, and Mary Sue Henifin
1983   *Office Work Can Be Dangerous to Your Health.* New York: Random House.

Sterling, Theodor D., Elia Sterling, and Helen D. Ward
1983   "Building illness in the white collar workplace," *International Journal of Health Services* 13(2): 277–287.

Sternbach, Richard A.
1964   "The effects of instructional sets on autonomic responsivity," *Psychophysiology* 1(1): 67–72.

Stevens, Robert, and Rosemary Stevens
1974   *Welfare Medicine in America: A Case Study of Medicaid.* New York: The Free Press.

Stevens, William K.
1988   "Diarrhea kills surprising rate of U.S. young," *New York Times*, December 9.

Stewart, David C., and Thomas J. Sullivan
1982   "Illness behavior and the sick role in chronic disease: The case of MS," *Social Science and Medicine* 16: 1397–1404.

Stimson, Gerry, and Barbara Webb
1974   "Obeying doctor's orders: A view from the other side," *Social Science and Medicine* 8A: 97–104.
1975   *Going to See the Doctor.* London: Routledge and Kegan Paul.

Stone, Deborah A.
1979a   "Diagnosis and the dole: The function of illness in American distributive politics," *Journal of Health Politics, Policy and Law* 4(3): 570–591.
1979b   "Physicians as gatekeepers: Illness certification as a rationing device," *Public Policy* 27(2): 227–254.

Stout, H. R.
1885   *Our Family Physician.* Peoria: Henderson and Smith.

Straus, Murray A., Richard J. Gelles, and Suzanne K. Steinmetz
1980   *Behind Closed Doors: Violence in the American Family.* New York: Doubleday.

Strauss, Anselm
1975   *Chronic Illness and the Quality of Life.* St. Louis: C. V. Mosby.

Struck, Miriam
    1981   "Disabled doesn't mean unable," *Science for the People*, September–October: 24–28.

Sudnow, David
    1967   *Passing On: The Social Organization of Dying*. Englewood Cliffs, NJ: Prentice-Hall.

Sullivan, Mark
    1986   "In what sense is contemporary medicine dualistic?" *Culture, Medicine and Psychiatry* 10: 331–350.

Sullivan, Walter
    1983   "Autopsies show 1 in 4 diagnoses were wrong," *New York Times*, April 28.

Suls, Terry, and Glenn S. Sanders
    1988   "Type A behavior as a general risk factor for physical disorder," *Journal of Behavioral Medicine* 11(3): 201–226.

Susser, Mervyn, William Watson, and Kim Hopper
    1985   *Sociology in Medicine* (third edition). New York: Oxford University Press.

Suter, Steve
    1986   *Health Psychophysiology: Mind-Body Interactions in Wellness and Illness*. Hillsdale, NJ: Lawrence Erlbaum.

Sutherland, Allan T.
    1981   *Disabled We Stand*. Bloomington: Indiana University Press.

Sutherland, Prudy
    1987   "I want sex—Just like you," *Village Voice* 32(14): 25.

Svarstad, Bonnie L.
    1976   "Physician-patient communication and patient conformity with medical advice," pp. 220–238 in D. Mechanic, ed., *The Growth of Bureaucratic Medicine*. New York: Wiley.

Syme, S. Leonard, and Lisa F. Berkman
    1976   "Social class, susceptibility, and sickness," *American Journal of Epidemiology* 104: 1–8.

Syme, S. Leonard, and Jack. M. Guralnik
    1987   "Epidemiology and health policy: Coronary heart disease," pp. 85–116 in S. R. Levine and A. Lilienfeld, eds., *Epidemiology and Health Policy*. New York: Tavistock.

Szasz, Andrew
    1983   "The reversal of federal policy toward worker safety and health," *Science and Society* 1(Spring): 25–51.

Szasz, Thomas S.
    1970   *The Manufacture of Madness*. New York: Dell.

Taussig, Michael T.
    1980   "Reification and the consciousness of the patient," *Social Science and Medicine* 14B: 3–13.
    1987   *Shamanism, Colonialism, and the Wild Man: A Study in Terror and Healing*. Chicago: University of Chicago Press.

Taylor, Frederick
    [1911] 1947 *Principles of Scientific Management*. New York: W. W. Norton.

Taylor, Kathryn M.
    1988   " 'Telling bad news': Physicians and the disclosure of undesirable information," *Sociology of Health and Illness* 10(2): 109–132.

Taylor, Rosemary C. P.
    1984   "Alternative medicine and the medical encounter in Britain and the United States," pp. 191–228 in J. W. Salmon, ed., *Alternative Medicines: Popular and Policy Perspectives*. New York: Tavistock.

Telles, Joel Leon, and Mark Harris Pollack
    1981   "Feeling sick: The experience and legitimation of illness," *Social Science and Medicine* 15A: 243–251.

Terkel, Studs
    1974   *Working*. New York: Avon.

Thoits, Peggy A.
    1983   "Dimensions of life events that influence psychological distress: An evaluation and synthesis of the literature," pp. 33–103 in H. B. Kaplan, ed., *Psychosocial Stress: Trends in Theory and Research*. New York: Academic.

Thompson, Edward P.
    1966   *The Making of the English Working Class*. New York: Random House/Vintage.

Thygerson, Alton
    1976   *Safety: Concepts and Instruction*. Englewood Cliffs, NJ: Prentice-Hall.

Tipton, Steven M.
    1982   *Getting Saved from the Sixties: The Transformation of Moral Meaning in American Culture by Alternative Religious Movements*. Berkeley: University of California Press.

Todd, Alexandra
    1983   "Discourse in the prescription of contraception," pp. 159–187 in S. Fisher and A. Todd, eds., *The Social Organization of Doctor-Patient Communication*. Norwood, NJ: Ablex.

Tolchin, Martin
    1988a   "Changes urged in payments to doctors," *New York Times*, September 29.
    1988b   "Curbs on tuition for doctors raising fears for care of poor," *New York Times*, July 25.
    1988c   "Length of average hospital stay drops 22%," *New York Times*, May 25.
    1988d   "Shift on Medicare to hurt hospitals in the inner cities," *New York Times*, October 19.
    1989a   "Concern over the costs of malpractice liability," *New York Times*, November 5.
    1989b   "Hospitals give record pay rise to attract nurses," *New York Times*, March 26.

Totman, Richard
    1979   *Social Causes of Illness*. New York: Pantheon.

Townsend, John M., and Cynthia L. Carbone
    1980   "Menopausal syndrome: Illness or social role—A transcultural analysis," *Culture, Medicine, and Psychiatry* 4: 229–248.

Trostle, James A., W. Allen Hauser, and Ida Susser
    1983   "The logic of noncompliance: Management of epilepsy from the patient's point of view," *Culture, Medicine, and Psychiatry* 7: 35–56.

Trotter, Robert T., and J. A. Chavira
    1981   *Curanderismo: Mexican-American Folk Healing*. Athens: University of Georgia Press.

Tudiver, Sari
    1986   "The strength of links: International Women's Health Network in the eighties," pp. 187–214 in K. McDonnell, ed., *Adverse Effects: Women and the Pharmaceutical Industry*. Toronto: Women's Educational Press.

Tuller, David
    1989   "The 90's occupational epidemic," *San Francisco Chronicle*, June 12.

Turner, Bryan S.
    1977   "Confession and social structure," *Annual Review of the Social Sciences of Religion* 1: 29–58.
    1982   "The government of the body: Medical regimens and the rationalization of diet," *British Journal of Sociology* 33(2): 254–269.
    1984   *The Body and Society: Exploration in Social Theory*. Oxford: Basil Blackwell.

Turner, R. Jay, and Samuel Noh
    1988   "Physical disability and depression: A longitudinal analysis," *Journal of Health and Social Behavior* 24: 23–27.

Turner, Terence
    1980   "The social skin: Bodily adornment, social meaning, and personal identity," pp. 112–140 in J. Cherfas and R. Lewin, eds., *Not Work Alone: A Cross-Cultural View of Activities Superfluous to Survival*. Beverly Hills: Sage.

Turner, Victor W.
    1968   *The Drums of Affliction*. Oxford: Clarendon.
    1969   *The Ritual Process*. Chicago: Aldine.

Twaddle, Andrew C.
    1981a   "Sickness and the sickness career: Some implications," pp. 111–133 in L. Eisenberg and A. Kleinman, eds., *The Relevance of Social Science for Medicine*. Dordrecht, Netherlands: D. Reidel.
    1981b   *Sickness Behavior and the Sick Role*. Cambridge, MA: Schenkman.

Twaddle, Andrew C., and Richard M. Hessler
    1986   "Power and change: The Swedish Commission of Inquiry on Health and Sickness Care," *Journal of Health Politics, Policy, and Law* 11(1): 19–40.
    1987   *A Sociology of Health* (second edition). New York: Macmillan.

U.S. Bureau of the Census
    1984   *1980 Census of Population*, volume 2, Subject Reports: Occupation by Industry. Washington, DC: Government Printing Office.

U.S. Congress, House Select Committee on Aging
    1984   *Quackery: A $10 Billion Scandal*. House Report No. 98-435, Washington, DC: Government Printing Office.

U.S. Department of Health, Education, and Welfare
1972   *The Health Consequences of Smoking: A Report of the Surgeon General.*
          DHEW Publication No. (HMS) 72-7516. Washington, DC: Government Printing Office.

U.S. Department of Health and Human Services
1980   *Summary Report of the Graduate Medical Education National Advising Committee.* DHHS Publication No. (HRA) 81-651. Washington, DC: Government Printing Office.
1984   *Health, United States, 1983.* Hyattsville, MD: National Center for Health Statistics.
1986   "Birth, marriages, divorces, and deaths for 1985," National Center for Health Statistics, *Monthly Vital Statistics Report* 34(12): 1–12.
1987   *Health, United States, 1986.* Hyattsville, MD: National Center for Health Statistics.
1989   *International Classification of Diseases.* Public Health Service, Health Care Financing Administration. Washington, DC: Government Printing Office.

U.S. Department of Labor
1981   "Workers on Late Shifts," *Bureau of Labor Statistics* September Summary: 81–103.

Verbrugge, Lois M.
1985   "Gender and health: An update on hypotheses and evidence," *Journal of Health and Social Behavior* 26(3): 156–182.
1986   "From sneezes to adieux: Stages of health for American men and women," *Social Science and Medicine* 22: 1195–1212.

Verbrugge, Lois M., and Frank J. Ascione
1987   "Exploring the iceberg: Common symptoms and how people care for them," *Medical Care* 25(6): 539–569.

Verbrugge, Lois M., and Deborah L. Wingard
1987   "Sex differentials in health and mortality," *Women and Health* 12(2): 103–143.

Vogel, Virgil
1970   *American Indian Medicine.* Norman: University of Oklahoma Press.

Volicer, Beverly
1977   "Cardiovascular changes associated with stress during hospitalization," *Journal of Psychosomatic Research* 22: 159–168.
1978   "Hospital stress and patients' reports of pain and physical status," *Journal of Human Stress* 4: 28–37.

Wagner, Melinda Bollar
1983   *Metaphysics in Midwestern America.* Columbus: Ohio State University Press.

Waid, William M.
1984   *Sociophysiology.* New York: Springer-Verlag.

Waitzkin, Howard B.
1971   "Latent functions of the sick role in various institutional settings," *Social Science and Medicine* 5: 45–75.
1979   "A Marxian interpretation of the growth and development of coronary care technology," *American Journal of Public Health* 69(12): 1260–1268.

1983a "Health policy and social change: A comparative history of Chile and Cuba," *Social Problems* 31(2): 235–248.

1983b *The Second Sickness: Contradictions of Capitalist Health Care.* New York: The Free Press.

1984 "The micropolitics of medicine: A contextual analysis," *International Journal of Health Services* 14: 339–378.

1985 "Information giving in medical care," *Journal of Health and Social Behavior* 26: 81–101.

1989a "A critical theory of medical discourse: Ideology, social control, and the processing of social context in medical encounters," *Journal of Health and Social Behavior* 30(2): 220–239.

1989b "Health policy in the United States: Problems and alternatives," pp. 475–491 in H. Freeman and S. Levine, eds., *Handbook of Medical Sociology.* Englewood Cliffs, NJ: Prentice-Hall.

Waitzkin, Howard B., and John D. Stoeckle
1972 "The communication of information about illness," *Advances in Psychosomatic Medicine* 8: 180–215.

Waitzkin, Howard B., and Barbara Waterman
1974 *The Exploitation of Illness in Capitalist Society.* Indianapolis: Bobbs-Merrill.

Waldron, Ingrid
1976 "Why do women live longer than men?" *Social Science and Medicine* 10: 349–362.

1983 "Sex differentials in human mortality: The role of genetic factors," *Social Science and Medicine* 17(6): 321–333.

Wallston, Barbara S., S. W. Alagna, B. M. DeVellis, and R. B. DeVellis
1983 "Social support and physical health," *Health Psychology* 2: 367–391.

Walsh, Diana Chapman
1987 *Corporate Physicians: Between Medicine and Management.* New Haven: Yale University Press.

1988 "Toward a sociology of worksite health promotion: A few reactions and reflections," *Social Science and Medicine* 26(5): 569–575.

Walters, Vivienne
1982 "Company doctors' perceptions of and responses to conflicting pressures from labor and management," *Social Problems* 30(1): 1–12.

Ward, Martha C.
1986 *Poor Women, Powerful Men: America's Great Experiment in Family Planning.* Boulder, CO: Westview.

Wardwell, Walter I.
1972 "Orthodoxy and heterodoxy in medical practice," *Social Science and Medicine* 6: 759–763.

1982 "Chiropractors: Challengers of medical domination," *Research in the Sociology of Health Care* 3: 207–250.

Warner, Richard
1986 "Hard times and schizophrenia," *Psychology Today,* 20(6): 50–52.

Warnock, John W.
1987 *The Politics of Hunger: The Global Food System.* Toronto: Methuen.

Waxler, Nancy E.
    1980   "The social labeling perspective on illness and medical practice,"
                pp. 283–306 in L. Eisenberg and A. Kleinman, eds., *The Relevance
                of Social Science for Medicine*. Dordrecht, Netherlands: D. Reidel.
    1981   "Learning to be a leper: A case study in the social construction of
                illness," pp. 169–194 in E. Mishler, L. AmaraSingham, S. Hauser,
                R. Liem, S. Osherson, and N. Waxler, *Social Contexts of Health,
                Illness, and Patient Care*. Cambridge: Cambridge University Press.

Weber, Max
    [1904] 1958   *The Protestant Ethic and the Spirit of Capitalism*. New York: Charles
                Scribner's Sons.
    [1922] 1963   *The Sociology of Religion*, trans. E. Fischoff. Boston: Beacon.

Weeks, John R.
    1986   *Population: An Introduction to Concepts and Issues*. Belmont, CA:
                Wadsworth.

Weil, Andrew
    1983   *Health and Healing*. Boston: Houghton Mifflin.

Weil, Andrew, and Winifred Rosen
    1983   *Chocolate to Morphine: Understanding Mind-Active Drugs*. Boston:
                Houghton Mifflin.

Weinstein, Henry
    1985   "The health threat in the fields," *Nation* 240(18): 558–560.

Weir, David, and Mark Shapiro
    1981   *Circle of Poison*. San Francisco: Institute for Food Development
                Policy.

Weiss, Jay M.
    1972   "Psychological factors in stress and disease," *Scientific American*
                226(6): 104–113.

Weiss, Kay
    1983   "Vaginal cancer: An iatrogenic disease?" pp. 59–75 in E. Fee, ed.,
                Women and Health: The Politics of Sex in Medicine. Farmingdale, NY:
                Baywood.

Wertz, Richard W., and Dorothy C. Wertz
    1979   *Lying-In: A History of Childbirth in America*. New York: Schocken.

West, Candace
    1983   " 'Ask me no questions . . .': An analysis of queries and replies in
                physician-patient dialogues," pp. 75–106 in S. Fisher and A.
                Todd, eds., *The Social Organization of Doctor-Patient Communication*.
                Norwood, NJ: Ablex.
    1984   *Routine Complications: Troubles with Talk Between Doctors and Patients*.
                Bloomington: Indiana University Press.

West, Patrick B.
    1979   "Making sense of epilepsy," pp. 162–169 in D. J. Osborne, M. M.
                Greenberg, and J. R. Eiser, eds., *Research in Psychology and Medi-
                cine: Social Aspects, Attitudes, Communication, Care, and Training*, Vol.
                2. New York: Academic.

Westley, Frances
    1983   *The Complex Forms of the Religious Life: A Durkheimian View of New
                Religious Movements*. Chico, CA: Scholars Press.

Wethington, Elaine, and Ronald C. Kessler
    1986   "Perceived support, received support, and adjustment to stressful life events," *Journal of Health and Social Behavior* 27: 78–89.
Whiteis, David, and J. Warren Salmon
    1987   "The proprietarization of health care and underdevelopment of the public sector," *International Journal of Health Services* 17(1): 47–64.
Wijkman, Anders, and Lloyd Timberlake
    1984   *Natural Disasters: Acts of God or Acts of Man?* Washington, DC: International Institute for Environment and Development.
Wilford, John Noble
    1988   "Common operation aimed at strokes faces new questions about safety," *New York Times*, February 11.
Wilkes, Michael S., and Miriam Shuchman
    1989   "Pitching doctors," *New York Times Magazine*, November 5.
Wilkinson, Richard G.
    1986a   "Income and mortality," pp. 88–114 in R. Wilkinson, ed., *Class and Health: Research and Longitudinal Data*. New York: Tavistock.
    1986b   "Socio-economic differences in mortality: Interpreting the data on their size and trends," pp. 1–21 in R. Wilkinson, ed., *Class and Health: Research and Longitudinal Data*. New York: Tavistock.
Willen, Richard S.
    1983   "Religion and law: The secularization of testimonial procedures," *Sociological Analysis* 44(1): 53–64.
Williams, Rory
    1983   "Concepts of health: An analysis of lay logic," *Sociology* 17(2): 185–205.
Willis, Evan
    1983   *Medical Dominance: The Division of Labour in Australian Health Care.* Sydney: Allen and Unwin.
Wohl, Stanley
    1984   *The Medical Industrial Complex.* New York: Harmony.
Wolff, Harold G.
    1968   *Stress and Disease.* Springfield, IL: Thomas.
Wolinsky, Frederick, and Sally Wolinsky
    1981   "Background, attitudinal, and behavioral patterns of individuals occupying eight discrete health states," *Sociology of Health and Illness* 3: 31–48.
Woodrow, K. M., G. D. Friedman, A. B. Siegelaub, and M. F. Collen
    1972   "Pain differences according to age, sex, and race," *Psychosomatic Medicine* 34: 548–556.
World Bank
    1987   *World Development Report, 1987.* New York: Oxford.
World Health Organization
    1981   "Self-help and health: Report on a W.H.O. consultation," Report Number ICP HED 014, 6484 B, Copenhagen: World Health Organization.
Yago, Glenn
    1985   "U.S. lacks transportation policy," *In These Times* 9(15): 7.

Yelin, Edward
    1986   "The myth of malingering: Why individuals withdraw from work
                in the presence of illness," *Milbank Quarterly* 64(4): 622–649.
Young, Allan
    1976   "Some implications of medical beliefs and practices for social an-
                thropology," *American Anthropologist* 78(1): 5–24.
    1978   "Mode of production of medical knowledge," *Medical Anthropology*
                2: 97–124.
    1980   "The discourse of stress and the reproduction of conventional
                knowledge," *Social Science and Medicine* 14B: 133–146.
Young, James H.
    1967   *The Medical Messiahs*. Princeton: Princeton University Press.
Zborowski, Mark
    1952   "Cultural components in response to pain," *Journal of Social Issues*
                8: 16–30.
    1969   *People in Pain*. San Francisco: Jossey Bass.
Zola, Irving K.
    1966   "Culture and symptoms," *American Sociological Review* 31: 615–
                630.
    1982   *Missing Pieces: A Chronicle of Living with a Disability*. Philadelphia:
                Temple University Press.
    1983   *Socio-Medical Inquiries: Recollections, Reflections, and Reconsidera-
                tions*. Philadelphia: Temple University Press.

Author Index

Subject Index